TWELVE PATIENTS

TWELVE PATIENTS

LIFE AND DEATH AT
BELLEVUE HOSPITAL

ERIC MANHEIMER, MD

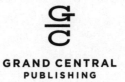

GRAND CENTRAL
PUBLISHING

NEW YORK   BOSTON

Grand Central Publishing
Hachette Book Group
237 Park Avenue
New York, NY 10017

www.HachetteBookGroup.com

Printed in the United States of America

RRD-C

First Edition: July 2012

10 9 8 7 6 5 4 3 2 1

Grand Central Publishing is a division of Hachette Book Group, Inc. The Grand Central Publishing name and logo is a trademark of Hachette Book Group, Inc.

The publisher is not responsible for websites (or their content) that are not owned by the publisher.

Library of Congress Cataloging-in-Publication Data
Manheimer, Eric.
Twelve patients : life and death at Bellevue Hospital / Eric Manheimer.
    p. cm.
Includes index.
ISBN 978-1-4555-0388-9 (regular)
1. Bellevue Hospital.   2. Hospital patients—New York (State)—New York—Case studies.   3. Hospital care—New York (State)—New York—Case studies.
I. Title.
RC31.N5M36 2012
362.1109747'1—dc23
                                                                        2012005513

For Diana

Contents

TWELVE
PATIENTS

The One-Strike Law

The view from my office at Bellevue Hospital looks north up the East River. The south side of the UN building rises like a thin polished band, and it cuts through the arc of the 59th Street Bridge that reaches east over Roosevelt Island and then to Queens. On the southern tip of Roosevelt Island, I can make out the skeleton of the smallpox hospital now in ruins. FDR Drive pulses with white lights heading south as I look out at seven o'clock on a still-dark morning. Red taillights string north in the dark evenings as people head back to the outer suburbs locked in their cars.

The old Bellevue psychiatry building, now a men's homeless shelter, frames my window on the left. The building is stained with water and neglect. Just to its right is the New York University School of Medicine with its laboratories, classrooms, and hospital beds. Hidden beyond the construction site exactly in the middle of my view is a small white tent. The site had been our northern parking lot until September 11, 2001, when air-conditioned freezer trailers were moved in and surrounded by a chain-link fence. Guards monitored access. The remains of the dead from 9/11 were brought to be identified, their DNA measured against the DNA extracted from toothbrushes and clothes. It reminded me of the ZAKA in Jerusalem (the Hebrew acronym of an Israeli organization that aids disaster victims), who came to the site of a suicide bombing wearing their tzitzis and collecting brain matter and fingers into plastic bags for burial, so that the souls of the dead would be able to join their people when the Messiah came.

The tent is still there as I look out my same window eight years later, though the refrigerated trucks and guards are gone. The view is being progressively obliterated. The Economic Development Corporation has taken over our north-side parking lot and leased the area to a California company to build a biomedical laboratory building. I figure I have about another three months before the UN disappears completely, and with it the medical school, along with the old psychiatry building *cum* homeless shelter.

When most people hear "Bellevue" today, they picture an old-fashioned insane asylum—but that is just one aspect of this city-within-a-city where I spend my days. For aficionados of *Law & Order* or *Nurse Jackie*, Bellevue is synonymous with psychotic killers perpetrating random acts of violence. But Bellevue is the oldest hospital in the country, 275 years old. It is also arguably the most famous public hospital in the United States. The first maternity ward, first pediatric ward, first C-section—Bellevue is full of firsts. Its public sanitation programs date back to the Civil War. Yellow fever, tuberculosis, typhoid, and polio epidemics were brought under control here. Famous for psychiatry, Bellevue also pioneered child psychiatry with the first inpatient unit complete with a public school for children. Two Bellevue physicians won the Nobel Prize for heart catheterization. The first cardiac pacemaker was developed at Bellevue. So was the early treatment of drug addiction.

Today, the hospital continues to work at the cutting edge of public health issues—HIV, lethal flu, potential terrorist epidemics. Bellevue also has a hundred-bed prison unit to care for prisoners of Rikers Island, the largest prison complex in the country. As part of the city hospital health system, we look after the needs of all New Yorkers—from Park Avenue to the tenement housing of recently arrived Fukienese immigrants, survivors of torture, and everything in between. With thirty thousand discharges and half a million visits in our hundred-plus different outpatient clinics, we see the effects of global problems often before most people know the problems exist: outbreaks, violence, climate change, tobacco, drugs, and the fast-food industry. We are known for many things, in particular our emergency room. If a cop gets shot in Manhattan, his first choice is often Bellevue. If a diplomat gets attacked at the UN, he gets taken to Bellevue. If an investment banker goes into cardiac arrest, his limo driver knows where to take him. If New York is a microcosm of the world, then the doctors of Bellevue are on the front line. We are a vibrant institution that moves to the same rhythms as the city we serve.

Where in colonial times there was a farm named Belle Vue now stands a vast hospital complex of several thousand beds with seven thousand employees, and several thousand new New Yorkers being born every year. The modern campus sits in Kips Bay, a few blocks south of the United Nations, flanked by First Avenue to the west and the FDR Drive snaking along the East River. The northern boundaries are the aforementioned men's homeless shelter spun out from the old psychiatric buildings, and an intake center for kids in crisis; both were parts of the original sprawling hospital campus. The southern boundary runs into a nursing school and the Manhattan Veterans Hospital on 23rd Street. For the past 150 years, Bellevue has also been the teaching hospital for the New York University School of Medicine.

I arrived at Bellevue in 1997. After seventeen years as a physician at Dartmouth, I was ready to be back in New York and in public health. As a child growing up in the Bronx, I used to accompany my father, Dr. Robert Manheimer, as he made house calls at night. A rheumatologist and internist at Montefiore for more than fifty years, he took me on night rides in the family's baby-blue Peugeot with an adjustable spotlight to find house numbers on Gun Hill Road or the little-known alleyways off the Grand Concourse. The sounds, smells, and rhythms of medicine entered my primitive brain's limbic system. I had no choice. Though I loved everything else—history, languages, archaeology—medicine was my passion.

In the 1970s, when I was a medical student at Downstate, in Brooklyn, the city went bankrupt. Crime rates escalated. The city saw gigantic unemployment, a crack cocaine epidemic, racial tensions, and escalating economic and social disparities. As I made my way to pathology class Monday morning, the Brooklyn morgue was lined with bodies. The late 1970s, when I was a resident at Kings County, a huge public teaching hospital in central Brooklyn, were also crazy times for New Yorkers. The city was homicide capital of the world.

Son of Sam was one of my more infamous patients of the time. There was nothing we had not seen after years working through all of the services, each with its own building on the campus. We had no on-call rooms, so we slept on empty stretchers. There was no air-conditioning, so in the summer we brought several extra shirts to change into. We would meet at midnight in the break room for peanut butter sandwiches and trade a CT scan for a barium enema before going back to battle. After ten years I had seen almost everything.

After a physician was stabbed to death in the parking lot of the hospital by a crack addict trying to rob him of five dollars, I answered an ad in the *New England Journal of Medicine* for a job in New Hampshire.

I met my wife, Diana, at Dartmouth—she was a young professor with Canadian parents and had been raised in Mexico, where her dad worked as a mining engineer. Diana's work encompassed the world of the arts, theater, performance, literature, and politics, and I was seduced by it from the beginning. From her early childhood in Parral, Chihuahua, a dusty mining town whose only claim to fame was that Pancho Villa had been killed there, her family had moved to Mexico City. In 1997 I followed Diana back to New York City, where she was offered a position at NYU. I, like a true homing pigeon, started working in the city public hospital system again. Bellevue completed my inner circle, which consisted of Diana; my son, Alexei; and our daughter, Marina.

Looking down out my window, I see a corrections van, "New York's Boldest" stenciled on the side, pull outside the "Blue Room" (holding pen) between the emergency room and the adult psychiatric emergency room, which goes by the acronym *CPEP*—that is, the "Comprehensive Psychiatric Emergency Program." The occupant of the van must be a high-value prisoner from Rikers Island—seven police and corrections vehicles surround it. The vehicles stop just below my window, and the corrections tactical squad members emerge in full body armor, carrying battlefield-level weaponry. They survey the perimeter, then create a human corridor through which two corrections officers (who must be captains, judging by their starched, formfitting white shirts) escort the shackled prisoner. He is Latino, with dark disheveled hair and a wispy beard, wearing the standard baggy orange jumpsuit. His skin is tattooed everywhere I can see. Blue, black, green, and red. His neck, arms, and hands.

He looks up toward my window. Las Maras have arrived in New York. They are one of the deadliest gangs. Their signature is extreme violence, no holds barred, unsentimental murder and mayhem. Their initiation rights involve peer beatings and an initiation murder or *asesinato*, as it is called in Spanish. Many of them grew up undocumented in the street gangs of Los Angeles, and were later deported as teenagers and young adults—some to El Salvador, where their parents had fled from the horror of civil war, and some to other countries of origin they had never known. Now they were back, more lethal than ever, with a spiderweb network of drug trade from Colombia and Peru all the way to Los Angeles and Long Island.

This guy's hands and feet are bound with metal chains; another chain connects the hands and feet, and everything is connected to a strong leather belt around his waist. Is all this security to protect him from a rival gang that wants his territory, or is it to prevent his gang from helping him escape? This transport moment is the vulnerable point—he can't escape from Rikers, though someone could kill him there. Given the gang's power and codes, however, that's unlikely. The guards push him into one of the cells in the Blue Room.

"*¡Hola, jefe!*" Patty, my executive assistant, walks in around eight a.m. and startles me out of my thoughts. "You have a full schedule today."

"As opposed to every other day?" I ask.

"*¿Quién te manda, jefe?*" she rejoins. "You are your own taskmaster. So today, the UN Secret Service folks are coming in to make sure we're ready for the upcoming General Assembly meeting next week. God forbid they take a shot at one of those world-leader types and he ends up here. The Mexican minister of health will pop in to discuss health care for Mexican migrants." She goes down the list and finishes with: "By the way, Budd called down from the prison health unit asking if you would run up to say good-bye to Juan Guerra, who is to be discharged on compassionate release."

I pause, speechless. "He's finally going home? I can't believe it."

"Don't believe it till you see it, *jefe*. You know how things are around here."

Juan Guerra going home—unbelievable.

"I'll go see Guerra before the UN guys come—I'll be right down. Get them some coffee and donuts if I'm late, *por favorcito*."

The first thing I ever noticed about Juan Guerra was his neck, which I recognized from twenty-five yards away.

I was making rounds with Budd, the lead physician on the nineteenth floor. Rail-thin, six foot six, Dr. Budd Heyman was an internist with a long history of working in correctional medicine from the Tombs, Manhattan's prison adjacent to Chinatown. An indefatigable advocate for the disadvantaged, he knew that the game of life could change quickly for anyone and the only difference between the rich and his patients was that the rich had options. We usually began at one end and walked our way around. Even if the patients weren't in their cells at the start of our rounds, they would magically appear by the time we got there. There was too little going on in prison to miss the opportunity to talk to someone new. There were twenty-five men, between the ages of seventeen and seventy-three, who had been there for as little as a few hours or for as long as five months plus. The corrections officers at their posts were a reminder that they were still prisoners, even though they wore hospital gowns. The gates were solid metal and locked; there was no decor and no color. Mesh screens covered all the windows.

With the guards, the gates, the IDs, more gates, it's hard to "drop in" on that unit, and I am a drop-in kind of doctor and medical director who prefers to be on the floor rather than behind my desk. You get a feel for a unit. People in the know can actually size up a hospital in a few hours just by walking around it, talking to people, asking questions. You get a clear sense of what's going on. You don't need ten inspectors spending two weeks crawling through policies and procedures. A few sentinel scenarios tell you if the hospital is a Potemkin village or the real deal.

Guerra was a slight man under five foot eight, thin, with hospital-issued pajamas and slippers, short-cut pepper-gray hair, and a short goatee. And a neck I would know a mile away. The swelling told the full story immediately. I could anticipate every question, issue, side effect, treatment option, and alternative. I had no idea what his personal story was, where he was from, where he had been, or what his life trajectory had looked like so far. But I certainly had a fair sense of what his future possibilities might be. The left side had four golf ball–size tumor-filled lymph nodes that stuck out and left the skin over them stretched taut. They weren't giving him any pain or interfering with his swallowing. He was thin but not gaunt and had a glass of water in his hand. His disease was advanced, and his chances of making it very slim. I wondered in what way I, as a physician, could have a positive impact on Guerra's dwindling life.

Many physicians do not get into the boat at all and stay on the shore. Many become obsessed with lab values and the rituals of the white coat and stethoscope, the computer now safely between them and the patient so that hardly a glance is necessary before they can be off to the next. For this type of doctor, the loss of a patient is a narcissistic blow. It activates a primal fear of loss. It represents a deep professional failure. It makes a sham of what medicine is supposed to do. Regardless of the regimens, treatments, expenses—regardless of other specialists brought in, the surgeries, secondary options, drug trials, and rescue chemotherapies, the futile treatments themselves are a symptom of the physician's inability to accept an ending. The doctor becomes frozen, protecting the illusion of power. But the illusion is untenable—it goes against the laws of physics. Everything dies. Nothing touches the inescapable outcome that is entropy itself. The Second Law will prevail, it always does, the house never loses.

I hesitated before approaching Guerra. Something else held me back: I was recovering from the same exact disease. My own treatment for SCC, or squamous cell carcinoma, from a peanut-size lesion near my right tonsil, had started on a Monday in mid-October a year earlier and finished with a final dose of radiation therapy and chemo in early December. The complications and recovery were still fresh. I had had a neck node that wouldn't quit, that sat out the radiation and the chemo nearly to the end and then finally collapsed in a couple of days. Would his collapse? Would mine stay collapsed? Would his fate foreshadow mine? Seeing his neck created an anxiety in me I didn't like to admit to myself and certainly couldn't share. It's painful to see your own worst fears made real and immediate in the person in front of you. It's not simply a matter of the empathetic *This could be me*. It's more like *This could very well be me sometime soon*. I pushed the thoughts as far back as they would go. I understood what lay ahead of him in a way no healthy physician could.

I walked over to him, holding out my hand: *"Buenos días, soy médico, parte de tu equipo de médicos en el hospital. ¿Tienes un ratito para platicar?"*

Patty is ushering the two Secret Service men into my office through the front door as I enter through the back. I intended to see Guerra first thing this morning, but was stopped in the hall by one of the chiefs telling me there was a problem in an operating room. Figuring out a solution has taken the best part of an hour, and I need to get back. I ask Patty to find out what's happening with Guerra ASAP, and then greet the two men.

They are standard government issue. Beefy, short haircuts recently clipped, cheap gray suits off the rack, plastic white earpieces with a cord disappearing down their necks, and the omnipresent clipboards. The president and other heads of state are due to meet at the UN next week, so these men are here to check the hospital security and trauma and cardiology readiness, as Bellevue is the receiving hospital for heads of state. They are here for a walk-through, very hands-on. As part of the emergency-management system, we rehearse a variety of different activations such as biological attacks, mass trauma, and dirty bombs. I make them coffee with my new espresso machine that Diana gave me. A box of Dunkin' Donuts has miraculously materialized on the polished wooden conference table. This is not the quiche-and-Perrier crowd. Even though they come every year, we always go down the same checklist.

Randy, the senior Secret Service officer, says, "You have 24/7 in-house trauma attendings?"

Check.

"Dedicated trauma operating room?"

Check.

"Examples of current emergency escalations?"

"We had a gunfight two weeks ago with three cases in the trauma slot and in the OR in a few minutes," I responded. "Rival gangs involved in narcotics turf warfare. Fifty units of blood and product for the cases. We can access an enormous quantity from the blood bank and sister hospitals quickly."

Randy looks up and smiles: "Like Maryland. Except their business is car crashes, not the knife and gun club. Do you have helicopter access?"

Check.

Jim, the junior guy, texts on his BlackBerry throughout the meeting. We schmooze comfortably and eat donuts as they complete their paperwork.

We then take the walk around the central administrative hub of the intensive care unit (ICU), where a safe space is secured in the event a high-profile politician or diplomat comes in with trauma or another life-threatening condition. I stop to introduce them to Maria, the secretary to the surgical intensive care unit, and the chief resident on neurosurgery. I look in on the fifteen members of the trauma team that surrounds the bed of a young woman who lies in a coma after her motorcycle was hit by a distracted octogenarian behind the wheel. She was launched into a low orbit that caused multiple cranial fractures, internal bleeding, and swelling that killed all tissue above her brain stem. The doctors are carrying out some of the tests we relied on completely before the age of CT scans. Do the pupils react to light? Are they equal in size? Do you see doll's eyes moving together when you rotate the head to one side and the other? She has fine features and long dark hair. For an instant she reminds me of my daughter, and I look away. They are around the same age. Too painful to think about.

My cell phone goes off, and I check it as I walk the Secret Service men to the elevators. It's Patty—the Mexican minister of health has been delayed at the mayor's office. We have a meeting to discuss the partnership that Bellevue has developed with the Mexican consulate to provide health care for the influx of documented and undocumented Mexican immigrants—more than five hundred thousand of whom live in the greater metropolitan area alone, and twelve million in the United States. I ask her to call me when he arrives.

She assures me she's on the Guerra case. "*Jefe*, thought you'd like to know that Dr. Faruz is waiting here to see you. I told him you're busy upstairs but he says he'll wait. He wants to complain to you about..." I pray for patience and hang up.

"A happening place," says one of the Secret Service men.

Juan Guerra is going home—unbelievable. After half a life in prison, his throat cancer might actually save his life. Maybe. I think back on my earliest discussions with him, a fifty-nine-year-old man born in New York of Dominican parents.

As a child in the Bronx, Juan Guerra had made several lengthy trips to the Dominican Republic, first living on a ranch, riding horses near the Haitian border, and later in the capital city, Santo Domingo. Timing was everything, Guerra had told me. And his timing had always been terrible. Coming of age when Vietnam was exploding like a grenade with the pin pulled, his lottery number had been 11 and he went to war with the neighborhood. This was not a Crawford, Texas, neighborhood with street names like Harvard and Princeton Place. There was no question of a deferment for an injury or conscientious objection or a family that could stash him safely in the National Guard to ride out the waves of Hue that would bring the nightly death counts onto living room televisions across the country. Guerra and his family knew he was the one who would always be caught. A black cat had walked across his mother's path when she was pregnant, he said.

Guerra had served in Vietnam in a combat unit, though in fact he was in Cambodia ferrying U.S. troops illegally into the border areas to find and destroy Vietcong storage tunnels. What he didn't know was that not all the risks in the army were booby traps in the jungle or black-pajama-clad locals who might be soldiers, sympathizers, or just villagers trying to survive one side or the other depending on the time of the day. What he didn't know was that a pure white powder would claim his future and, in many ways, remake him into another person before he was twenty-one years old.

He came back, like many in his unit, addicted to heroin, and for the next thirty years tried dozens of times to kick the habit, relapsing regularly. He was caught in possession of drugs, sent to Rikers and occasionally upstate for longer sentences of over a year, and put on parole again and again. The last time he was sentenced to prison was for being fifteen minutes late for a meeting with his parole officer. His adult life post-Vietnam had been one extended coda with the Department of Corrections of New York State. It was like his second family—maybe even his first at this point. He had a wife and a son whom he missed terribly and who'd supported him unconditionally through thick and thin over decades, an aging mother and father, and an extended family in the Dominican Republic. In fact, a lot more than many non-felons could claim.

Guerra and I had talked about this often over a hospital meal at his bedside. I asked him why he would make such bad decisions knowing the consequences—and how the police needed to make their arrest quotas. These were minor drug offenses, possession or selling tiny amounts of methadone. How could he take the risks?

He said that he was an addict and had been one for thirty-five years courtesy of the U.S. Army. His entire social network was made up of addicts, dealers, and minor neighborhood drug types who couldn't get any type of employment.

"I made a lot of bad decisions and pay the piper every time. After a certain point it doesn't matter. You will get picked up and charged with someone else's crimes since they know you cannot say no and you plead down so you don't have to go upstate."

"So can't you play it extra safe, knowing that?"

"I need methadone. Once the clinic shut me out, paperwork they forgot to file. They told me to come back in five days. I had to choose between withdrawal and getting some drugs to tide me over. There is no slack. You do anything not to withdraw."

Guerra paused, then continued. "A year ago I was arrested for walking Tiger off a leash. He weighs four pounds. He is my grandkid's Chihuahua. It was the end of the month and the rookie needed to fill his quota. The senior cops all laughed at the rookie for such a stupid arrest. I went to prison and they laughed at him.

"Doc, try living in the stop-and-frisk world of the NYPD. Just for a week."

"How does your family take it?"

"*Es una locura.* And why my wife has stayed with me for over thirty-five years. Who knows! She knows hard time with her brother for the real bad stuff. Mine is petty stuff and I am faithful and I love her and our kids. Our world includes prison time and probation and the likelihood you will be back again."

After his latest incarceration, Guerra's disease was diagnosed, and he began his treatment with radiation therapy. Every morning at ten thirty the guards would escort him per protocol in handcuffs and leg shackles through the metal gates to the elevator bank for supplies. They would go down to the ground floor and walk out to the Blue Room. He would wait there until a prison van arrived to take him three blocks north to the basement of the university hospital. Two officers would escort him to the radiation therapy area. He would be unshackled and assisted onto the table, where he would lie back on the thin metal gantry covered by a sheet.

The technician would fasten the plastic gridded molded mask over his face and screw it into the table. His throat was burned raw by the radiation treatments. Two circles of hair loss on the back of his head marked the radiation fields. To relax him during the procedure, a nurse injected him with Ativan, a sedative to take the edge off the anxiety and discomfort of being locked down on a metal table with stomach acid lapping up his esophagus, the nausea from the chemotherapy threatening spontaneous spasmodic vomiting. His stomach tube dangled down the table, almost touching the floor.

Very few people in the United States know that the largest penitentiary system in the country is in New York City. For most, Rikers Island exists simply as a TV set. Only the guards who go there and the prisoners and their families have a clue about the scale and operational routines of the place. There are eleven prisons on Rikers, an island about the size of Central Park, a short distance from the takeoff corridors of LaGuardia Airport. The only access is by a bridge from Queens that is heavily controlled by the Corrections Department. Family members, lawyers, guards, and prisoners are ferried back and forth in vans and buses to the eleven prisons, infirmaries, and miscellaneous outposts on the island where thousands of people are warehoused out of society's view. There is a supermax prison for the extremely predatory and violent prisoners, a prison for women with room for their infants (if the women have the capacity to care for them), and a prison boat when the census gets extremely high. A smattering of high-value prisoners, such as the corrupt cops and Madoffs of the world, are kept segregated—otherwise, imagine.

The general population of Rikers consists of short-stay prisoners awaiting trial or sentencing, or prisoners sentenced for under a year. Longer terms are served in more than sixty upstate prisons holding more than fifty thousand prisoners, most of them from New York City. The state legislature in Albany has lobbied hard to bring prisons to the poorer rural communities in the northern reaches of the state, providing economic benefits to dying industrial communities. The fact that prisoners are separated from their loved ones and the fragile human ecosystem that sustains them when they finish their time is an "externality," an unfortunate side effect. It's an economic and social cost that is not factored into the "benefits" of rural development and keeping society safe thanks to the mass incarceration model. The rotating prison door of re-incarceration is good for certain businesses.

After I reach 19 South, our med-surgery prison unit, it takes me

about ten minutes to make it through the elaborate security appara-
tus run by the Department of Corrections. Metal detectors, sequential
electronic gates, and a Plexiglas-enclosed lookout monitored by several
officers dressed in blue uniforms review all incoming and outgoing
activity in this hospital prison. I call Patty to tell her that I will now
be incommunicado, and then place my cell phone in a mailbox-size
locker and pocket the key, supervised by a seated, attentive corrections
officer.

"Gate," I shout. A very large guard approaches slowly and without
affect, dangling a huge key in his hand. He lets me into the unit without looking at me—his eyes floating to some invisible place right over
my head. When I finally enter, I am really in Corrections' space. This
is not a civilian universe, though we have made an effort to bridge the
cultures of medicine and corrections, to achieve a balance of security
and a health-supporting environment. As I enter the conference room,
Juan Guerra looks up and smiles. He and his twenty-two-year-old
son are in deep conversation. His wife, a lively, strong woman, looks
worried.

This dingy "conference" room at least offers a modicum of privacy and, most important, some freedom from the constant barrage
of noise, the shouting, the bright fluorescent lights, and the call for
"gate" that punctuate the air like a slap in the face as nurses, aides,
doctors, corrections officers, pharmacy techs, dietitians, therapists,
administrators, supervisors, regulators, and wardens make their way
in and out of the unit. Still, the windowless room is depressing with its
dead color, the echo of metal on metal, the scratched Plexiglas, and the
omnipresent guard in the corridor outside.

I am glad to see Guerra looking relatively strong. He is about to get
up when he sees me. I urge the family to go on. I pretend to look for
something in the chart to give them time to speak.

"The *pandillas* [gangs] are death for you, *m'hijo*. You have to make
a choice soon, or it will be made for you." Guerra waves me into the
room, but I step outside the door and signal that he should take his
time.

"My friends are who protect me," his son says.

"That type of protection is a death trap."

"Without them I am dead."

"Then you will go to the DR this week and stay with Tio Juanito," Guerra's wife interjects. "We used to leave Santo Domingo to avoid Trujillo and his butchers, now I have to send my son home to avoid the gangs here."

"Tio Juan's is bullshit. I am too old for horseback riding and cleaning the stables and driving a tractor."

"When I was your age it was the Lords or the army," Guerra says.

"So what are you saying?"

"I am saying, Javie, that for you it is the same choice."

Javie laughs. "The army will save me? Look at you!"

"Learn from me. You go in, you enlist and choose carefully who you hang with, and you stay away from drugs—nothing in the vein, up the nose, nothing. You do that and the odds shift right away."

I sense a pause and lean my head back in the room. Javie looks at me straight in the eyes without anger or hostility. He knows I am on his father's side. After decades of being in and out of the system, Guerra has learned to use his smarts and humor to get people to help him. He is not completely powerless, even though he has cancer and is in prison. He is trying to teach his son to survive in what suddenly strikes me as a nearly hopeless situation.

Guerra stands up, a bit shaky, and introduces me to his family as the "*mero mero*" or *the* man who would help explain his treatments. We shake hands and trade the *bachata* CDs we've both brought, the rhythmically contagious music from the Dominican Republic. In fact, Juan Guerra and I like to joke about his *tocayo* or namesake, Juan Luis Guerra, one of the most popular *bachateros* in the world, who sells out Madison Square Garden in an hour.

Juan Guerra's family has visited him in jails and prisons from New York City to the upper reaches of New York State near the Canadian border. They have sustained him and, in a way that is not immediately obvious, he has sustained them. I lay it out slowly and carefully, what to expect from the chemo, the radiation, the fatigue, the pain medications, and so on, taking a lot of time for questions, drawing diagrams and a time frame on pages ripped out of my black-flecked notebook. The treatment will take another two months, and the recuperation another four months after that. To return to a sense of well-being takes at least a year—really two years. During that time, quarterly surveillance in the form of PET scans will determine his future (or if he will have one). The disease and the treatment will test the whole family's limits—they will need as much backup from family and friends as they can muster.

Guerra blocks me when he thinks I am saying too much. It's interesting because I thought he hadn't been paying too much attention, but he has taken in everything and has been weighing it against what his wife and son can handle. I am struck by his subtle calibration of his family's ability to handle stress in its protean forms.

For years, I had been at the tail end of discussions about compassionate release for terminal prisoners, those who were so ravaged by disease that they posed no threat to society regardless of their crime. Guerra, who had never committed a violent felony and was struggling against a life-threatening disease, was a good candidate for release.

Humanity dictated that people like him could and should spend their last days with their families. The hard-line punitive thirty-year-plus political environment demanded time served without mercy. Many patients, unfortunately, had no family left and many families were dysfunctional remnants, incarceration's other silent victims. For others, this basic social unit proved remarkably durable. Most patients released under the compassion rubric could not walk. Others had progressive neurological diseases and couldn't breathe without oxygen being forced into their lungs. Most had only a few weeks or a month to go. Still many critics of the humanitarian program clamored for revenge—"Let them rot in prison and die alone!"

But I can't help but think of the old expression: If one is intent on revenge, one should dig two graves. One for one's victim and one for oneself.

Why was Guerra still in limbo regarding compassionate release? Yes, he was a recidivist and still addicted to heroin. He had a possible terminal disease with a generous 30-plus percent chance of a cure. It was all numbers, statistics, and probabilities. The treatment was protracted; if he could complete it, he had a chance. If he could not, then he had no chance and the inexorable growth and expansion of the cancer would kill him in a year max.

We'd filed the papers for compassionate release with the prosecuting attorney, a recent Harvard Law School grad (as she let me know in the first three minutes of our conversation), and we attempted to call her office a dozen times without a response. Finally, I called on connections. The husband of one of my attending physicians was a prosecuting attorney with a bright political future. He was eventually successful in getting his colleague to return my call.

She was tired, grouchy, and clearly did not know much about the case in question. This was not a highlight of her day. The scorecard for her life after the DA's office was about putting prisoners behind bars, not letting them out. That was her ticket to partnership and a lifetime in elite legal circles. I got that, so I put my argument in terms of not compassion, which would have netted zero results, but rather cost efficiency. Juan Guerra's care in jail would cost $350,000-plus; he had a wife and son and a stable home situation. I also reassured her that the Guerra case would not come back to haunt her as she moved up professionally. Guerra's Vietnam War record and the fact that he had no felonies for weapons possession or violent acts of any kind were predictors in his favor.

We still heard nothing for well over a month. During that period I would pop in to talk to Guerra from time to time, to check his neck and mumble reassuring nothings. He was losing weight, losing hair, and, indomitable as he was, beginning to lose hope. He was not angry talking about prison or his life. He did it half laughing and with a partial smile. It was life as he knew it. The prison routines, the judicial system, the court-appointed lawyers, the shitty food, indignities, risks and violence, gangs, protection were all kept in a part of his brain he shared only occasionally. The trick was appearing confident and not vulnerable when he spoke of his life behind bars. This was survival strategy number one. Knowing how to wait. But now, of course, waiting was not a survival strategy. Hope was not a plan.

As I leave the conference room to go back to my office, Budd finds me. "There's been a glitch," he says.

"No!" I say, surprising even myself by the tone of surprise in my voice.

"Yes." Budd's matter-of-fact tone does not hide his frustration. "Apparently the clerk faxed in the wrong form and the lock-them-all-up-for-life guy in Albany got wind of the release so it's all touch and go now. We can't release him without the right document. We'll have to get the right one signed ASAP if he's going home."

"Guerra doesn't know. Can you stall a bit?"

"Yes, we'll have to. Let me figure something out."

"Okay. I'll be back up later. Call me if you know anything."

"'Kay. Later."

Getting out of the prison unit is a lot easier and faster than getting in—if you're a doctor and not a prisoner, of course.

I check in with Patty to learn that the Mexican minister of health has been delayed. I climb the two flights of stairs to the male psychiatric ward to take a look. Some patients sit at the round tables in a large room chatting with the aides, nurses, and doctors or sit quietly by themselves or pace. Coffee and cartons of apple juice and packages of cookies have been handed out, like a break at summer camp. Uniformed guards stand at both entrances. There are about thirty patients, mostly black men, a few whites, and some Hispanics. They are schizophrenic, bipolar, depressed, anxious, suicidal, schizo-affective, and have personality disorders. Many have been abused, many are ex-felons, many have drug problems, some have AIDS, and many have all of the above.

The psych ward brings up a memory of my medical school training years in Brooklyn.

A twelve-year-old had been found in the psychiatry emergency intake room by a clerk, who noted that he had been there for several days sitting in the same chair. The boy was wearing a pull-down gray winter hat and sunglasses. He was brought into the triage area for questioning. When the nurse removed his hat and sunglasses, the bruises around his head—black eyes and a swollen-shut right eye—made it clear in a microsecond what the issue was. His story emerged in stages over weeks. His mother and her boyfriend would tie him to the steam heating fixture in their apartment. He was fed from two dog bowls on the floor, one for water and one for dog food. He was beaten if he cried and if he didn't cry. He was whipped and watched this couple smoke crack. His mother would bring up other men for ten dollars. He would whimper and they would beat him. One day they dropped him in front of the hospital. After he was admitted, we fed him ice cream, candy bars, McDonald's hamburgers, Rice Krispies, and anything else he wanted. Then he was sent to the ACS, Administration for Children's Services, for disposition to a family that would look after him. That was it.

Today he would be forty-six years old. I was twenty-four when I met him. I have never gotten the image of his baby face out of my mind. Every time I see a bruise, I see his face. Was he in the prison ward? Was he in a unit like this somewhere, having orange juice? Was he alive?

Many if not the vast majority of the individuals in the psych unit were subjected to extremities of violence themselves as children. If there is a laboratory experiment in how to create people at the margin of functionality by eliminating all resources and social supports, education, medical care, and community involvement, these are the guinea pigs who have been dumped out of their cages and turned loose on the streets. The prosecuting attorneys lock them up in the city's penitentiaries, and we treat them for the medical and psychiatric problems that flourish in the hothouse atmosphere of a prison system. In forty years, that system has gone 180 degrees from rehabilitation to punishment, without regard for the long-term self-inflicted collateral damage.

My cell phone rings, and Budd's name appears on the screen. "Nothing yet. The Guerra family is getting agitated."

"Okay. We're working on it."

I decide to go back up to the prison unit until I hear from Patty. I want to be useful to Guerra and his family and smooth over the discharge. Plus, I remind myself, I have other patients there that I need to talk to.

I see Marlene Scott, the head nurse for over twenty-five years, bending over a file at the nurses' desk. A middle-aged, diminutive Afro-Caribbean woman, she emanates calmness and authority. The escalating curses of a patient being wheeled to his room/cell down the hall behind her do not even seem to register. She looks up and smiles at me. "Budd's in with a patient."

We reminisce about the old prison unit in the administration building at Bellevue, before the new hospital was built. No one wanted to go there. It was made of wide-open wards typical of the time. Kings County, where I trained, had the same setup. Everyone was in one big room with only curtains to protect their privacy. And the curtains didn't work! On my first day as resident, I was on rounds and tried to pull the curtain shut. Dozens of baby cockroaches fell on the patient's huge cirrhotic abdomen filled with tense ascites, fluid from a scarred and marginally functioning liver. His yellow hue was the same as the stained sheets. He didn't move when the roaches scrambled off him onto the bed.

I ask her about Guerra. "No news," she says, "but they've got a whiff of the problem. It's hard for them, after everything they've been through. The possibility now that he won't get out seems more than they can bear."

"I'm going to see him now."

She decides to walk with me through the unit to the waiting room. As we go, she tells me about a retirement party a few weeks earlier at Bellevue where a woman spoke of her first job on the prison unit when she was eighteen. She had called a prisoner by a number. Her supervisor asked her to step outside. He told her this was a human being and to call him Mr. Jones. She never forgot that lesson. She used it as an example of the many contradictions that crop up in trying to treat people as human beings in systems that degrade their humanity.

I see Guerra's wife speaking intently to her son. I wonder for a second who comforts her.

I put my hand on Guerra's shoulder and assure him we're working on the release. Guerra just shrugs. "I was an idiot to hope. What a *pendejo*!" He looks old. In prison, everyone looks ten to twenty-five years older than they are, except the teenagers.

I check my watch and go to the nurses' station to call Patty. No beeps, so that's a good sign. She picks up immediately and tells me something has come up in the Mexican consulate; the minister is delayed again. He will make it in by late afternoon. He'll call. She got the Guerra release files again and hand-delivered the right form back to the prosecuting attorney's office. She wants me to call them to expedite it, sign it, and return ASAP. They won't pay attention to her.

My beeper goes off several times and I retreat to the nursing station for a phone, a computer, and a modicum of quiet. Medical Director Ed Fishkin from Brooklyn's Woodhull hospital is on the line about our lack of ICU beds and their inability to transfer three patients who have been waiting for more than a day. A young woman has falciparum malaria after returning from Southeast Asia. And she is in her third trimester of pregnancy and cannot breathe. We need an ICU bed and a team from high-risk OB, pulmonary, and critical care medicine right now.

The next call is from my daughter, Marina, inviting me out to dinner at a small bistro on First Avenue, our usual place when Diana is out of town giving a lecture. Marina was back after a post-BA year studying in Israel and was settling into a new job in Midtown. Sometimes the five of us would go out, including my son, Alexei, who lives in Brooklyn with his wife, Gladys. Diana complained that all the best family dinners happened when she wasn't around, but she understood and appreciated the family support system.

After getting an ICU bed, I make a call to the prosecuting attorney's office and tell her assistant about the urgency. I promise to email the attorney. I put in a few words like "justice" and "the American way" and "my friend at the *New York Times*" in the hope of hurrying this along.

I report in to Patty.

"*Jefe*, I have a turkey sandwich on your desk for when you get back down here." She then puts through my voice messages—all routine except the one from Diana sending me hugs and kisses from Santiago, plus she's found me the perfect novel by Faciolince and pulsating *vallenato* recommended by her friends in Colombia. Our long-standing tradition from her innumerable travels: She finds the most interesting book everyone is talking about and the CD that you can't live without.

I wind my way back through the gate and pick up my cell phone, then head back to my office. Too late I remember that sanctimonious Dr. Faruz is waiting. He'd been in several times in the past couple of weeks already, complaining that another department was poaching on his area. As new technologies have developed, several departments (not infrequently with a monopoly source of income) have been losing ground on what they see as their immutable rights to turf. Interventional cardiology with catheterization has reduced the volume of bypass surgeries dramatically worldwide. There are medical winners and losers in the financial game. This is why Faruz was waiting for me, though inevitably the tensions would be expressed in terms of quality and patient safety, competency, and so on. I was not sympathetic. Times change, new procedures come online all the time. Departments that try to hold on to things using technical and bureaucratic stratagems to control their monopolistic practices are not just hurting themselves. In the long run, they limit the institution's ability to stay vibrant and adaptive and will ultimately hurt our patients.

I'm not in the mood for Dr. Faruz—I just want my turkey sandwich.

As I put my hand on the back door to my office, I hear my name called from behind. Beth, the head of the forensics unit, is on her cell phone and waves at me to wait. She listens intently into the phone. When she hangs up, she asks me if I have some free time to go with her to CPEP to see a new prisoner who was brought in recently. I think about my sandwich, then look at my phone and see that Patty has moved the appointment with the Mexican minister of health until the end of the day. I think of Dr. Faruz and turn to follow Beth back down the stairs to the ground floor.

We wind our way through the back corridors and are stopped by a phalanx of corrections officers. There are the usual officers in blue with holstered guns, but now there are also many in white shirts and the entire area is blocked off from every direction. We see a single prisoner being led between a squadron of blue and white shirts in front of us down the hall from the Blue Room to the CPEP entrance.

He's the prisoner I saw come in early this morning from my office window. He is shuffling in his leg shackles. He looks over at us since we are the only non-guards in his field of vision. He is totally expressionless. His eyes are alive, but he gives away nothing. His tattoos are obvious now, even more chilling since they cover every inch of exposed skin except the front of his face. His neck bears the letters *MS* and a number *13*.

Las Maras Salvatrucha. The Maras are leagues away from the Crips and Bloods. They're relatively new to New York. I am familiar with them from my trips to Chiapas, the southernmost state in Mexico near the Guatemalan border. The Maras prey upon undocumented immigrants fleeing north. They will steal and extort everything. They will cut off arms, disembowel, or behead someone for nothing. When the Maras are sent to prisons, they take them over, organize them, terrorize the guards, and train their fellow inmates in their particularly vicious brand of violence.

CPEP, where the Mara gang member is taken, is a very controlled space. New York City police and hospital police stand right outside the doors and glass windows. The many staff members inside this prison wing are used to dealing with all kinds of difficult situations, particularly violent and unpredictable patients. "Tako"—as he is nicknamed according to his file—swallowed some silverware at the supermax prison on Rikers, and needs some X-rays and a surgical consult. We have to observe him for a couple of days while things work their way through his system and out the other end. This is a fairly common practice, and we call the patients "swallowers." Inmates use this little trick as a way to get off the island and break up the boredom. Our Mara friend says nothing. I'm glad to get out of there and thank my colleague for taking me down with her, though I will have Maras *pesadillas*, nightmares, for a few weeks afterward.

I head back to my office as my beeper goes off. Budd. I call up.

Guerra isn't eating. Won't allow anything in the tube, either. His wife and son are beside themselves. I say I'll be up.

Late in the afternoon, the ritual of getting into 19 South is compounded by the rush for elevators, the waiting, pushing, shoving off all those in a hurry to go up or down. After I make it to the floor, Budd takes me to Guerra. He looks gray. If anything, he has aged since this morning. He looks up at me, weary, and looks down at his shoes again, bent over as he is with his shoulders on his knees. His wife and son look alarmed.

"What's up?" I ask him.

"I'm sick, Doc."

"How come you're not eating?"

"I'm afraid to throw it up. It'll hurt."

"You have to eat, Guerra, or you're going to get weaker. You need all the strength you have for this. We will use the stomach tube now exclusively to feed you, so no worry about swallowing at all. You will reteach yourself how to swallow when you're stronger. Your throat muscles will learn again."

He looks at me. "It doesn't matter."

"Guerra, don't give up now. You'll be home soon. You have to save your strength for your treatment. Don't make it harder for your wife or for your son."

Guerra looks up again, and stares at each of them.

"Okay. Bring it on." His wife attaches the syringe to the plastic outlet on the tube that dangles from just above his belly button—her first time feeding him, and pours in the Ensure. He holds her hand as the liquid goes in.

"Good," I say. "You'll both have to learn how to do the feedings and look after the equipment. It's not hard. You'll get the hang of it. Small amounts six times a day and slow feeds overnight by the pump. That's it."

I smile at them as I leave.

Back in my office, I put on some music and make myself a coffee. I email Patty for an update, but ask her to give me a few minutes if possible. I sit and look out the window, and am suddenly furious. Why is someone like Juan Guerra treated the same as the Mara? When did mental illness and petty drug possession offenses become equivalent to major crimes? The psychiatric patients need mental health care, Guerra needs cancer treatment at home with his family, and "Tako" needs to be locked away in the supermax—not that imprisonment will deter him from continuing the terrible things he's done. There are now at least tens of thousands of Maras and their deadly offspring spread from LA to Long Island. Do we really need to finance an incubator for more? Why are so many people, with such a wide range of problems, sent to prison as the one-size-fits-all solution?

If our goal as a society is to lock people up and throw away the key, then there is a genius to the three-strikes laws. If the goal is to make us feel safer and to create a society that is healthier and more productive, then we have failed miserably.

I pull my thoughts back to the present when Patty calls. Guerra's papers have been signed and he is being released within the hour. She also tells me that the young woman in the SICU with a severe brain injury from her motorcycle accident has died. Normally Patty wouldn't call me about this, but the body was left in the room for six hours before being claimed by the medical examiner, headquartered just a block north of the hospital. The family flew in from Italy, not only bereaved but irate over the lapse. They are saying they won't be able to get their daughter home for a proper burial. I tell Patty I'll phone the parents and apologize profusely after speaking with the attending and getting details from him. The *ministro de salud* of Mexico has arrived, she adds, and will be up in five minutes. I look at the building encroaching on my view, the steady thread of cars heading north on the FDR. One of them will soon have Juan Guerra in the backseat with his wife and son on their way to the Bronx and a future they can't anticipate. Will he even complete the treatment? This thought starts to burrow its way into my brain. I reel it in and turn off the heart-aching fado music of Dulce Pontes as I get up to greet Mexico's minister of health.

CHAPTER 2

Tanisha

The walk from Bushwick in North Brooklyn had taken several hours. Ice-cold air and slushy snow on the streets had the effect of another dose of adrenaline for Tanisha. She had climbed down the fire escape outside the window in her room when commercial garbage trucks were making their predawn rounds. Her hands were freezing against the oxidized and flaking bare metal that scraped raw the skin on her palms. Three flights down and then a fifteen-foot drop to the sidewalk. By the time she was at the bottom and hanging from the rusty bottom rung, her five-foot-one frame left her with a mere ten-foot controlled fall. It was four o'clock in the morning, and the streets were empty. A flickering streetlight reflected off the snow and ice. She could see the barbershop sign as she hung for a few seconds. The lights of a 24/7 Bodega "El Amanecer" on the corner were nearly hidden in a cloud of steam from a sidewalk vent. She let go and dropped, hardly making any noise when her Converse All Stars hit the cement. She remained in a crouch, rubbing her ankles, for a few seconds.

Tanisha was sixteen, pretty, with braided hair that hung to her mid-back. She had bundled herself in several T-shirts, a sweater, and an extra-large Yankees sweatshirt along with jeans layered over pajamas. She headed toward Myrtle Avenue a few blocks away, carefully scanning the streets. A few lone cars drove past her as she made her way, her breath turned white. She was glad it was freezing, unlikely anyone would be hanging outside.

She had stayed too long at this foster family's apartment. She knew it from her placement there exactly four weeks ago. The caseworker from the Administration for Children's Services had taken her in a car with another worker. It had been her twelfth foster care placement, almost one a year since she was born in Kings County Hospital sixteen years earlier. They had arrived in the late morning and a middle-aged woman opened the door, smiled, and welcomed them inside. Tanisha had dropped her guard slightly when the woman, Letitia, spoke with a Spanish accent. It had brought her back momentarily to the one foster placement that had been a home to her several years earlier.

The warmth of the apartment—the radiators that had no controls— and the steamed windows made it seem almost friendly. The case-workers had stayed for over an hour, talking with Letitia, introducing Tanisha, and helping unpack the small backpack of what remained of her worldly items. She had a few changes of clothes and a small zipped bag for her toothbrush and hairbrush. The senior caseworker Anna had given *la puertoriqueña* Letitia two plastic pillboxes and gone over the instructions for the timing of the medications and possible side effects. There was a sheaf of papers she had in a plastic binder. She gave Letitia a copy of some documents and asked her to sign and date a form. The workers turned to Tanisha, who was sitting quietly at the dining room table, came over to give her a hug, and told her she would be fine here and they would be by to visit in a few days.

The problem started that night. In the late afternoon, Letitia's daughter had come home with her boyfriend. They put on the television and ate pizza while talking and ignored Tanisha after a perfunc-tory introduction by Letitia, who promptly left to do some errands. The boy was around twenty and lived upstairs and didn't appear to notice that Tanisha was even in the room.

It was after midnight when Tanisha was in bed. She had left the window open a few inches since the only way to control the tempera-ture was to let in some cold air. She heard the window scraping against the frame and saw a sneaker and leg enter the room, followed by the young man from the afternoon. The light from the street made it clear who he was even in the shadows. He slid the window down, looked over at her, and took out a switchblade.

This wasn't the first time Tanisha had been raped, violated, or abused in foster care, but she had decided it would be the last time.

She said nothing to the family the next morning after they banged on the door to the bathroom as she showered under near-boiling water for fifteen minutes to cleanse her mind and body. The window didn't have a lock. She jammed it shut that morning and rigged a wooden bar so that it could not be opened. She also took a knife from the kitchen and kept it at the side of the bed. She heard rattling at the window a few nights later, again after midnight. The young man came over several days a week, and one night she noticed that the piece of broomstick keeping the window secure was gone. It was time to get out.

When she got to Myrtle Avenue, she turned right under the elevated train. She had gotten directions on the walk to Manhattan from a friendly counterperson at the White Castle all-night diner. "You go to Myrtle," he'd said, pointing out the window, "and make a right turn. It is another fifteen minutes until you hit Broadway. There is another elevated train there and you make another right turn. You just walk the length of Broadway and stay under the elevated train. It runs right into the Williamsburg Bridge. You can't miss it. You are practically in the East River. It is another world there. You are in another country." He smiled enigmatically while handing over two hamburgers and french fries "on the house, *chica. Suerte*, good luck."

By the time she got to the hundred-year-old bridge it was past five a.m. and the streets were starting to fill up. At first she was anxious, but she could hear the trains squealing overhead. The early-morning risers were going to work. Bundled up against the cold, they barely gave Tanisha a glance, walking quickly to the steep stairs to the M train platform or ducking into the coffee and donut shops that lined Broadway in a shadowy sunless netherworld. She knew she was near the bridge when several men walked along the early-morning streets of Williamsburg in long black coats and round brown fur hats with white socks. She had heard about this group of Hasidic Jews, the Satmars. They ignored her and spoke among themselves in a guttural foreign language. An orange school bus idled at the corner, plumes of white exhaust exiting the rear like a surreal post-apocalyptic beast. The door opened and long black coats and fur hats got inside.

It took Tanisha awhile to find the pedestrian walkway across the bridge. She waited until a group of middle-aged workers, black metal lunch pails in hand, started across and trailed them by fifty feet. They would be her safety net to the other side. The morning was sparkling clear and very cold. The wind whipped through her layers. She tucked the hood tightly around her head and put her hands underneath her armpits. Traffic was picking up. Red taillights zipped by. Tugboat lights headed north up the East River toward Roosevelt Island. Sparkling yellow lights from Manhattan stretched as far to the north as you could see. Once she was across the bridge, she was in known territory. She had been "placed" on the Lower East Side two years earlier. There wasn't a block, bodega, or pizza shop she didn't know in the area, from Delancey Street to 14th Street. Avenue C in Alphabet City had been her home base. It would be good to be out of a Brooklyn she was unfamiliar with—each neighborhood a crazy quilt of angled streets, different languages, street gangs, drug dealers, hustlers, hipsters, and old folks sitting on their stoops. You had to have your wits about you and stay in your safe zone or it was a game park.

As Tanisha wound her way past the midpoint of the bridge and began the downward slope into Manhattan, her thoughts changed into Spanish. She was back in the house of her *abuelita*. Mama Lola as her family called her and *abuelita* (little grandmother) as the six young girls called her, wards of the state in foster care in a group home run by Mama Lola and her adoring husband, Hugo. He drove a livery car or gypsy cab fifteen hours a day, as the price of gasoline had inched its way up and cut into his weekly take-home pay. *Abuela* always said her husband "was an exception to Dominican men. He has one wife and one family, and he is a loving man. I found the one in my town."

As her legs carried her down the slope, she ran through in her mind the families and group homes she had lived with over the years since she had a memory. Of her mother she had no recollection, and there virtually no information was shared with her or perhaps known. All Tanisha knew about her mother was that she was a Latina drug addict; crack was her drug of choice. She had several other children all in foster care removed by ACS. She had left Tanisha when she was a child with some "crack sisters," and a neighbor called 911. After the police arrived and found a six-month-old girl in a filthy rug, they brought the baby to St. Barnabas hospital in the Bronx. ACS was notified and traced the mother to the Rose M. Singer women's prison at Rikers Island. They worked through the legal system to have Tanisha removed permanently from the mother's custody given her long record of drugs, abandonment, and prostitution. Tanisha's mother had been a victim herself of a mother who had been a gang member, drug user, and petty dealer who didn't actively abuse her children so much as neglect them. *Feral* was the term ACS used in a report that had been shared with Tanisha by a social worker when she was a young teenager. Tanisha had no idea what feral was. She had thought it was an animal, a pet tiger.

The Smiths were the first family Tanisha remembered. They were a black Jamaican couple with six youngsters under their care. Tanisha was four years old. They were benign with the children. There was food on the table, and the kids were bathed and kept clean, dry, and warm. They slept in one large dormitory room with the door open. The husband came home from driving a city bus and sat in front of the television and slipped a bottle of rum out from a brown paper bag. His personality went from quiet and calm to an animal growl with a few sips of the brownish liquid. Tanisha could still hear his voice penetrating the walls and the open door, "Get your fucking ass in here, bitch. Get your fucking ass right in here." The yelling, cursing, screaming, door banging, and throwing would cease around midnight, when he could be heard snoring. The thunderous snores were punctuated by long apneic pauses when he ceased to breathe altogether. And then the rumble would begin again after some horse-like snorts. The kids would finally get to sleep between nightmares and bed-wetting. One day a dozen ACS workers showed up at the apartment with several official white vehicles idling in the street. The children were all packed up and taken away. Two workers accompanied each child. Mrs. Smith was nowhere in sight. Mr. Smith was driving his bus. They were all taken to a large shelter somewhere in Brooklyn.

By the time Tanisha was seven, she had been in seven different residential homes and foster families, plus a few shelters and ACS distribution facilities. She remembered her first hospitalization as she reached the bottom of the bridge and kept walking down Delancey Street. She stopped in a Dunkin' Donuts on the north side of the street. This was an old hangout, and she was glad it was still here after so many years. There was already a line in front of the counter where some Indian women presided over the coffee and donuts. She settled in a window seat warming up for a few minutes. At age seven she had become unmanageable. The foster family had called 911 when she attacked another foster child who hit Tanisha and called her a bitch. Something had flipped and continued to flip without any warning signs.

She would be fine—then suddenly hypervigilant. Something would snap, and later she had no recognition of what had happened. Except that some adults were holding her down, sitting on her, injecting her buttock with Haldol that put her to sleep or left her extremely dopey, in a dream-like state. She had once been taken to an emergency room at the local hospital. After hours of sitting on a stretcher with a bored woman in light brown scrubs looking at her, reading the paper, and talking to her boyfriend on her cell phone, she was admitted to the inpatient pediatric unit. The other kids had diabetes, pneumonia, influenza, epilepsy, asthma, and mental retardation. Tanisha remembered the doctor who talked to her two days after she was admitted. He took her into a quiet room, with a social worker taking notes at his side. There were toys in the room. Tanisha was asked if she wanted to play with the toys or draw. She refused to talk to the man, who looked bored and tired. She was hungry and asked for food. They said after she drew them a picture. She sat and waited them out. After a month on the unit, visited by social workers, psychologists and the occasional psychiatrist, and ACS workers, she was transferred to another foster family.

A succession of families followed, interrupted by shelter stays when the families disintegrated in a shower of police calls, domestic violence, drug dealing, and ACS investigations. As Tanisha pushed out the door of Dunkin' Donuts and headed north, she thought she glimpsed a man she had pushed to the back of her mind but could never forget.

She kept an eye out for him instinctively. A habitual roving third eye. There were many times when she thought she saw him in a crowd, on the subway, on a bus, or across the street. She was always prepared to lose herself, make herself disappear, or if necessary take her own life.

The Brown family had been gregarious and welcoming. The children, all four of them, were teenagers, well dressed and well behaved. The house was spotlessly clean, with old but well-maintained furniture that shone after being polished every week. The children did their homework in the evenings and then were allowed some television time before going to bed. Chores were divided up evenly and listed in rotation on a board in the small kitchen: garbage, dishes, laundry, bed making, tidying up, washing the kitchen floor. It all seemed too perfect. Tanisha's symptoms had been better, and she didn't have a "flipout" more than a couple of times. Lester Brown liked to read to the children at night. After a few months he had asked Tanisha if he could read her a special story. His wife was in the bedroom with a migraine and had taken a sleeping pill. He and Tanisha were in the living room alone with a reading light on, a blanket covering them. He placed Tanisha on his lap and opened Dr. Seuss. He whispered in her ear and she felt something hard between her legs as his breathing accelerated and he moved rhythmically. She had sat totally still as the large man panted in her ear then clutched her to him in a spasm that seemed to last forever. He made her change her pajamas before he put her into bed, whispering, "You are my favorite, Tanisha. We will read together again, just the two of us. Let's keep this our secret."

Tanisha pushed open the doors to the ACS intake building just off First Avenue at six thirty a.m. The building was just north of the main entrance to Bellevue Hospital and part of the original sprawling hospital complex. The morning shift was starting to stream in through front doors. The rectangular silver food carts were jockeying for position on both sides of the avenue. Delivery trucks were triple-parked, and an FDNY ambulance hung a hard right turn down to the main emergency room entrance. She was patted down for drugs and weapons and then fed and bathed. The senior administrator knew her well and stopped by to welcome her. After six hours of evaluation and innumerable phone calls, two workers took her to the Bellevue emergency room.

The child psychiatric emergency room had bright colors, flat-screen television sets, and a glass-enclosed nursing station. A nurse and health tech escorted Tanisha into a private exam room. They asked her to undress and gave her some hospital-issue pajamas to wear on the unit. They told her she could have her own clothes back later. The aide searched her carefully and discreetly as she handed her the tops and bottoms and a bathrobe. This wasn't a new routine for Tanisha; she had been through it half a dozen times before. In her own mind she had run out of options and had to find the safest place possible.

I was having lunch with Francesca Durat, the on-call child psychiatrist, when she was beeped urgently to the emergency room to see the new admission. We had been deep in a discussion of her experiences with childhood trauma. She was French Algerian, and we had been talking about her years working in the *banlieues*, or immigrant ghettos ringing Paris. The populist anger, economic deprivation, racism, and religious intolerance that had led to riots in the suburbs of Paris resonated loudly in post-9/11 New York City. The overhang from a decade of foreign wars, failure to resolve immigration issues, globalization's domestic effects, and the growing unemployment and inequality was creating combustible domestic politics here, too.

We walked back to the child unit together, and I asked if I could sit in on the intake interview. Tanisha showed no emotion when I shook her hand and asked if she minded if I sat in with Francesca. She nodded okay, looking me directly in the eyes. It made me feel vulnerable. This sixteen-year-old, five-foot-one Dominican Haitian teenager with a thick Bellevue chart from multiple hospitalizations, evaluations, emergency room visits, and psychological testing was rapidly sizing up the two adults in the room who would be evaluating her and making some determination about her future. I switched roles with Tanisha and felt the weight of her "chart" on all of us, the caretakers over her lifetime. What secrets, tragedies, and small mercies were buried in its pages?

I had canceled my afternoon and asked Patty not to put through any calls unless they were true emergencies—and even then to come down and get me, since I turned off my phone and beeper. The consultation room was a corporate back office, a cell with a windowed door leading to an outer vestibule. We sat there for nearly three hours while the psychiatrist tiptoed into Tanisha's life.

She was very smart with a sharp wit and gradually became more spontaneous and talkative. Monosyllabic answers gave way to short responses.

"Why did you run away from the foster home in Bushwick?"

"I did not run away. I left of my own free will at a time of my choosing. I never ran."

"Sorry, I didn't mean run away in that way. Why did you leave?" Francesca practically whispered this time. She was getting quieter and softer as Tanisha was getting more assertive. It was as if there were a scale in the room for affect or emotion. As Tanisha heated up, Francesca turned down her emotional volume.

Carefully calibrated, Tanisha responded, "ACS has sent me to so many shitholes, with so many assholes that want to fuck with me or fuck me. Just who should you be interviewing?"

Tanisha did not blink for a long time. She held us in her gaze and kept us there. This was not a usual kid in crisis who was melting down in a rage-fueled episode of "acting out," cutting herself, homicidal, or suicidal. You could feel her intelligence in the small room. She had a special-education plan or IEP that had put her in small classes with other "disturbed" adolescents. Most of the kids in these special programs had low to normal intelligence; many were severely retarded from drugs or alcohol in utero, and many from sheer intellectual deprivation. Socially isolated, the parents of many of these children were themselves marginally literate. The level of stimulation in a home was limited to shouts, obscenities, and a 24/7 blasting television.

"I do have a plan to kill myself," she answered in response to another question from Francesca.

"What is your plan, Tanisha? Have you had these thoughts recently?"

"Doctor, I have had a plan for a long time if things don't work out. If I cannot get out a back door. I won't tell you my plan, then it wouldn't be a plan, would it? I mean it wouldn't be my plan, it would be our plan. I don't have hardly anything at all in my life. Every time I get moved in foster care I lose half of my stuff and the other half gets ripped off. Like I have nothing except what I have in my head. If that motherfucker had made it into the room again I would have killed him or myself or both of us. That is for fucking sure."

After a few hours of conversation with Tanisha, I felt spiritually dehydrated. Like everything had been sucked out of me. It was like watching an accident over and over again in slow motion. Kids like Tanisha are trapped. They will die, and there is nothing you can do to save them. You cannot keep playing that script over in your head without hurting yourself. I had gone through her chart before going in the room and had a sense that a form of soul death was foretold for this young girl. What were her chances of making it out the other side of childhood emotionally intact, considering what she had been given?

Tanisha's diagnosis at admission was provisionally depression with suicidal thinking secondary to PTSD or post-traumatic stress syndrome. There were a million social risk factors listed in the diagnostic categorization. Every box was checked off. She had not been given her medication by her "family." She made it clear she wouldn't have taken it under any circumstances, since the medications made her feel worse and gain weight. She had been on an anti-depressant and an anti-psychotic medication used to "augment" or improve the effectiveness of the anti-depressant. I had seen the drug advertised on television, in popular magazines, and on the subway.

PTSD is a diagnostic category that emerged from the Vietnam War. In the 1970s when the war was grinding its way to a close, the range of symptoms seen among returning vets did not fit other categories of mental illness. The cluster of symptoms was not just depression, not simple anxiety, not only related to the use of drugs or alcohol. The PTSD complex included flashbacks of the traumatic events, extreme vulnerability, irrational fears, nightmares, depression mixed with anxiety and rage. Vets were placed on cocktails of prescription medications—with mixed results—as the diagnosis became widely accepted and many millions of dollars were invested by the federal government to understand the syndrome or "disease" better. PTSD was made an "official" disease in 1980. This is twenty-seven hundred years after Homer described the effects of war on warriors in his majestic *Iliad*.

Recently the category was being refined to fit kids who had been subjected to violent and abusive events. Some kids who witnessed parental abuse and violence or had been physically or emotionally abused became emotionally unhinged. Tanisha lost control of her emotional regulators. She couldn't think her way out of a flash emotional discharge. Her emotional centers were "hijacked." Ordinarily children learn how to control their emotional states. This is one of the major tasks of childhood. When kids are subjected to trauma during vulnerable developmental periods that make them children and not mini-adults, they miss the development of emotional control. This emotional dysregulation flows through many childhood disorders. It is almost a universal symptom.

Tanisha described a fleeting anxiety—what she called her "third eye"—continuously scanning the environment for dangerous people. They could be anywhere, her experience had taught her. "They look just like you, Doc. How do I know you are not one of them? You can't tell by just looking at someone. The worst shit has happened to me from the most smiling, most friendly, let-me-help-you-out-young-lady bullshit ones. In fact, they are the ones I worry about the most. They want you. They want you to like them and they disarm you. Man, I been there and done that and never again doing that. I have an alarm detector, a regular LoJack for that shit." Then, when it got activated, she said, "I don't even remember what happens, it is so fast. I am being pulled off someone or in the hospital injected with one of your latest and greatest medications and then I just go to sleep for a whole day. I have no idea what goes on when it hits me."

I left to go back to my office. The back stairs to my office are down the hall from the emergency room. Yolanda from the Organ Donor

Network spotted me before I saw her. "*Qué tal*, Dr. Eric, how are you?" she boomed, carrying a cardboard tray of coffees and croissants.

"What's up, Yolanda?" I asked. "You are not here for good news?"

"You heard about the kid, Ignacio?"

"I haven't heard anything, Yolanda. I've been locked up for hours with a patient and had my cell phone off." I remembered and reached down to fiddle with the buttons.

"Kid wearing iPod earbuds leaned too far into the path of an oncoming Q train."

I knew the story from a middle-of-the-night phone call from Jamila, the night administrator, whose calm and sonorous Middle Eastern accent took the edge off even the worst events. I realized what all the activity was in front of the family waiting room down the hall and now could make out sobbing more distinctly. The young man had never felt anything, and his heart was strong and beating when the ambulance picked him up. They had controlled the bleeding with pressure, then radioed ahead and brought him to the trauma slot.

My meetings with city leaders the next morning had been scrubbed— they headed to Albany in a shiny black SUV to lobby against the looming cuts to the public health system—so I walked down to the child psych emergency room. Tanisha was sitting having breakfast dressed in street clothes: skintight blue jeans, a long-sleeved tan T-shirt, and black Converse sneakers with fire-engine-red socks. She was talking to another girl, a late-evening admission, who was showing her a grade school black speckled notebook. She looked up and saw me through the glass in the nursing station. I nodded a hello, which she ignored and went back to eating and listening to the girl.

Coming into the emergency area, I had passed through the cramped waiting area past a fashionably dressed middle-aged couple. While waiting to get into the nursing area, I had said good morning, introduced myself, and asked if I could get them anything. The wife was attractive, with sharp-cut stylish dyed-blond hair and wearing a dark gray business suit. She gave me a weak, tense smile but said nothing. Her husband stood up and shook my hand. His tailored Italian suit fit his trim body like a glove. They were clearly exhausted. In a deep voice, he looked me directly in the eyes and began thanking me for the excellent care his daughter, Emily, had received overnight. I gave them my card if they needed anything during the hospital stay and showed them where they could get a cup of coffee two hallways down to the left.

Ingrid Thomason, the social worker, was in the nursing station writing up her report from the night before on the new admission, Emily Abeloff. I pulled up a chair on wheels next to her. Ingrid was a polyglot thirty-five-year-old who had spent several years in Rwanda and other centers of genocide in Francophone West Africa before decamping at Bellevue. She had just returned from her honeymoon in Mali with her Senegalese psychologist husband, and I congratulated her. We shared an interest in the music mix from the griots of Mali infused with Cuban Son and traded favorite CDs. The concerts were fantastic affairs that continued into the wee morning hours and sold out the first day tickets went on sale.

"Your patient Tanisha has taken up with Emily. They were up most of the night talking and writing. The nurses suspended the bedtime rules since the other kids were watching a movie together and it was more like camp here than a psychiatric emergency room for once."

"What's up with Emily?" I asked.

"Sixteen years old, same age as Tanisha, transferred from Methodist Hospital in Park Slope last evening at the family's request. Her parents called 911 when she told them she was filled with suicidal thoughts and they couldn't leave her or talk her down. The nearest hospital from their brownstone is Methodist, which has only a small emergency room and a tiny pediatric inpatient unit. The parents called around and the private uptown units were full. Their neighbor is an NYU professor who knows you and he told them to transfer her here. Said their daughter would get the best psychiatric care in the city!" I made the connection. I could smell the barbecue and look into their backyard from my friend's house.

I nodded and started to ask her for more information when she went on. "She has a long psychiatric history with multiple hospitalizations and twice as many diagnoses. Evidently, she started to fall apart or decompensate when she was six years old. She was up all night, had tantrums, head banging, withdrawal into her room, and extreme irritability from minor provocations of everyday life. There were some family deaths, grandparents were killed in a freak car accident, that may have been triggers but nothing obvious. From what I can piece together, her first hospitalization was for depression and suicidality with a good response to SSRIs or anti-depressants. She had intermittent therapy for a few years and ended up in a pattern of a new therapist, a new diagnosis, and a new medication almost as an annual rite of spring. I am cataloging at least ten different switches over that many years." She handed me a piece of graph paper. The time line had columns and lists in her precise handwriting with arrows to medications and assorted treatment regimens. After looking at it, I asked Ingrid for her interpretation.

"Eric, kids in this developmental period have pretty non-specific symptoms. Their brains are growing and maturing like crazy. They don't have symptoms like adults. Depression in kids does not look like it does in adults, with depressed mood, sleepiness, a lack of enjoyment in life, decreased libido. Irritability is the hallmark symptom in kids. The kids' psychiatric illnesses are pretty undifferentiated, and sometimes hard to tease out. One kid will turn out to have major depression, another schizophrenia, still another a personality disorder, and the last will outgrow everything. The worst mistake is to assume these little humans are little adults. They're not. Adult rules do not apply here."

"And trauma, Ingrid? A common denominator?"

"For the kids we see usually it is. But not always. Take Emily, for example. Her doctors have looked high and low for trauma, parental abuse, or sexual abuse, but many times that's not the case. There are other subtle issues like personality, coping skills, and environmental cues that we don't know about. Remember your biology: Kids are what their grandmothers ate!" She smiled and got back to business.

Through the window I saw a girl about ten years old accompanied by a young female psych tech approach the two teenagers at the table.

She had been watching them from a seat outside her room where she had sat through a fifteen-minute "time-out" for a mini tantrum when she refused to get dressed for breakfast. The two girls looked at her as she spoke to them. They then made room around the table, and the tech pulled up another chair and brought some paper and crayons. In a few minutes she was hunched over her project. Tanisha lent her some pencils, and Emily started talking to her.

The picture that emerged of Emily was a pre-pubertal girl with a pretty average upper-middle-class life, who developed fluctuating or exaggerated emotional highs and lows in first or second grade. Then over the years she was diagnosed with depression, anxiety, histrionic personality, schizo-affective disorder, eating disorders when she suffered from anorexia and bulimia, conduct disorder, borderline personality disorder, and manic depressive disorder plus a handful of other "disorders" from the *DSM*, or *Diagnostic and Statistical Manual*, psychiatry's bible for the last thirty years. Equally impressive was the list of medications in another column with dates connected by arrows to the disorders, as well as a list of psychiatrists, psychologists, and psychiatric social workers she had seen in a decade of peripatetic therapy throughout the city of New York. The list of medications included all the SSRIs I was familiar with and a few I had seen on television ads but didn't know anything about. Ritalin and long-acting stimulants, anti-psychotics from Abilify to Seroquel to clozapine, and a long list of anti-anxiety medications in a broad range of dosages from short to long acting. Emily was also taking a variety of other medications for allergies, mild asthma, abdominal pain, menstrual cramps, and migraine headaches, along with birth control pills.

I watched her through the glass. She was so young. As she sat drawing with Tanisha and the younger child, I found it hard to believe that she'd been medicated for most of her life. In fact, watching them, I was struck once again by how very difficult it is to grow up in our environment. Both of these young women thought actively about dying, about taking their own lives. Money did not cushion all blows.

For Emily, the problem maybe consisted of too much "care" rather than too little. The kinds of therapies she had received were as diverse as her diagnoses and medication lists. There was a prominent Freudian Manhattan psychoanalyst. There was a Jungian analyst, a psychotherapist, three different psychologists who specialized in personality disorders, one who taught Cognitive Behavioral Therapy (CBT), and another Dialectical Behavioral Therapy (DBT), a third specializing in neurocognitive testing, and a fourth at the bottom of the page involved in investigational work with a new treatment group modality for personality disorders at Columbia. The social workers included therapists from Brooklyn to Queens, Manhattan's lower reaches, and its northernmost enclaves near the Cloisters. I was totally baffled by Ingrid's list—and at the same time it gave me a deeper insight into Emily's problems and her parents' frustrations, hopes, fears, and feelings of hopelessness and helplessness in the face of the diagnostic and therapeutic overkill. There was another column labeled "misc" for miscellaneous. This column included gynecologists, internists, neurologists, gastroenterologists, pulmonologists, acupuncturists, Chinese herbalists, and some I couldn't interpret.

I arranged to attend a group meeting on 21 West, the inpatient adolescent unit, a few days later. The floor is for kids only, in the middle of our 350-bed psychiatric hospital within a hospital.

The head nurse, Jane Tyler, unlocked the unit for me and then locked me in when I went through the gray double metal doors. She put her finger to her lips and waved me over to her, whispering, "We are just starting the unit daily meeting. Come in and join us." She pointed to an empty seat between the art therapist, Julie, and a young skinny Chinese boy whose age I could not guess. Twelve? Fifteen? He sat quietly drowning in the folds of his hospital gown, looking down at his hands in his lap.

We went around the room for introductions. A 21 West unit head nurse ran the meetings. She was firm and established rules of politeness and respect that were repeated in unison. At the same time she was tuned in to every gesture and emotional nuance in the room. Tanisha and Emily sat next to each other opposite me. They each had black speckled notebooks in their laps. They opened them during the meeting. They appeared to be reading from them or taking notes from time to time.

In the middle of the meeting a boy named Tyrone, who appeared to be eighteen from his size, began shouting and stood up in the middle of the room. He felt one of the other boys had looked at him and said something disrespectful. Several behavioral health aides got up at the same time and surrounded him. One RN left the room and came back three minutes later with a psychiatrist, Tom Tregerman. When Tyrone saw the psychiatrist, he looked at him and started to explain what had happened. At the same time he relaxed, put his arms down, and walked with the physician from the room. Tom was the one person who had an immediate calming effect on Tyrone. He was enormous for his age and had caused serious property and bodily damage to another patient and an aide during a flash outburst. As I remembered Tyrone's "story," his childhood had been like living in *Apocalypse Now*.

Tyrone talked about his father all the time, asking when was he going to come and visit? When did he call? Did he know the phone number and address of the hospital? Those of us who knew his story understood that the father had abandoned him as a small child. He and his mother lived in poverty, and the father failed to provide child support. His visits, when they happened, were short and unannounced. Tyrone lived for them. He was on the waiting list for the state hospital. There had been too many failures sending him home and to alternative "residential" homes in the archipelago of child and adolescent facilities. What was his future? His life trajectory? Next stop adult psychiatric unit, or Rikers Island, or a mix of both? You didn't need to be a soothsayer to see into the future.

The part of the brain that processes emotions and perceived inputs like fear into rapid bursts of hormonal outputs is called the amygdala or emotional regulator. It's the part of the deep ancestral brain that responds directly to environmental signals, premonitions, and threats. The conscious neural connections to protect this part of Tyrone's emotional brain from being directly activated were poorly developed, perhaps destabilized by childhood trauma or even stress in utero as a developing fetus. The external environment offered no stabilizing or mitigating relief. The hope of his team of therapists was that routines and predictability, rewards for positive behavior, and careful schooling under reliable supportive supervision could start to rebuild the missing pieces. Create a mini scaffolding to build upon. He desperately needed to be cared for and loved. The moving pieces on our units, the staff rotations and shift changes, vacations, and absences for illnesses, made it all seem confusing and reproduced the most profound emotional activation in him, rejection. The state hospital would be a short-term "solution" in this situation. Drugs would calm his behavior, and he would be looked after in a reasonable environment in central Queens.

I caught up with Tanisha a few days later in PS 37, the inpatient school for kids. This New York City school is at the opposite end of a long corridor from the adolescent psychiatry unit. All of the classroom windows look out onto the East River. She was sitting in a social studies classroom with three other teenagers. The top of her head half covered a notebook. Mr. Vargas waved me in and introduced me to the class. I sat next to Tanisha and asked, "*¿Qué tal, Tani? ¿Cómo va el diario?* How are you doing and what's up with your diary?" The kids were encouraged to journal and use art to express themselves. They used the large pads and colored pencils and crayons to share something about themselves. We reviewed the art as part of the forensic evidence of the kids' emotional "temperature" at daily rounds.

The drawings were posted around the units and exhibited in the hospital's giant atrium. Like outsider art, art from untrained, non-professional artists, some of it was spectacular. It was the amygdala speaking truth to power. And some of the most provocative art came from patients who could not verbalize what was going on in their heads. I had gone to outsider art exhibits in New York where the best work was by hospitalized patients forgotten in long-term facilities. Martín Ramírez drew exquisite and intricate pictures of interiors full of trains on used brown grocery bags. The recluse Henry Darger created erotically charged internal fantasy worlds of a depth and richness and erotic sensibility that gave you pause. Cracks in the wall. How to interpret the subtle signs from the kids' hidden worlds? What did the newest diagnosis, conduct disorder, mean? An authorization to use Zyprexa?

Tani. That's what she was called on the unit; her *abuela* had called her Tani. "I am writing about my life. Besides, I am finding things I had forgotten. Places where I had lived and people who I knew but had been buried someplace. I have seen some strange stuff. You guys think I am making it all up."

"You know, Tani, we hear and see some unbelievable things that kids cannot make up. I don't think there is one thing you have shared with us that we don't believe. Not one. You really amaze us with how well you look after yourself. We know your suffering has been real."

"Well, maybe sometime I will share this with you. You told me you keep a journal. You always have that little black notebook with you in your pocket. I see you taking it out and writing in it. What do you put in there?"

I took it out and let her thumb through it. "I have a hundred of these notebooks. I have been writing down my thoughts and the odd things, connections that I know I will forget. Like a vivid dream that wakes you in the morning and then vanishes."

"The stories that *Abuela* told me come back in dreams. Like last night I was riding a horse bareback in the countryside. Going to the next town to get some milk for a baby I helped deliver, and the mother's milk had dried up. I was terrified the baby would die before I got back. *Abuela* was a midwife. She told me many times there wasn't enough food for everyone. They pretended to eat. She said in Haiti, just over the border, they were so poor they ate dirt. They made it into patties, cooked it, and ate it. Just to fill their bellies. She said so many babies died over the border they stacked them in the morning like wood and at the end of the day a man would come and put them on a cart and take them away."

My mind drifted to my time as a medical volunteer in central Haiti, in the Artibonite Valley. The neonates did die, a lot of them. The ones with tetanus were hard like cordwood. Their tiny emaciated cadavers frozen in a death rictus. Their ribs like grinning teeth. They were stacked and taken away by a man with a cart. I didn't know where they went.

We sat and talked until the bell rang and the class was dismissed. The kids moved to music and art class two doors down at the southern end of the corridor. "I am drawing my dreams as I write about them," she said as she packed up her stuff. "I will give you the one I have been working on this week."

The kids were escorted down the hall by a tall well-groomed black man wearing a suit and a yellow tie with a lovely smile. "Okay, kids, let's get to it. Music and drawing. Work and fun to be done. Dr. Manheimer, you are welcome to join us. We do some great stuff in here."

Tani pulled out a large drawing from her personal stack. Chagall would have been proud. "I had a dream I was on the farm in the DR, the Dominican Republic. All of the animals were talking like humans, just like us. Many were half humans and half chickens," she said, pointing to one peculiar beast that had the head of a chicken and the body of a man but also had wings and was floating through the air. The yellows were mixed with reds, blues, and purples. An enormous moon eclipsed the sun so only a sliver could be seen. Animals and people floated by. A silver-haired woman rode a horse in the center with a man behind her. His arms were wrapped around her. "You can keep this, Dr. M." It was beautiful and dream-like. There was no anger or rage in the picture. Everything was in harmony. The center was holding. The couple, clearly Tani's *abuela* and her *marido* or husband, were the force holding everything in orbit as they moved around, floating in the ether. Something clicked at that point. I made a connection and wrote a note in red ink in my black notebook with the picture secured under my arm. I took the elevator down to my office.

Patty buzzed me on my cell phone as I was checking my email on the BlackBerry waiting for an elevator. The Abeloffs, Emily's parents, were in the office. Of the dozens of emails that had accumulated, a couple stood out.

I apologized to the Abeloff family for my lateness as we settled in the office. Emily had been with us for over two weeks at this point. There had been family meetings and a miscellany of private discussions. I thought they wanted to transfer her to a private hospital in the suburbs, or perhaps a bed had opened at one of the private hospitals in the city, maybe even McLean in Boston or the Hartford Retreat.

"We want to thank you for the care our daughter has received on

21 West." Ariel Abeloff took the lead this time. Her face was different. It wasn't frozen with fatigue and resignation.

"Dr. Adrian spends hours with us. She patiently walked us through the entire course of Emily's illness. The multiple diagnoses, the hundred and one treatments, and the one-inch stack of medications." She paused for a moment and looked at her husband. "For the first time we have a handle on the issues both for Emily and for us." I listened.

"We felt paralyzed and infantilized. Out of the blue, Emily would burst into a rage, cut herself, or threaten to kill herself. She was anorexic and bulimic. Some of it felt contagious from other kids in her school. New symptoms, more doctors, additional tests and specialty referrals. We didn't know what to do, or how to help her. We became passive and accepted all of the expert opinions. Even though many were contradictory and there was minimal communication among the therapists, if any. We felt we didn't know anything and became more confused."

I said, "We are overspecialized and now there is 'plausible deniability.' I mean, no one is in charge."

"Things would be calm for a few weeks and we'd rejoice inwardly that we were finally on the right treatment plans, that we'd found the magic bullet, that Emily would get better. We kept an eye on her, and tried to help her and reduce tensions, often by giving in to her most ridiculous demands. 'Why can't I smoke pot in my room? It helps keep me calm.' *Oh, okay then.* Anything to keep her calm. 'I need shopping therapy. It makes me feel better.' *Well, anything to make her feel better!* 'I bought a five-hundred-dollar dress on impulse. Maybe I have an impulse disorder. Or maybe mania?' We felt powerless. Even the 'remission' was part of the illness. Then the next crisis would arise and the whole cycle of hospitalization, doctors, meds, and fear began again. We begged the doctors for a diagnosis. Wasn't there some new pill we could try? Would she ever have a normal life?" She went on for a full fifteen minutes before she paused for a breath. I was dumbfounded. Here I was thinking that I would be called on the carpet for a litany of complaints, from the food to the lack of soft sheets on the bed. Her husband sat quietly and let her have the floor.

"For the first time in ten years, we have an honest interpretation of what happened to our family. We understand that while Emily has an anxiety disorder, let's call it that, and has a very hard time regulating her emotions, a lot of her symptoms are learned. They can be unlearned. She became a grab bag of every imaginable disease. Labels were put on top of labels. She was kidnapped by the system. The medical system and the drug companies. We let her be kidnapped. We are going to get our daughter back. We understand it is going to take time and we have a lot of work to do here. We have to unlearn our reactions, too. We also get that we have been part of the drama. We know we are not innocents." I thought about the cycles of actions, reactions, overreactions that Ariel Abeloff described, where no one had a footing. Who was leading whom in this dance? Parents losing their moorings as parents. A loss of confidence. I saw it clearly in some home visits with social workers in family therapy. Strengthening the parents to be able to parent and take back the home was a critical issue. Sometimes all of the agencies' involvement and the threats of investigation or loss of their children eviscerated parental authority. Now who was in charge?

"It is also not simply a question of money. What is sold as the best care by reputation or well-meaning friends is equally confusing. We lost our common sense somewhere along the way. We were overwhelmed by the constant episodes and treatments. We took refuge in our careers—it was the only place where we felt some control. All this has had a corrosive effect on our relationship. John and I blamed each other—if only you hadn't been so strict or if only you'd been home. Why do you take her shopping every time she wants something? Had we done too little? Or too much? We felt bad and guilty all the time. We have to get ourselves back as well." She finished all at once and the room was quiet. I didn't know what to say—or if I should say anything at all.

John started, "We came here out of desperation a few weeks ago. When Emily ended up at Methodist, our neighbor Glenn said he had emailed and then phoned you about a kid who had Emily's diagnosis and treatments and asked what you recommended." The "kid's" case was not unusual at all. The feelings of helplessness are common, too.

A kid's symptoms can be a proxy for both parents' and society's issues. Society and culture and genetics all create symptoms. "'It is time for a time-out' is what Glenn said you said. Figure out what's what and whose job it is to control it." The two of them had gotten it out and looked relieved, a lot different from my first glimpse of them sitting in the emergency room. It was going to be a long haul for all of them. But it was not hopeless.

I really didn't say anything for the forty-five minutes they were in the office. A few mutterings, maybe a musing about experts and specialty knowledge. How tricky kids were as their brains developed. Every child manifested behaviors that could be called malfunction if we proceeded to medicalize every behavior. Is anorexia a psychological disorder or a social one? Is a child who is beaten or abused crazy if he bites back? Behaviors need to be understood within the larger pattern of the family and the society. Parents all make mistakes; that's what parents do. But feeling guilty does not help. If anything, it makes everything worse. I walked them to the elevator bank, shook their hands when the doors opened. We agreed to talk some more.

Emily and Tani were from opposite poles of the universe. A product of abandonment at birth, Tani had ricocheted like a pinball around a system desperately trying to find a safe haven. In her sixteen years, she'd had a couple of loving experiences between forced death marches in enemy territory. Emily was picked up by a car service and driven to her private school, then sat down to dinner overlooking a backyard with a Bach clavichord playing in the background. And yet barely out of first grade she was melting down and unable to regulate her emotions. Her parents had desperately tried to find the missing love, the missed signals, the early intervention that might have changed the course of their history, all in vain.

Two social workers from child psychiatry, Ingrid and Ana Reid, were sitting in a booth sipping coffee when I sat down across from them. Ingrid's description of Emily and her pedigree of doctors, diagnoses, and medications had led almost directly to the intrinsic problem—disentangling the skein that had enveloped the entire family. Illness, they would discover, serves everyone in a family; it focuses attention and resources. The family seemed committed to understanding and working through that. Emily was being released tomorrow.

Then Ingrid turned to Tani's case. She was determined if nothing else to make sure Tani did not have another experience in another foster home that reproduced the horror stories.

There was one glaring exception in Tani's list of tribulations, and that was why I had asked Ingrid and Ana to join me for breakfast. They told me as they developed a file on Tani that when *Abuela* Lola died three years earlier after her long bout with breast cancer, the kids who lived with her and her husband had been picked up by ACS and scattered around Brooklyn. The husband had fallen ill shortly after her passing and been diagnosed with lung cancer. Within ninety days of Lola's death—his other half of forty-plus years—he was dead himself. Their nine children were busy taking care of their own children, trying to make a living scratching something from the hardscrabble Brooklyn tarmac and concrete. One was a cop, another an electrician; a daughter owned a beauty parlor; and on and on. *Abuela* Lola's eldest daughter, Lila—as Ingrid and Ana remembered—was the anchor of the entire group, in many ways the key. She had been sent by her mother to nursing school in Santo Domingo, the capital of the Dominican Republic, and then to New York City for a U.S. degree. With the earnings from her work at Maimonides hospital, she had brought every sibling to the city, and then her parents. The siblings all recognized her as the direct descendant of Lola, the matriarch, *la mera mera*. She was the chosen one and had earned both their respect and clan leadership.

"Why don't we contact Lila. She seems like the real deal. Tani was a part of the family and maybe, just maybe she will be willing. Even better, maybe she will understand that this is Tani's chance, maybe her only chance to become part of a family." I was pretty emphatic, and they looked skeptically at me while picking at their scrambled eggs.

"Eric, you are dreaming. She is not a foster mother, she is not licensed, does not have any legal standing here for one thing. And obviously, why would this woman—three years after the death of her parents, with responsibilities for her children and grandchildren plus her husband, who works like a burro—take on a kid who is ancient history?" Ana let me have it. "It is ridiculous, silly, and a waste of time." I waited until she chilled out. Ana was rational, 99 percent correct in my experience, and utterly dependable. It did leave open the one-in-a-hundred chance that it might work out. I felt those were better odds than we'd find at a state hospital for zombie-eyed Tanisha. She certainly still had the life force. She was creative, was energetic, and had writing and art skills that showed insight and depth.

The odds were the problem. There would be attempts to violate her again under the right—or really, wrong—circumstances. She would kill someone or go down herself. You certainly did not have to be prescient to appreciate her depth of rage despite her successes on the unit. Her three-hour walk on a freezing winter night to the receiving center of the new ACS building on First Avenue proved her determination. She knew she would be held there safely, fed, and given some warm clothes. She also knew she would probably be sent to Bellevue for evaluation and admission. She had been taking it day by day. But not entirely. She had been counting on us to fight for her. She had done what she could to engage us in her battle. We were the only extended family she knew in the city. We were a safe zone—the most trustworthy thing Tani had going for her. We could not let her down.

I pulled out my black notebook and opened to a page where I had printed in large box letters "LILA!!!" And then "TANI????"

I stopped by to see Tani and the 21 West team at least weekly. The irony was that with the state hospital option on the table, the pressure to discharge was gone. There was a long line and fewer beds every year. Between cuts from Albany and a long-overdue move to bring kids in the juvenile justice system closer to their parents, capacity was shrinking. Tanisha might have to wait for a year. I brought her black notebooks with thin black ribbons to mark the page; some had blank pages for her drawings, some graph paper for writing. When a notebook was filled with her small fine handwriting mixed with sketches and full drawings in pencil or black ink, she would give it to me to read and to lock away so they wouldn't get stolen.

I would go through them very slowly. It was painful to read them. Halfway through one book she switched into Spanish, rather than her

Spanglish or vernacular English. She entered into her other self completely. No shadow here lurking. *Abuela* had created the one safe and
trusting space in her life. This wasn't multiple personality disorder,
but dissociation for survival. But here there was a kid with a life and a
home—half of it imaginary, but all the more real.

Ana, my social work conscience, emailed me one day to call her as
soon as possible. I broke off from rounds and found a quiet place to
make a phone call. "Ana, what's up?"

"Ingrid and I have talked to Lila Pagan, together. She wants to meet
with you. She says she knows you. I will send you her cell. Sorry, you
are the social work department now. We have taken it as far as it can
go. Let's hope that this is the one-in-a-hundred chance. Then it is 100
percent."

I was startled and very jittery. This was too much for anyone, too
much responsibility. I was used to all kinds of issues and trauma, death
and dying, organ donor calls, blood, and cardiac arrests. The heart
and soul of a teenager was something else. If I fucked this up, there
would be no place to hide.

"*Señora Lila Pagan, soy el Dr. Eric del Hospital de Bellevue.*" Lila
said she was a Dominicana who spoke poor English, was embarrassed
by her English despite the decades she'd spent in Flatbush. "*Yo sé, Doctor, yo sé bien. Esperaba su llamada.*" She'd been expecting my call.
We talked in generalities for a few minutes and agreed it was necessary
to meet "*cara a cara,*" face-to-face. I told her I had a meeting in Brooklyn in two days and would be honored to visit her at her home if that
worked out for her. "*Por supuesto, Doctor. Mi casa es su casa.*" Kings
County had opened their new psychiatric building and I was getting
a private tour from the director of psychiatry, a friend of mine. It had
been a long time since I had worked in G Building—all the way back to
the Son of Sam era. I could still recall the weight of the heavy key that
let you into and out of the units.

Since I was making extra stops, I took my own car to Clarkson
Avenue. I went on my tour then spent another hour catching up with
my colleague in psychiatry, trading a little gossip and sharing some
war stories. For lunch the burrito truck on the corner had the biggest

line so I made a beeline and ordered *"un poco de todo"*—a little bit of everything platter—sipped my Snapple, and decided to walk to Lila's apartment, an easy twenty-minute trip in the bright sunshine.

The apartment building was well maintained and looked like a hundred others I had passed on the way. The area was slowly gentrifying. It had the telltale signs, with increasing numbers of the Haredi, ultra-Orthodox Jews, spilling over from Crown Heights and young women in skintight jeans pushing designer strollers speaking into the earbuds hooked to their iPhones. "The Bean" coffee shop sat comfortably adjacent to a Latino bodega. I could sniff the impending Starbuckification. Like a heavy hint of rain, you could smell and feel it before it happened.

I buzzed Señora Pagan from downstairs and was buzzed in immediately. The apartment was on the second floor of a four-floor walkup. A middle-aged woman greeted me with an open door, music filtering from around her, and an easy smile. Her hair was blond and the roots were gray. It was swept to one side. Her makeup and clothes were perfect. The living room was just as meticulous. I could see heavy wooden furniture, dark rugs, a TV off to one side, and heard several-generations-old *bachata* music on a CD player. I recognized *"Muero contigo,"* a classic tune by Rafael Encarnación, and remembered what Tani had told me about Lila's mother. As she lay dying, she wanted the music on all the time, because she would dance in her head, even if she couldn't move. Lila had looked after her and ensured that she was the center of the universe until she turned ashen and her skin was ice cold.

"Dr. Eric, we know each other. I met you years ago at Bellevue, first in the coffee shop and then after my mother's operation." I thought back and tried to fix Lila and her mother in my mind, but nothing came up. *"Lo siento, Lila, mi memoria me falla.* My memory fails me."

"I heard you were very sick yourself," she said quietly and knowingly. I had not expected that the neural networks transporting news of my life traveled to the amygdala of central Brooklyn.

"First we met in the coffee shop. Danny was serving both of us across from each other. He told me you were *el jefe,* the chief, and I apologized and interrupted your lunch to ask a favor." Lila smiled easily and widely. I started to remember a little about the long-ago lunch. Her mother needed surgery for a major problem. It was elective yet it was not elective—meaning that you would die without the surgery, and you had a high percentage of dying with the surgery. I had brought up the case with Greg, the head of cardiovascular surgery. He had personally sewn in the double valves and bypassed the diseased coronary arteries. She'd had a rocky post-operative course but then one day turned the corner. A few days later I saw her walking down the hall with her son on one arm and on the other a daughter. This was Lila, that Lila from many years ago. "You helped my mother. What can I do for you?"

She made me a thick espresso from a silver stovetop aluminum coffeemaker and loaded a tiny cup halfway with sugar. She set a plateful of cookies and cakes on the table. We both took our seats, and she listened intently as I began to talk.

"So Tanisha or Tani has one chance left as best we can determine." I pulled out the drawing she had given me a few months earlier. It covered most of the table; we moved the plates and cups to the sink. "This is one of her dreams of Mochi in La Republica. Your mother's hometown and where you grew up before coming to New York City. Tani has adopted the stories and the town and the animals as her own. She has dozens and dozens of stories, names, people, events, miracles, births, funerals, crazy people. She knows more about *el cabrón Trujillo* and his henchmen than anyone I know, myself included. It is as if your mom were an oracle and Tani, her amanuensis. She took copious notes in her head and never forgot so much as a flavor. She is now writing it down and putting it into pictures, into art." I stopped, exhausted from the emotional drain of communicating everything I needed to—not forgetting anything and yet not overwhelming Lila. I had to be fair about all that Tani had been through. Lila was an adult who had lived in the real world and had no pretense.

"You cannot live without love, Eric. It is not possible. Animals need to be loved, and especially people. People don't need money to be successful. There is a lot of confusion today about this. My family all lives within three blocks of this apartment. My mother and father lived across the street. We saw each other all the time and stayed in touch constantly." Her phone had gone off at least fifteen times during the visit. She would check the number and hit Hold. Only when her husband called did she say, "*Mi amor*, I will call you back after *el doctor* leaves." Her philosophy was very simple and direct: You loved other people and were loved back. Both were necessary. She was explaining to me how her world worked.

I had my brown leather briefcase with me; I had left it with my jacket in the living room. I got up now and brought it to the kitchen table. I took out a black journal and put it on the table. "*Lila, Tani ha estado escribiendo un diario de su vida. Ya van cinco tomos.*" Tani wrote a diary of her life; she has completed five of them. "*Por favor*, this journal is about her time with *Abuela* Lola. Her memories of the life your mom lived in DR, the tales she told to the children living with her. Her philosophy and the life she passed on is all in this book, handwritten in Spanish. I borrowed it from Tani and told her I wanted to share it with a very special person who would understand it and keep it to herself. She has shared her journals with me as she completes them. What I know of her is what she has written. Much more than what she has said. I think life has been too painful for her to say it out loud even to people she is starting to trust, even a little. We all leave her."

We sat across from each other and didn't say anything for a few minutes. Lila looked at the picture, the colorful animals flying across a sky darkened by an eclipse of the sun. She saw her mother and father in the center of the picture and pulled it closer to her.

"Dr. Eric, I will read it and then talk to my husband. I understand what you are saying. And I understand what you are asking. We are a poor family. We don't have a lot. Except one another. My husband works all the time and worries about our expenses and our health. He is a good person and loves his children and his grandchildren."

Our conversation drifted to the neighborhood and how much it was changing. The apartments were going co-op, and Lila was worried about the future of rent control and the New York State legislature, but she liked the safety and the variety of families that were moving in. "I feel more Jewish than ever before," she said with her usual smile.

"I used to see Rabbi Schneerson being driven around on his way to visit people at Downstate hospital. He was a wonderful man and a real community leader. Look at how the community has grown." She had moved over to the window and parted the white gauzy curtains while looking down on the street. "You know, it doesn't matter really which religion you believe in. There are many religious people who cannot love anyone or accept love from anyone."

At that point we both moved toward the door. I grabbed my coat and my ancient brown leather briefcase. We hugged at the door and she kissed my cheek. "*Voy a llamarte, Eric.* I will call you, don't worry." I retraced my steps to Clarkson Avenue, where I'd parked across the street from the large campus of Kings County Hospital. I'd spent ten years here learning how to become a doctor. It all flooded back to me as I unlocked my car and paused for a few moments looking up and down the streets that were increasingly less familiar. The new buildings' red brick hadn't had a chance to weather, and the glass-and-metal entrances were surreal. I took my time driving down Flatbush Avenue and over the Manhattan Bridge. The traffic was heavy, the potholes merciless on my aging Volvo, but I savored just being in Brooklyn, another time zone, another planet in the galaxy of New York.

Back at the hospital, I met with the child team and let them know I had met with Lila Pagan privately in her home in Flatbush. Briefly I went over the visit, leaving out most of the details. More than anything I did not want to raise anyone's hopes that the Pagan family could or would be able to take on the responsibility of becoming foster parents for Tani. In addition to making this decision, they would have to go through the process of applying to be foster parents and enter into a long process of interviews, background investigations, and multiple home visits by social workers before being accepted. They were an intact family, emotionally connected, financially not desperate, and had a physical home that was appropriate. There was also a record of the *abuela*'s care and dozens of kids over many years well looked after. The system had almost seventeen thousand kids in foster care in New York City at any one time. There were thousands entering and leaving annually. Many kids had impossible needs.

The system at the moment had "seized up," according to one social worker I had talked to about Tani. A mother had left a very young child with her younger boyfriend. The baby had been bludgeoned to death. Aside from the criminal investigation, there had been a cover-up. As one of our Bellevue kids commented, "I would rather get beaten by my own parents than my foster parents." I knew if Lila was going to accept this, it would not be for the money. It would be for her the memory of her mother and for Tanisha. Or not at all.

A month passed. One day as I was finishing up lunch across the street from the hospital at East Bay, an alternative Greek diner, my cell phone vibrated and then starting ringing. Lila's name came up. I waved to the group and took the call in the space between the double entrance doors. "*Dr. Eric, habla Lila.*"

I pushed into a corner of the closet-size space. My own hearing was really compromised; my family was pushing me to get hearing aids. "Lila, how great to hear from you," I practically yelled into the cell phone. She wanted to meet with me. My offer to come to her house again was politely turned down. Her son, the police officer, was going to drive her to Manhattan, and she would be there this afternoon at three.

"*Por supuesto*, of course, Lila, that is perfect. Mezzanine Room 30. We will be waiting for you."

We were waiting in my office at two thirty. The head of child psychiatry and the social worker Ana. We were nervous and made some small talk about the new child psychiatry unit that was going to be built since St. Vincent's hospital had closed, leaving a huge gap in city beds for kids in crisis. I made espressos for everyone, and we ate chocolates from a clear plastic box labeled "ORGAN DONOR NETWORK NEW YORK CITY." Lila was on time and came in the room with her son Enrique, the New York City cop, in uniform. Patty ushered them in and shut the door quietly.

After polite hellos and hugs I introduced the group to the Pagan family and asked them to sit. Lila had a shopping bag that she put on the table. First she took out the black journal I had left with her, and then Enrique put a heavy large rectangular package on the table wrapped in heavy paper surrounded by bubble wrap and taped carefully.

Everyone was completely quiet, waiting patiently for Lila and her son to lead us where they had planned to go. "Doctors, we have had almost a month to read the journal and share the information with all of my brothers and sisters, all nine of us and husbands and wives. In fact many came over to my house to read the journal out loud to one another. It never left my sight, I assure you." She looked at me. "The painting, *el cuadro*, we took the liberty of having framed with glass to protect it. All of the children wanted to see it and touch the animals." I got a scissors from my desk and handed it to Enrique, who slowly and methodically cut the layers off protecting the *cuadro*. When he was done, he put it up on its side and sat it on the arms of an empty chair at the end of the faux-marble conference table. The other doctors hadn't seen the picture before. It was elegant with a simple wooden frame and a gray border around another narrow band of white.

Lila continued. "From the journals, we learned things we didn't know about my mother. The stories were all about her childhood. Many of the episodes, if not most, we knew by heart ourselves. We lived them and were in many of them. Tanisha must have memorized them almost word for word since they are the way my mother would talk and how she would tell a story." She was animated now and had engaged all of us completely. I felt a lot lighter. My heart stopped beating so hard.

"I didn't know my mother had gone to Haiti and brought some babies back to DR. They had been abandoned after birth and needed families. I mean, we all went back and forth across the border, we were only a few miles away and there was all kinds of buying and selling. My father made money selling cans of gasoline when things were difficult. And many families came across the border desperate from starvation and the Tonton Macoute under Papa Doc, who were like Trujillo's henchmen, butchers.

"She used to say, 'What is a border? These are people just like us, but they have no trees on their side since the *caciques* have cut them down and sold them to the United States. They have flayed the country alive'—she would use the expression *despellejar*.

"Tani used my mother's expressions in her Spanish. It was like reading my mother's journal, though she couldn't possibly have written one since she only could write and read a little. We had Sunday dinner at my house and we read some passages together, everyone came over. Just my brothers and sisters early so we could talk together. My husband took some time off from his livery to sit with everyone." Lila slowed a bit.

"I asked them all about what you requested we do as a family for Tanisha. Everyone remembered Tanisha. She disappeared with the social worker after my mother passed on. All of the kids were gone. We picked up the pieces of our lives after the long illness and got back to our husbands and wives and our children." I wasn't sure if she thought we felt bad about her. We certainly didn't. It never occurred to us. The kids were moved constantly for a million different reasons. Tani had the record as far as any of us knew. The world of foster care could be a monster, hard, painful, with both wonderful people and predatory sociopaths.

"My mother would have taken Tanisha in with her. If this happened and you had approached Lola, she would have taken her to live with her without further discussion. She loved Tani, and it is clear from the journals and the picture that Tani loved her and felt completely that she was her *nieta*, granddaughter. We will do the same as my mother and take her into our family." She said it matter-of-factly.

I heard her say it before she did and started to get up as she was finishing her sentence. I walked over to her and we hugged for some time. I shook hands with and hugged the burly New York City cop sitting next to her. The doctors and social worker, too, hugged Lila and her son, then gradually made their way out of my office back to the twenty-first floor.

The details were not insignificant, but they were really beside the point. There was nothing that we could not finesse, manage, catalyze, push forward to make this happen. Tani would stay with us on 21 until the paperwork had gone through and the Pagans had been made her official foster parents. That would also give them all time to get re-acquainted. We could keep her in a holding pattern on the unit waiting for a "bed" at the state hospital. In the meantime there was school-work that we would supplement with more writing and lots of art-work. There would be no intermediary placements. She would go from the one place she felt safe into another place I knew in my heart would be her permanent home.

I stayed in my office for some time after walking Lila and Enrique to the elevator bank. It was my job to tell Tani what had happened. First I took down some pictures and hung up her Chagallesque flying animals. I put her black journal under my arm and walked toward the express elevators to the twenty-first floor.

CHAPTER 3

Sunrise to Sunset

Frank Sinatra was not what I felt like hearing. His *Greatest Hits* album filtered through the jet-engine noise of the Varian linear accelerator at nine o'clock on a sunny Monday morning, October 13. I preferred Steely Dan and made a note to bring *Aja* or "Black Friday" the next morning. A middle-aged Latino radiation technician, who had converted from merengue to mild-mannered U.S. love songs, hit the Play button. He wasn't just my deejay. He was also my radiation therapist, and he had bolted my head onto the hard metal gantry that would slide first upward and then backward into an overhead arc, sending high-energy electrons into my head and neck.

The black formfitted mask covering my face was a plastic rectangular grid that had been heat-melted onto my profile two weeks earlier. My name was printed in black Magic Marker on the outside silver metal frame, "MANHEIMER, E." It was mine and only mine. It sat on a shelf with dozens of others, like fencing masks at a Midtown sports club, waiting for their owners to claim them. I was about to receive my first radiation treatment for throat cancer. That afternoon, I would start my first round of chemotherapy. It was happening. And I was stunned, in shock, and exhausted.

Alexei, my older child, had called the night before to tell Diana and me that his wife, Gladys, was in labor. Even though it was the night before my first cancer treatment, Diana and I got in the car and drove to the hospital. We pulled into the empty south parking lot at Bellevue around ten p.m. I showed my ID to the guard in front of the main elevator banks, and he waved us through. Alexei and our daughter,

Marina, were anxiously waiting in the hall of the maternity ward for us and for the new arrival as the stages of labor progressed.

Gladys was smiling, though clearly in pain. We held her hands. Esther, Gladys's mother, had come up from Washington, DC. The nurses on the floor were helpful and very pleased to see me. They were happy that my family was delivering at the city hospital where they worked and received their own care. The fact that Gladys was from Douala, the mercantile city of Cameroon in Francophone West Africa, made it even sweeter. The many Haitians among the nurses switched from their native patois to upscale French. We were now part of a larger diasporic family of displaced persons. On the delivery floor where babies were born, the precise details didn't matter.

For Diana the long-awaited day of the baby's birth would have been perfect…had it come at a better time. The waiting grew intolerable. At one in the morning, I told Diana I had to go home. My first treatment, a few hours away, consumed my thoughts. We said good-bye, Diana grudgingly but understanding, me impatient to be gone. The fluorescent lights and incessant beeping of the labor and delivery areas were making me nauseous. Our kids pretended to be okay with our heading home and promised to call as soon as the baby was born.

Bolted to the table, willing myself to keep my eyes open, I thought about what had happened to me. How had I gone from being a doctor to patient in just a few weeks? A month earlier, I was in Morelos, Mexico. Diana and I were at the end of a late-summer vacation. This was rainy season in central Mexico: biblical late-afternoon downpours and hour-long lightning displays that would take out our neighborhood transformer and with it our electricity for several days. Rolling thunder ricocheted between the craggy vertical cliffs of the Tepozteco. Eagles and hawks drifted in the updraft. We had come to Tepoztlán over many years revisiting Diana's deep childhood roots. We made this stretch of ten-thousand-foot mountains and volcanoes our parallel universe. At our house, the shadows danced, the water streamed off the roof. I sat on the terrace wrapped in a sweatshirt and baseball cap. As summer drew to a close, I knew there was something wrong with my throat.

I returned to work after Labor Day and was immediately drawn into the dramas and emergencies that populated the round-the-clock routine of a big-city hospital. We had two patients in our emergency ward who had been declared brain-dead, and the families were making decisions about organ donation. Our ICU was full, and cardiac surgery transfers were being delayed. A stream of department chiefs wanted to meet and walk down the F-Link at lunchtime to the café where I always did a "business lunch."

By September, I had a swollen yet discrete lymph node in my right neck. I outlined the node gently with the pads of my fingertips. It was soft and unattached to any surrounding muscles or tendons, or to the thyroid gland. I looked at the node in the mirror. It looked back at me, round, smooth, two centimeters in diameter, feigning innocence. That evening I went through my mail. A fresh copy of the *New England Journal of Medicine* came with the stack. A "State of the Art" review article on "Head and Neck Cancer" was listed in bold black type halfway down the cover page. My diagnosis was in hand courtesy of the U.S. Postal Service. I sat by myself in the living room and by the ebbing northern light read through the article line by line.

Unconsciously, I shifted gears. Splitting my personality neatly in half, like the hemispheres of my brain, I buried myself in technical jargon and Kaplan-Meier survival curves. Like my Russian and Romanian ancestral burial grounds, I had an apparently infinite cellar in my head that teemed with childhood demons, maternal warnings about the inevitable next pogrom, warnings issued before I could walk; and with demons from a medical career, dead patients who were more alive in their graves than they ever were in life.

The raspiness and voice fatigue sent off an insistent internal buzz. I ran through the range of diagnostic possibilities and came up empty.

Except for cancer.

It never occurred to me to ask *Why me?* There was no anger and no regret. It was a fact of life. I knew the details—up to a certain point—of what had to happen next: I had to get started on therapy, and quickly, to prevent progression of the disease and to prevent the abyss of anxiety that lay beneath my conscious awareness from overwhelming my family. I knew what I didn't know. The extent of the hole I was going to enter was uncertain. No one could lead me there or prepare me for that part of the journey to come. I would have to go there mentally alone.

As a physician, I knew all too well that a delayed diagnosis would allow the tumor stage, size, and metastatic status to change—and each bit of growth would drop my survival rate by 25 percentage points like a plunge in the stock market. I had seen it happen for breast, lung, ovarian, melanoma, and other cancers. Ordinary symptoms, a negative exam, a reassuring comment, a trial of medications, a pat on the back, and delayed follow-up equaled a recipe for disaster for many patients. I didn't consider my diligence luck. I have a suspicious nature.

The biopsies were simple and painless. Guided by ultrasound, the needle found the liquid center of the node, and the blood-tinged fluid was hurried off to the pathology lab. My doctors' faces were expressionless, the waiting room full of anxious couples. The secretary wanted to update my insurance information. I walked out plotting the next steps while shifting into autopilot.

I stopped at the East Bay diner on the way back to Bellevue to deliberately linger in solitude in the few minutes I had before the diagnosis was official. Like a guilty man waiting for the deliberating jury's verdict, I had a finite period before hearing my sentence. Before my colleagues in pathology peered into their microscopes and found the traitorous cells with a Rorschach nucleus of inkblot mitotic spindles in disarray. Before the ICD-9 official diagnostic codes entered the computer system. Through the large windows fronting First Avenue the red-brick men's shelter, Bellevue's former psychiatric hospital, sat in moldering decay, littered with garbage, water stains resembling stalactites hanging from the window edges. Ageless bearded black men with long dreadlocks loitered on the corner bumming cigarettes. Their grocery carts overflowed with scavenged high-tech backpacks and bulging transparent plastic garbage bags. The collected detritus of New York City's excrescence of garbage oozed from its pores, piled in front of the condos and co-ops in Kips Bay.

It was comfortable inside, familiar waiters, the owner chatting behind the register, a buzz of conversation. I sat sipping coffee by myself, brooding over where I was heading and what would follow. The diner filled up with hospital staff in their multicolored uniforms, a brief pause from the Brownian motion of the eight-hundred-bed hospital a block away.

My cell phone vibrated on my belt. I didn't recognize the number. When I answered, Dr. Kepal Patel came on the line. He told me the biopsy had come back. I had cancer. Squamous cell carcinoma. We talked for less than one minute. I called Diana, who answered before one ring. She knew what was coming—the diagnosis, that is. But not what was coming over the next year. That was unknowable. Very quickly, I had to tell my family, friends, and colleagues. Autopilot was where I would live for the next three weeks, until the therapy began.

The walk from the diner to my office can take five minutes or an hour depending on whether I take the long loop around the Belle-vue campus—not to mention greeting everyone I see and performing the small negotiations and acknowledgments that are at the heart of the small city that is this public hospital. Today I took the long loop, down First Avenue, past the nursing school and the emergency vehicles strewn out on the access road. I had been through many conversations with patients and their families about death and dying. Now I would be having a variation of that conversation with myself. I had lived through the Kübler-Ross fiction about the stages of death, defining for several generations a reality where there were often not stages, just a Munchian scream. The idea of "the good death" had been attractive and provided a lodestar for my own behavior toward my patients. But finally, as Montaigne said, it was useless to "worry about death, it will take care of itself. Worry about life, that needs management."

I had thought of death often. I had read about it and dreamed about it. My greatest fears were Holocaust survivor fantasies that tormented me and my family, and had been handed down directly to my daughter. Marina's identification with her chosen tribe went back to the destruction of the Second Temple and the replays of diasporas upon diasporas. "Countries don't love you," my mother had warned. "Collect passports, you never know when you may need them," she added as a practical note. Her worldview included death, dying, killing, and being both the hunted and the hunter. My way of dealing with the stress of mortality on a daily basis was to bury it for another day. If it wasn't exactly the elephant in the room, then it was a smell somewhere in the basement that wouldn't go away.

I believed that everyone feared death. That mortality petrified everyone. That very few would go gently into the night. And that those who did had reached a state of radical acceptance or had their souls stolen by their disease—the one gratuitous positive thing a terminal illness might offer. The soul would be kidnapped slowly, allowing the disease its final victory lap. Now, as I walked the long way around, I was scared shitless. But I had my methodology: I would focus on the here and now. Tasks that had to be completed. Lists to be made and checked off. Supplies to be purchased, people to be notified. My soul would have to wait for another day.

Secured to the radiation table, replaying the events that had brought me here, I became hyper-alert to everything that went on around me, despite the din from the radiation machine. Music is my drug of choice, and my body was rejecting Ol' Blue Eyes. Dominican *bachata* was my anti-depressant. *Vallenato* from Colombia an intravenous hit of an amphetamine stimulant. Bach meditation in the lotus position. Piazzolla's jazzy tango journeys to the pleasure of longing and short-circuited desire. Qawwali Sufi chants by Nusrat Ali Khan hypnotically induced trances that erased consciousness. Dylan, of course, aspirin and penicillin, the all-purpose poly-pill appetizer, dessert, or main course. Time ticked by slowly. Trifling delays were magnified. Idle chitchat among the staff about girlfriends and last night's baseball game annoyed me.

Squamous cell carcinoma, SCC, was well known to me from decades of contact with patients. It would not have been my first choice at the Bureau of Tumor Assignments; nor would I have guessed it in a million years for me, as it usually showed up in heavy smokers and drinkers. *I am fucked* is the first thought that crossed my mind. The SCC had lodged in my buccal mucosa. My entire aerodigestive tract was vulnerable: trachea, esophagus, the whole works. "Cancerization," Nick, the head and neck specialist, had called this as he explained the radiation treatment designed to attack the entire area. That was a new word for me. So it wasn't *Why me*, but *Why this particular disease?* I could have been sipping aged tequila or hundred-dollar-a-bottle single-malt Scotch and drawing in deeply on fragrant Cuban cigars for the last thirty years while looking at the snow-covered volcano Popocatépetl from the terrace in Tepoztlán. At least then there would have been a reason.

Squamous cells were common skin cells or lining cells of the mouth or reproductive organs whose DNA had gone independent of all controls. They were resistant to treatment if not removed surgically, but slow to metastasize or spread beyond their original rogue cell. All it took in my case was one cell that had gone "viral." That's what cancer is: A rogue cell replicates, unresponsive to the internal signaling system that tells it to stop. If untreated, the errant cell duplicates relentlessly and eventually spreads through the lymphatic system to regional lymph node collection centers, where the independent cells continue to reproduce and spread again. Cells then escape into the blood and are carried to the lungs, bones, and brain, where distant metastases will flourish. Different tumors have their own predilections for different areas.

The most common SCC cancer is cervical—at the cervix, or opening of the uterus. If a Papanicolaou (Pap) test picks up a case, then freezing the tumor cells or a surgical approach is curative. Unscreened populations of poor women delay diagnosis, leading to a miserable death. The discovery of the relationship of the HPV virus and cervical cancer and the subsequent development of an effective vaccine was scientific medicine at its best. The endless debates over the vaccine, however, have been politics at its worst. The issues of affordability and dissemination, false fears of the vaccine having some connection with autism, and teenage sexuality quarrels were raised by opportunistic politicians who ignored history. Vaccines work. Think of polio, tetanus, and measles.

SCC had changed a lot in recent years. It wasn't confined to alcoholics and tobacco abusers. Younger patients with no risk factors were presenting to physicians and dentists. A teenage girl in the hospital with this disease had a metastasis to her foot. She didn't respond to chemotherapy and died rapidly. We were stunned by this new incarnation of an old disease. It defied the smug thinking of the careful, clean-living, safe-sex-practicing among us who equated cancer with bad habits, lifestyle excess, personal (ir)responsibility, or a suspect genetic pool. Cancer is never neutral. It's fully loaded when it comes out of society's closet—an unmitigated failure next to the current complex heroic ideal of survivorship through a valiant "fight" or a valiant death. The reality is much more complex and nuanced.

I knew this disease well but didn't know its newest incarnation. No one did, really. But I knew I did not want SCC.

As I lay on the table, I reminded myself that daily doses of radiation were just one part of the assault on my cancer. The course of treatment had come together quickly after the diagnosis. David Hirsch, my surgeon, looked at Diana and me. He said I had cancer but that I would be fine. We sat in his office at the university hospital.

"This cancer is not only treatable," he said, "it's curable."

We would hold on to those words like a life raft as I went further and further into the treatment.

From then on it was all about percentages—75 percent chances of survival—and numbers; Stage II cancer, three lymph nodes involved, five radiation treatments a week for seven weeks, three rounds of chemo, the number of pounds I could afford to lose before I became too weak to withstand treatment. Nick had insisted that keeping myself as strong as possible would be the most important part of the support. "A patient's prognosis isn't determined only from his cancer staging and treatment. His Karnofsky score is the most tightly related to a good outcome."

Now, I knew about Dr. Karnofsky, and I knew about his score. This wasn't the only disease where your ability to tolerate the treatment was based on your ability to wash, shower, dress, and walk to the bathroom by yourself. With too much weight loss, there wouldn't be much of you left to treat. The last thing I wanted was to become what we called a "Harvard Death"—the treatment was a success, but the patient died.

It was all numbers. No one counted the months of agony.

Cancer care is a team sport. David was directing traffic and pulled everyone together. He would email, text, and call me regularly, including office "drive-bys" and home visits. David asked Diana if she had any questions. She was scared but I knew she both liked and trusted David. That was my main concern. We were going to be in for a long and difficult haul and I would need to depend on her utterly in a few weeks for every aspect of my life. Her supports would be our team of doctors, our kids, family, and friends.

Bobby, my internist, had been a friend since second grade. We used to walk to school together. He checked in daily and called Diana regularly to clarify any questions about my progress. Nick wrote the computer program for my cancer and coordinated my visit with my new oncologist, who was a platinum specialist. Within a couple of weeks there were audiologists, dietitians, nurse practitioners, counselors, gastroenterologists, cardiologists, neurosurgeons, psychiatrists, hearing specialists, radiologists. The workup to begin the treatments was dizzying. I made lists, wrote in my journal, kept my appointments on my usual calendar jammed in between medical board meetings at the hospital, family meetings, rounds in the intensive care unit, emergency phone calls, and pushing my usual thousand and one projects forward. I had planned to work for six weeks and then take a couple of months off. By the second week of treatment, I wouldn't be able to swallow my own spit.

I had entered a new world, the Cancer World, and it was bringing me down. The small treatment rooms in the cancer center, the artificial light, the white coats, linoleum floors, the patients in the waiting room, pastel colors, coffee pod machines with multiple flavored brews, bottles of apple juice, Internet access, the blood drawing room, old *Vogue* magazines, the plaques of donors' names on everything, plastic wrist name bands for every visit. People who knew you looking away feigning deep thought, ostensibly respecting your privacy. Slips of paper stuck on the walls announced cancer support groups. The cushioned seats on the elevators foresaw the needs of those too weak and weary to stand. Cancer was built into the very structure of the building, everything thoughtfully arranged and controlled by architects and decorators. It made me feel banished to a new dead place. *Life, where are you hiding?*

Nick handed me off to the supervisor of the radiation treatment program.

I hung up my suit jacket, white shirt, and red silk tie and lay on the table as he approached me with a needle and some ink. The three tattoos on my chest assured perfect alignment with the radiation beam. He pressed the needle into the ink several times as a small round tattoo in the middle of my breastbone emerged.

Many years earlier I had joined a friend, the son of Auschwitz survivors, at a reunion they hosted near Nice. The survivors were flown in from around the world. Sipping drinks and overlooking the harbor full of yachts and the sparkling reflective waters of the Mediterranean, guests reached out with tattooed forearms for a drink or a canapé. Dozens of languages swirled around the flowered terrace, lit with candles, as a soft breeze lightly salted the air. My tattoo was a more subtle cancer identifier that identified me with another group of sufferers.

After placing the ink on the table, the technician turned around holding a mask with both hands. It had a metal rim the shape and size of a human head; joining the sides were black plastic strips at right angles from north to south and east to west every half inch. He fitted the mask over my head and used a screwdriver to fasten it into the table. Then with my eyes closed he brought the hair dryer over the front of the plastic latticework and heated it while pressing it with his hands into my face, so by the end of the "fitting" it was a perfect replica of me. My own personal death mask. There were rows of them on shelves in this same room with other names from Huang to Castro and now Manheimer. Lying on the table, I craved to get unbolted.

Two days later in the hospital minor surgery suite, a narcotic drip left me amnesiac while my gastroenterologist threaded his endoscope into my stomach and punched a hole anteriorly just above my belly button. A clear soft plastic tube was threaded through the new opening and secured with a small balloon. The three feet of tubing would be my lifeline for many months.

Fear stalked me when I wasn't busy. I was worried I would never be able to work again. It would come over me sitting in my office or sitting at home with Diana and when I lay in bed with the lights out. Death would take care of itself. It always did. It was living, the idea of being sidelined on disability—that was the torment. Too weak to do anything useful but not so weak that I would leave this terrestrial existence. Caught in a limbo world. I had always been absorbed by my work. I defined myself by it and was criticized for it. It extended everywhere. My office on the mezzanine floor at Bellevue was part of a greater dynamic creative project. It led from history and fiction, to a fascination with evolution and the environment, into the back-country of Latin America to the rhythms of international music and leisurely dinners with family and friends over bottles of wine and food expertly prepared and generously shared. If all that went away, and I was reduced to a homebody dripping cans of Ensure into a plastic umbilical cord, I would be better off dead. I didn't have the character or the charm to write novels blinking my eyelids to an amanuensis.

The PET scan is my pre-bout preparation before I can get into the ring with cancer. I check in, and a nurse comes out to greet me. She walks me to a small workspace in a cul-de-sac where she hooks me up to an IV. I change into a gown and lock my belongings in a locker. Then she shows me into the Quiet Room. The room is small and bare except for a reclining chair and a window overlooking 34th Street and directly into the windows of the apartments across the street. There is a small radio on the wall. The room is cold, and I wrap myself in three blankets. I know I will be having a PET scan every three months for some years. It is the test to monitor cancer patients. Like a mind reader, it can see things you cannot. Cancer cells you cannot feel. Sites they may be hiding in that are invisible to other X-ray tests. The test exploits the avid metabolic appetite of cancer cells for the simple sugar glucose, their preferred meal.

When I'm in the Quiet Room, my mind wanders all over my career, my diagnosis, the treatments, my kids, my friends, trips, sex, books, ideas, dying, and a slow death like a trickle, a drying streambed, a spent volcano, the remnants of a storm. Up until now I have had no time by myself between multitasking at Bellevue and this added measure of arranging a complex treatment regimen for myself. I arranged for other people's treatments. Transfers, tests, best doctors to see, second opinions, faxes and emails in Spanish from Latin America and Spain for advice, treatment options, new therapies, validation, ideas, assistance, reassurance, and everything in between. Time to discuss, explain, and meet with families. I did it yesterday, the day before, and the day before that. I did it at noon, in the afternoon, during dinner, and at two a.m. I arranged for heart transplants and sensitive psychiatric evaluations. I had done this for thirty years.

The PET scan takes a long time. Lying completely still on a hard thin table, strapped in, wrapped in a sheet, and covered with a blanket. I take off my watch first; my wedding ring will not come off and I don't want to take it off. I will be sliding in and out of a donut-shaped receiver that will measure the discharges from radioactive-tagged sugar molecules. The table is hard and my shoulder is out of position and beginning to hurt. I am tired after a long day. Has the tumor gone beyond the boundaries seen on the CT scan? That is the question. If so, then everything we have done is moot. The PET scan is the ultimate decider.

They finally unstrap me from the table, and I hang over the side light-headed from not eating. I walk back and get dressed in my suit and tie. I walk to the PET scan reading room and introduce myself to a young radiologist, the chief of nuclear medicine. I pull up a chair on wheels in the darkened room while he twirls the dials on the two large rectangular computer screens and I see my name and then my total body outline. My body is a light gray monotone, except my right neck. A confluence of black concentric overlapping circles and one deep black spot, like my inked tattoo, in my throat. There is the primary cancer and its mycelial threads into the adjacent lymphatic tissue. It is like a weather map on television with a storm center barreling up from the Caribbean. There are a few other flecks of black in my lung, but flipping up the CT scan clarifies that these are likely distant inflammations from long ago, immune system victories. The trail has gone cold except for the tumors we identified two weeks ago. I understand what I'm seeing and call Diana.

The world did not stop when I had symptoms. It did not stop when I had my biopsy, or the tests to get ready for my arduous treatment journey.

One of my friends was languishing with a big infarct at the university hospital's CCU. His left main coronary artery had ruptured a plaque and clotted off in the middle of the night. There was a young man who had blown an aneurysm in his cerebellum while visiting friends in Carroll Gardens in Brooklyn and been taken by ambulance to Woodhull hospital and then transferred to us; we quickly determined by physical exam and a CT scan that his brain was dead. He was the light of his parents' life. The tangle of abnormal vessels in his right temporal lobe had leaked before and been treated with small coils of metallic tubes to clot off the malformation. It didn't work. The family bled tears all night. I sat rubbing the mother's back and holding her and her right hand as she sobbed her way into and through her pain. I was numb. I held her and my own tears sat in the corner of my eyes. I involuntarily touched my right neck. The node was still there.

My email box was stuffed and I was having trouble keeping up since I spent half of my time walking back and forth to 34th Street now for appointments and consultations for myself. I had pulled into myself and was less communicative, less emotionally available at work and at home. Alexei and Gladys came over often to sit with us. Gladys was eight months pregnant with our first grandchild. Alexei, a graphic artist, would draw funny cartoons to cheer us up, and they'd bring flowers to brighten our apartment. Marina would cook for us and read to me. But I wasn't present. My withdrawal would continue involuntarily almost to a vanishing point. I dug into my work and arranging my treatments without giving much thought to the hard times to come. There was no psychological preparation possible at this point. It was happening too fast. Just as well.

And in the midst of everything, on October 13, I pressed the button marked "B" for *basement* for the first time as a cancer patient. Radiation therapy treatment centers are in basements, and everyone who works in a hospital knows what it means when they see you headed downward. There is nothing else in the basement. No patient services, no financial clearance, no psychological counseling, no library for patients, no patient advocacy offices, no administrative suites for the executives, no marketing or public relations, no conference rooms. The linear accelerators are large and weigh several tons each. The radiation therapy suites are windowless, artificially lit subterranean caverns. There are the ubiquitous plants and wood furniture to try to make it appear home-like and welcoming. The design created a camouflage of comfort, but I was not fooled.

The secretarial staff, I would learn, nominally gets to know you after a few sessions. Some pretended to recognize me and nodded between personal phone calls as Diana and I hunted for a couple of seats together between other patients. In the chairs around us, other patients were being treated for breast cancers, lung cancers, prostate cancers, metastases, bone tumors, and brain cancers. It wasn't hard to figure out who had what diagnosis. Wigs and scarves covered women's baldness. Others had decided it was a badge of honor; for others still, it's a time to suspend the vanity. The head and neck cancer patients had rounded hair loss at the backs of their heads and their beards from circumscribed radiation fields. There was no privacy among my fellow patients though everyone came in surrounded by a protective bubble. I looked through them, subway etiquette. Their thoughts were buried in impenetrable private spaces. The door opened for the next patient and the 747 *whir* of the Varian machines washed into the room, like the stifling humid heat on an August day. As the patients were called they were wheeled, shuffled, or limped into the linear accelerator rooms. This was a sub-basement after all. The room was about therapy, suffering, dying, reducing pain to manageable levels. Diana sat with me day after day, she never left my side, but we didn't talk when we were there. We got in and we got out. The less said the better.

My Frank-o-phile, Sinatra-dispensing Dominican radiation tech picked me up in the waiting room, led me to a changing room, and showed me where to leave my shirt and jacket and put on the standard hospital gown. Another patient was in the room changing back into his clothes and we nodded at each other, a quarter-inch inclination of our chins. He was skeletal; his clothes hung off his body as if he were a scarecrow. His considerable dignity remained intact. He took his time getting street-ready, checked himself in the mirror, ran a comb through the few strands of remaining hair, and walked out of the dressing room erect. From the cavernous echo of his cough and the darkened skin within the triangular radiation markings in black ink on his back, his lung cancer was advanced. You cured lung cancer with surgery if you were lucky; otherwise it was palliation, buying time and reducing pain. I had walked through this too many times with too many patients over too many years. What to do, how much to do, and when to stop were existential questions. There were no easy answers, no facile instructions, no algorithms to follow. Each case had to be hammered out face-to-face. Sometimes you got lucky; most of the time the house collected its money and went home.

I would see him three more times over the next two weeks and then he disappeared. I didn't speculate.

A few ring-a-ding-dings and one Nelson Riddle arrangement of "The Lady Is a Tramp" later, radiation was over. I dressed and picked Diana up in the waiting room. Back in my suit and tie, with my briefcase and laptop firmly in hand, Diana and I took the elevator to the sixth floor for chemo. The cancer center became our second home for the next few months.

The check-in at the desk was perfunctory. I looked normal and felt fine. How different it would be in two weeks. In a few minutes, an aide came to take us back into a warren of cubicles separated by head-high greenish tinged glass. The cubicles were rectangular; each had a recliner and a chair for a guest. There was a small rolling black stool for the nurse, a cabinet for supplies, a red plastic container for used needles, and a small TV that came out of the wall on an adjustable arm. A nurse welcomed me to the unit and made sure I was comfortable. We went over my identifiers, my diagnosis, and the treatments.

As I settled into the recliner with my suit jacket off and my sleeve rolled up on my left arm, a nurse chatted with me while expertly slipping in an IV and taping it into place. She drew some blood for the lab. Another nurse came in with a liter plastic bag filled with a saltwater solution and another, smaller bag—the size of a plastic lunch bag—with my name on it and "Platinum" on a white sticker. Both went through the exercise of double-checking everything, then hooked the platinum to the larger bag now running quickly into my vein. I also received an intravenous dose of steroids and some pills to prevent nausea.

Diana sat in the extra chair and worked at her computer, her home office for the duration of the chemo. I knew she was anxious to get to the hospital to meet Mateo and be with the kids. She talked about buying flowers on our way over. I, too, was getting antsy and decided to explore the unit. I unplugged the IV, rolled it into the main intersection where the nursing station was located, and began a circuit around the infusion center—one that I would come to make many times. There were old and young patients. Skinny and fat patients. Orthodox Hasidic Jews, Catholics, and agnostics. Those who looked like they were on their last legs and those who might have been just visiting, in street clothes, looking fit and trim. Nurses buzzed in and out checking in on everyone. One nurse whom I had known from her time at Bellevue came up to me. She had heard about my cancer and told me she would make sure I was getting the best care. I knew she had had lymphoma and been treated herself. The nurse taking care of me had lost her husband, the love of her life, to cancer. She had come out the other end and switched to the infusion center, feeling a tug of duty to give here what she had learned personally. And in some way it allowed her to continue to care for her dead husband. She had no self-pity, but there was a deep sadness behind her smile.

My oncologist stopped in about halfway through the infusion. She wanted to see how I was doing. The first day is a big day. The truth was that I was developing a metallic taste in my mouth. *Hello, Platinum, my old friend. You've come to talk to me again…* It had been years since I'd experienced platinum. When I was a resident-in-training on a rotation through the oncology wards, it was notorious. Patients on platinum would be in the hospital for weeks unable to move. Sedated patients lay in hospital beds without moving, unable to eat. They vomited at the slightest provocation. It was as if the ward were an ocean liner and all the patients had severe motion sickness. The ship was keeling sharply and the passengers were lying motionless on white sheets. Staff tiptoed in and out of the rooms without a rustle of the stagnant air. The chemo hadn't changed, but the newer anti-nausea medications made outpatient care possible.

I was nervous about where the chemo would take me, but the routine, the nurses, the location made it tolerable. I was surrounded by part of a family of people I had known for a dozen years. Privacy for me at this point was irrelevant. Being cared for by people I worked with and trusted outweighed any perceived benefits of a new institution where the relationships had to be negotiated and trust had to be built. These things took time and energy, both of which would be in short supply. At least I went into my diagnostic and treatment journey knowing the Virgils who would be taking me by the hand.

We finished up our first day on the sixth-floor chemotherapy infusion suite in the late afternoon. By mid-October the sun was setting earlier and the air was cooler outside, sweater weather. We gathered up our things, said good-bye to the nurses on the unit, went out to 34th Street, and treated ourselves to a cab to Bellevue, picking up some flowers on the way.

When we got to the obstetrical floor, we retraced our steps from the early-morning hours. Our family and its newest member were in the nursery. Mateo was nestled on Gladys's chest, a contrast in colors. Mateo was very white, and everyone looked on him in wonder. Esther stood next to us as we bent to kiss Gladys and the baby. "Don't worry," she reassured us, "he'll darken up." Diana laughed and cried. Alexei was obviously exhausted and exhilarated at the same time. His life had just changed completely. No more the guy in his twenties who did what he wanted when he wanted. He was married to a lovely strong woman, the mother of his son. Marina was thrilled, even though at the moment she could not foresee that this young boy would hang on her every idea as she took him through museums, zoos, and Washington Square Park, where he would play in the fountain. "Nini, Nini," he would be yelling every time he saw her, forgetting the rest of us. I held my grandchild, too many emotions to catalog moving through me. My family looked at me, expectantly. I smiled, weakly. I didn't want them to see I was frozen. I knew that the thoughts and fears and emotions swirling around me would confine me to my private space in the midst of a crowd. My thoughts were elsewhere as my family and friends and colleagues celebrated around me. They would be elsewhere for quite some time.

As the fall progressed, the combination of having my throat blow-torched by high-energy electrons and the chemo would force me to abandon my long-held antipathy toward medicating myself for pain. I learned to grind up narcotic pills and inject them into my feeding tube. I would soon have several narcotic patches on my arms, shoulders, or chest. I began wasting away. My weight, which normally hovered around 155 pounds, dropped to 123. When my renal function took a hit from the chemo, I had special liquid formula delivered in crates that I put in a 50cc syringe and slowly injected into my stomach tube every few hours.

At night, Diana and I watched the 2008 electoral campaign unfold in real time. We watched the five seasons of *The Wire*, me dripping Ensure into my tube, Diana eating cold poached salmon and sautéed spinach that she bought at the store. The smell of food made me sick, so we couldn't cook in the apartment. After the elections and Obama's victory, winter descended on the city. The days stretched out interminably. I had fevers every day, my muscles evaporated, and I fought to keep the feedings going, padding around the apartment like an animal in a cage.

I got weaker and weaker. When my white cells fell to near zero from the chemotherapy, I was hospitalized for sepsis. Marina would come and read to me every day. She sat on the edge of my bed and held my hand. Alexei would draw cartoons on the whiteboard reserved for nurses. Diana sat with me day in, day out. It didn't matter anymore. As I received blood transfusions and a drug to stimulate my white cells,

I decided that I had had enough treatments. I refused further radiation and chemotherapy. I lay in my bed and watched the events around me—the distress of my family, the helplessness of my doctors—without anxiety, comfortable that I had made the correct decision.

Where is it written that a good death is bearing gracious witness to the suffering caused by an errant cell that has exploded inside you? Isn't this meeting other people's expectations? Isn't there a time limit, a statute of limitations on expectations? In your final moments, aren't you free to pursue your own ends by the means you choose?

My doctors couldn't convince me to change my mind, but, luckily, Diana did. From my mental cocoon in the hospital bed, I could sense her at my side. "You're going to finish the treatment," she said softly. I did not have the energy, or perhaps the will, to disagree. She wheeled me down herself to finish my radiation treatments in the basement of the hospital.

Things did not get better anytime soon. Another hospitalization for implacable nausea and vomiting. I took myself off the narcotics and my withdrawal symptoms confounded everyone except Beverly, my nurse practitioner. "You are going through withdrawal, Eric. You tapered the narcotics too quickly." She handed me a new schedule and put me back on the patches. A few days later, I found myself on a stretcher rolling into St. Vincent's, where an emergency attending asked me who I was, where I was, and what date it was—none of which I knew—as he sutured my forehead.

Diana had left the room to make coffee when she heard a thud and found me unconscious in a pool of blood next to the bed. A CT scan showed four skull fractures and various intracerebral bleeds. I was transferred back to university hospital on the neurosurgical service, where they watched me for ten days. A cardiologist slipped in a pacemaker, deducing a long pause in my heartbeat from the chemo. The entire world slowly turned on an axis miles below my hospital bed. Any movement increased the rotation. I lay still. Morphine and Ativan erased thinking. A depression descended imperceptibly, a twilight without beginning or end in the dimmed lights and quiet of the nights, between the beeps and blood pressure checks, and took hold.

Night terrors invaded my sleep. In my dreams, I replayed the lives and deaths of my patients. I lived instant playbacks of wrong decisions, lives destroyed, raw fear. A dying patient had once told me, "In the dark night of the soul, it's always three o'clock in the morning." But now my treatment would leave me shaking, sweaty, and kicking. Diana rubbed my back to calm me and whispered my name. "It's all right," she would say, "you're all right." She would hold me as I went back to sleep. I don't know how or if she slept; she seemed alert to my every movement. I was living in a state of nightmares that could only be compared to status epilepticus—unending seizures.

By spring, I could shower by myself. The hot water sluiced over my skinny body. I still couldn't eat, but Diana took me to our house in Tepoztlán for my sixtieth birthday. I didn't want to go—I pleaded with my doctors to tell her I was too weak. They assured me that I could make the trip, that it might even be good for me. During the warm days on our terrace in Mexico, I began to eat again. I began to talk and even smile. By the end of the week, I was off the feeding tube.

Back in New York, soaping myself one morning, I felt a coin-size, slightly raised irregularity on my right outer thigh. Using a mirror, I detected a dime-size lesion with a steel blue lower edge. A melanoma. My dermatologist biopsied the lesion, and a few days later I was back in the hospital for a "deep and wide" excision; my right groin nodes were biopsied as well. By this point I was inured to cancer diagnosis and metastasis. Dan Roses, my surgeon, took out the stitches and told me I would be okay. He got everything. But I wasn't listening anymore. If death was coming for me then I was ready, if not exactly willing.

It took me at least two years to make it back emotionally. Persistence in the original lymph node picked up by a routine PET scan a year after successfully finishing the chemoradiation bought me a neck dissection. Nobody told us about this phase of the illness, and it's probably just as well. What is true is that even your doctors don't know the time it takes to partially recover. My survival strategy had been to withdraw deeper and deeper as the life force receded. All my unseen ties to outside life were cut. All my attachments fell away. This period was very painful for my family. I was an absent husband, an absent father.

Their own lives had been put on hold. Diana tried to keep a foothold in the normal world by preparing and teaching her graduate classes. Alexei and Gladys had recently gotten married and were expecting a baby. Marina was in her senior year at college yet spent much of her time looking after me. Now they tell me they remember very little of this period. From a running start we jumped off the cliff October 13, just when Mateo came squawking into the world.

Over many months that became years, I could see the attachments and the expectations returning. Invisible strands, gossamer-like, but strong as silk floating in the ether to be reattached. What I had now was the crystal-clear understanding and ability to make decisions about what was allowed back in and what wasn't. Only the deep, caring, loving relationships came back in. It had been very hard-earned.

It is a myth that cancer empowers you to witness the beauty and majesty of life. The gloss we try to put on suffering is that it offers us some insight—existential or otherwise—into life and its mysteries. That the sun is brighter and the air is clearer after a rousing contest with our corporeal being. That the relationships with our families matter more. That we learn to savor the small things in life, the colors, flavors, tactile sensations, a breeze blowing, the smells of flowers. That beautiful music resonates at a deeper, more profound level after we have been blasted from our mundane daily existences. That somehow out of the monumental task of being a cancer patient one deepens oneself and reaches into a repository of feelings, a depth of existence, a mode of being that was not previously expressed, that was hiding in plain sight, that but for the cancer might not have seen the light of day. It does occur. It can happen. But it is not the usual experience or the common one. People who were mundane are still mundane; things we found banal are still banal. As for the ties that bind, they can be loving and supportive or simply bind tighter still. There may be a window, a brief opening, a glimpse of an opportunity, a possibility, a path that could have been taken. There are the powerful social expectations of what cancer is supposed to feel like, what the "victim" is supposed to feel and express socially. I didn't have the strength or the good manners at the time to play the victim.

On October 13, 2011, we're at home, cooking and wrapping presents. Alexei, Gladys, Mateo, and new baby Zoe are coming over. Marina and her boyfriend are here. She is baking her special cookies. Lura sings in the background. We're happy and excited. We've bought flowers. The door opens and Mateo runs in. "Nana! Poppa! Nini!" It's his birthday.

CHAPTER 4

Beso de Angel

I could smell him before I could see him.

The heavy sweet smell hit me as I reached the end of the corridor. Dr. Kantor was waiting for me. He had called my cell phone a few minutes earlier as I was driving into the parking lot. I headed up to the tenth floor immediately. Maria, the secretary of the surgical intensive care unit, handed me the chart of Octavio Salcedo, the young undocumented Mexican who was behind the closed sliding glass door. His room was obscure, half backlit from a light behind the bed. A TV was on; the sun was coming up and streaking the sky the deep color of papaya. The orange light was reflected off the glass towers near the rectangular United Nations building. I could see Octavio's wife sleeping on two chairs next to him. He was hidden in the shadows in his bed. I could see his left foot sticking out from the sheets. There was no right foot.

Dr. Umut Sarpel, the attending physician, was from Turkey. The energetic young cancer surgeon with jet-black hair came down the hall with her chief resident, very dyed blond and very young, dressed in crisp white MD lab coats. Erika the social worker and Zita the head nurse quietly joined us, nodding good morning. We settled in to discuss Octavio, lying in the room in front of us. Red signs taped to the glass partitions warned that he was in "contact isolation," a no-touch containment zone. To enter, people had to don gowns and gloves to prevent germs hopping a free ride from room to room and patient to patient. Nurses and aides coming in and out during our discussion squirted white foam on their hands and wore disposable yellow paper gowns, face masks, and latex gloves in obeisance to the overlords from the bacterial world. With every swoosh open of the doors, a heavy humid smell washed over us.

My brain's limbic system registered the molecules from thirty-plus years of clinical medicine. I knew more from two inhalations than I would learn in the next thirty minutes. Putrefaction of dead and dying organs, tissue, flesh is singular and unmistakable. Scientific medicine peered into bodies with computerized millimeter-thin X-ray slices, giant whirring magnets that lined up protons in MRI scanners, and radioactive-tagged molecules that illuminated the footprints of altered enzymes and metabolism even before the landscape was altered. Paradoxically, physicians were losing the ability to connect directly with patients by doing an old-fashioned detailed history and a complete physical examination. The stethoscope connecting the ears of the doctor to the heart of the patient twelve inches away was more than symbolism. Any shaman worth his pesos knew that.

One whiff was enough.

"Mr. Salcedo...," Umut began in the classic medical case presentation. She was totally on target, parsimonious with her words yet hitting every key point. I would not have many questions to ask when she was done. "Mr. Salcedo is a thirty-two-year-old undocumented Mexican who has been living in Queens for the last five years. He developed swelling in his right groin a year ago. A biopsy revealed squamous cell carcinoma, and an extensive workup was done to look for the primary cancer. It was never found. An unknown primary. We have all of the documentation, X-ray results and summaries from the physicians at the local hospital. They did a colonoscopy, a CT scan, an MRI, an endoscopic look into the bladder, HIV tests, everything. Surgery was not promising, as the tumor had spread. Octavio was referred to oncology and radiation therapy, where he underwent a standard chemotherapeutic regimen of platinum for seven weeks, three doses two weeks apart and seventy thousand rads to his pelvis, daily treatments of two thousand rads for seven weeks. The tumor melted away, and he spent the next few months recovering from nausea, vomiting, radiation colitis, exhaustion, and weight loss, all treatment-related."

Futility. It was the single word that entered my mind. Metastatic squamous cell carcinoma was an unmovable object. Why overtreat? The fleeting response would be a Band-Aid on a five-alarm fire. The side effects from the treatment itself lasted months. Palliation, for God's sake, and a discussion about the end of days, how to spend it and where to spend it and who to spend it with. You could practically hear the mitotic spindles of the cancer cells splitting and dividing through the glass doors. I had heard this particular mitotic hum before.

"By the sixth month, he started to lose weight and started to ooze serosanguineous or bloody drainage from both groins. After several months of self-management, he reappeared at the clinic debilitated with bleeding from the right groin site—and while in the emergency room, the femoral artery exploded. A vascular surgeon attempted to stent the vessel unsuccessfully, and it was bypassed. This clotted off and his lower leg became gangrenous, requiring fasciotomies or long incisions down to his thigh muscle to relieve the pressure on his leg muscles and tissues from the swelling. At that point, their surgical team called us for a consultation-transfer. They had run out of ideas." Umut wasn't finished. I decided to let her go through the entire presentation without interruption and leave my questions for the end.

I got the picture and the sense of urgency from Umut's body language and her intensity. She was obviously desperate to do something for Mr. Salcedo and had run out of things to offer. Her skill set ran to complex tumors of the liver, pancreas, and biliary system. This often involved creating ingenious treatment options in complex sequences coordinated with other specialists. In Octavio's case, her sleeve was empty and she knew it. His disease was running wild. It had come out of nowhere, like a wildfire with a Santa Ana wind at its back. The cancer cells were doubling and growing, invading all the tissues around them at a prodigious rate. SCC usually advanced locally, like a ground army taking over adjacent territory block by block—in this case Octavio's pelvic organs, blood vessels, nerves, and bones. It was a bad actor. If you didn't get it early you never got it. I knew it well.

"Mr. Salcedo arrived here in an ambulance in septic shock—low blood pressure, acidosis, high white blood count, and tachycardia to 160. When he was stabilized we took him to the operating room and explored both groins. The tumor invaded everything from nerves to muscles, tendons, and blood vessels. The leg was gangrenous. To prevent another arterial blowout and a hopeless dead leg, the orthopedic surgeons disarticulated his right leg at the hip joint. There was nothing surgical to be done at this point." Cancer surgeons did not give up easily. They were creative in attacking tumors from their blood supply, radiation, local chemo infusions, and resections. A morphine pump was the only tactic left. Saturate pain receptors while the tumor killed its host.

"Okay. Now what?" I asked, looking at the semicircle of people standing in front of the room. Umut looked at Octavio through the glass. "He wants to go back to Mexico to die," she said. "He hasn't seen his family in six years. He has parents and three kids. He doesn't even know his two youngest sons."

I followed her gaze and saw the patient dozing in his bed. It was clear now why they had brought me in; what was not clear was what I was supposed to do about it. I looked around at all of them. The whole team was deeply invested in Señor Salcedo. Umut, Ken, Maria, Marilia the psychologist, Erika the social worker, Zita the head nurse. They looked at me and said everything without saying a word: *Your turn.* I pulled on a yellow paper gown, face mask, and gloves, and pulled open the sliding door. We went inside together.

The light was brighter outside by this time, and everything in the room was visible. "*Buenos días, Señor Salcedo y Señora Salcedo*, I am the head doctor. Your team has asked me to talk to you..."

I switched off the sound on the TV, telenovelas playing early in the morning on Spanish-language TV in NYC courtesy of Televisa. There were photographs of young children in small frames on a shelf, a pretty round-faced girl and two impish little boys. The room was large, comfortable, with magnificent views to the north that included the UN, the Empire State Building, and a broad swath of Midtown Manhattan. Liliana had been sleeping between two hard-backed molded plastic and metal chairs she pulled together next to the window, softened with folded sheets and blankets. She had on a few extra sweaters and gray baggy sweatpants with black sneakers. She was rumpled, and her face had creases and red streaks from the impression of the sheets she used as a pillow. She was totally alert now, shrugging off the night, and focused on my eyes. We looked at each other. I smiled under my mask and started talking in Mexican-inflected Spanish.

I shook Liliana's hand as she got up. She stood by the bed rails on Octavio's left and squeezed his hand as soon as she released mine. The first few minutes we talked about Mexico. I explained my Mexican connection to defuse any tension. Liliana smiled as I spoke, and I could see Octavio gradually coming around from his drug-induced semi-coma.

Octavio took all the cues from his wife. She was his lifeline to the world—that and the white button connected to the gray cord of the morphine pump. His luminous black eyes were sunk back deep in his head. He swiveled his eyes from his wife to me and back again as we talked. With what life force remained, he was willing himself out of the molecular tumor hailstorm that tracked every move he made. He made no movements, but it was clear there was an enormous effort under way to gain control.

Liliana did most of the talking at first. Between the infection Octavio had in his abdomen, the multiple surgeries, the open abdominal wound, the bleeding, the leakage, renal failure, and malnutrition, it would be unimaginable that he could do anything except focus his faltering attention on his wife and her comments about his children, his parents, and herself. "*Somos de Morelos, de Cuautla*, we are from the state of Morelos from the city of Cuautla," she said in a quiet voice.

I knew Cuautla personally, since Morelos was my home in Mexico as well. Our small house in Tepoztlán is a half-hour drive from Cuautla. I had adopted Mexico as my own many decades earlier, and my wife and I went there to escape from the world of work. Liliana's voice relaxed into a familiar chatter when she realized she didn't have to explain everything to me, that I understood where she was coming from. Any anxiety about formalities and making sense of what lay ahead fell away. Octavio interrupted, "*Doctor, conozco Tepoztlán muy bien. Cuando Kat, mi hijita, tenía cuatro años...*When my daughter Kat was four years old we would go there by bus, to Tepoznieves. Do you know Tepoznieves?"

"*Por supuesto*. It's my favorite place to buy ice cream in Mexico."

"Doctor, I would bring my daughter and my wife and we would walk the town and buy some *Beso de Angel*, angel's kiss, my favorite flavor. What flavor do you like from Tepoznieves?"

I thought a moment and then said, "*Zarzamora*, raspberry." He smiled broadly. The unexpected warmth and child-like vulnerability coming from this hulking body covered with a white sheet touched me instantly.

I asked Octavio why he had left Mexico six years earlier. He took a long time to answer. "My daughter asked me for a toy. She was four years old. *No había chamba*. There was no work. No jobs." Tears streamed down his eyes, and he took a long time to finish. The room was totally quiet except the insistent beep from the monitor, like a car alarm at two a.m. "I borrowed money and made arrangements for a coyote to meet me. I crossed the border and went to California on a bus." The deep humiliations and desperation of poverty had driven him at age twenty-six to leave his home and family, summed up in the streaks of tears on his face and the muffled sobs.

Maria, the Puerto Rican majordomo of our unit, translated quietly in the background for the medical team as we chatted. After a while it was clear Octavio was too exhausted to continue, and I asked Liliana if she would join me outside. The head nurse invited her into her office, then got her some coffee and a snack; I watched as the surgical team unpacked Señor Salcedo's abdomen and hip. The bandages were soaked in the nonstop bloody ooze leaking from his abdomen and pelvis. Umut dosed him from the narcotic pump and took out the last packing, which left exposed tissue, muscles, arteries, nerves, and cancer tissue, gray blobs of ill-defined tumor that bubbled up in all directions. She carefully cleaned out the wound with saline, patted everything dry, repacked the abdomen with white absorbent bandages, and bound it with Kerlix. I have had to develop a stomach for just about everything over the years and have seen almost every variety of assault on the human body, from knives sticking out of right ventricles to silverware protruding from various orifices. It wasn't the visuals of an abdomen ravished by tumor and surgery open to the world, but the smell of decomposition and decay that held me in its grip.

Smell's emotive power is without peer. I had learned the smell of patients with advanced liver disease and advanced renal disease. Different infections have their own special smells, from *Pseudomonas* to *Staphylococcus*. Dying tissue, teeming with the bacterial organisms that thrive without oxygen, give the aroma of putrefaction, of dying and death. There are trillions of bacteria in a normal body, about four pounds' worth. Many more than the normal number of human cells in an entire body. We need them to live and to function; our symbiosis with them is at the core of our being, from the mitochondrial power plants that colonized our cells a billion years ago to the bacteria that line our intestines. The balance between his former healthy body and the teeming organisms that lived within Octavio had changed. You could smell it.

By dead reckoning, Octavio had a few more weeks to live. His pain and anxiety could be controlled with a morphine pump, and a nurse could make his wound livable. If his tumor eroded into a blood vessel, then everything would conclude in a hemorrhagic spectacle worthy of a Quentin Tarantino movie. He could not sit up, and moving him would be awkward. He was a big man, two hundred pounds even after all the weight loss from malnutrition and minus a leg.

Umut volunteered to take him to Mexico. "Take him to Mexico? How would he make it?" I was taken aback. I added, for good measure, "And you don't speak Spanish and don't know the system. Turkish won't cut it in DF, Umut." I realized as I spoke that I was talking to a woman who had never taken *no* seriously her whole life.

Which is why she was standing there next to me, looking at me as if I were going to organize this final trip for the Salcedo family. I looked back. Her eyes did not blink.

"But we would need a lot of luck and preparation to make a trip," I protested.

"Yes," she agreed. But she did not back off.

"And who will pay for the transportation?" I asked, hoping to end the conversation.

"I will, if I have to," she said, "but you know better than I do that it costs considerably less to take him back home than to keep him here until he dies."

I looked at her. "Let me talk to Liliana," I said, hoping this did not commit me to the plan.

Liliana sat in a chair sipping a cup of Au Bon Pain coffee with an untouched chocolate-filled croissant on a paper plate. I asked her how she was doing. *"¿Cómo está, Liliana? ¿Cuentéme su situación aquí en Nueva York, en Queens?"* It didn't need much prompting for Liliana to tell me her story and how they'd ended up here at Bellevue. Octavio and she had known each other since they were teenagers. She was a little older than he was. After they started dating, they never went out with anyone else. They always expected to get married. Like all other young couples in their circumstances, they moved into the in-laws' house. She was twenty years old. Her father had died a slow, agonizing death from liver cancer when she was a teenager. Neither of them or their families had any financial resources. It was day-to-day, every day. Everyone worked at whatever job was available to pay the bills that kept coming in for rent, for food, schools, cell phones, electricity. Chicken or pork was a once-a-week treat. Tortillas with frijoles and green mangoes were the staples. The tiny bit left over went for an emergency fund for health care. Inflation in Mexico was very simple. You had to run faster every three months to stay in the same place as the peso bought less and the government removed its subsidies for corn, gas, and petroleum. It was a kind of slow torture. A quarter of a turn of the screw and then another.

Liliana wasn't particularly close to her own family and felt very welcome with the Salcedos, since Octavio's parents had known her since grade school. The Salcedo house was small—two bedrooms, a living room, a kitchen, and a small workroom filled with tools and parts for automobiles and appliances. Their plan had been to buy an adjacent empty lot and build their own house. Everyone lived with their parents now, Liliana said. No one could afford to have their own place.

Multigenerational housing in perpetuity. The jobs in Cuautla had dried up years earlier. Campesinos or small farmers from the countryside had poured into the market town after NAFTA destroyed much of the export agricultural business in the adjacent states of Puebla, Oaxaca, and Guerrero. So while there was some local economic growth, it was not rapid enough to meet the exploding demand from a countryside in economic collapse. The narco economy was just beginning to lap at the heels of Morelos. You could read about Ciudad Juarez and feel how lucky you were. "It's not happening here," I had heard frequently. Mentally, I would add *yet*.

Brigido, her father-in-law, had a very modest automobile repair shop that paid the basic bills. No one had new clothes, and the entertainment was television and *tertulias*, long talks, with relatives and friends who lived in the barrio and made rounds from house to house. Everyone helped one another in the network. Octavio had been an excellent auto mechanic and could repair anything. He had learned his trade directly from his father, but there simply was not enough work to go around. Octavio left for the United States when their daughter, Kat, was four. For five years, he sent money back. For many relatives it was the monthly *remesa*, or money sent back by relatives in the U.S., that kept them afloat. Octavio's sister, Barbara, received a hundred dollars a month from her husband, who also worked in Staten Island with Octavio as a house painter. This kept Barbara and their daughter Marisa in food and basics. They, too, had been living with her parents now for several years, since paying rent was out of the question. So they all lived together—the parents, the two women, and the children. Barbara and her teenage daughter shared a bed, clothes, and food; they held hands all the time and were like sisters-daughters-mothers *sobreviviendo* (surviving), she said.

The first time Liliana had come to Queens, she paid a coyote three thousand dollars. Octavio was lonely, and she decided to join him and work in the United States. They both worked and sent money home until their second child, a son, was born in the U.S. Then they couldn't afford to look after him with Liliana working, so she decided to go back to Mexico. She was pregnant, and their third child, another son, was born in Cuautla. Octavio had never seen him. Everything fell apart when Octavio got sick. She paid the coyote another three thousand dollars and returned to care for him.

Things went from bad to worse. First the lump in his groin, biopsies, waiting, more trips to the doctors, missed appointments, costly medicines, delays, and a diagnosis of a tumor that made no sense to either of them. None of the doctors at the local hospital spoke Spanish. They pieced together the health care that was offered, grateful for what they could get as things quickly spiraled out of control. At one point Octavio was using feminine napkins to stanch the oozing from both of his groins as he tried to continue working in the restaurant. He took dozens of Tylenol a day to deal with the pain. If he missed too many days, he would lose his work, and the years of stability and regular income would evaporate immediately. They lived in a small room in the attic of a private house off a cul-de-sac in a firemen's community. They knew that if they missed the rent, there were many other recent immigrants from Latin America who could replace them without difficulty.

The treatment took an additional toll. Early each morning they navigated a series of buses to get Octavio to the hospital for radiation, chemotherapy, and hydration from the nausea and vomiting. She watched him get weaker and fed him fresh tortillas sprinkled with coarse salt. She cooked them on her two-burner stove. They would be warm in his hands as he ate one after another. "He says he cannot wait to have the corn tortillas from Cuautla with chunky salt, his favorite, even more than *Beso de Angel*." She smiled. "If they had tortilla ice cream…" It was by sheer determination that she got him through the treatments. As the tumor receded, they were under the benign but false assumption that the disease had been cured. That was the time to buy a one-way ticket to Mexico, but of course as undocumented immigrants, they could not leave the country legally.

There were actually a few good months during which they celebrated the turn of events and tried to get Octavio's strength back. But the cancer suddenly reappeared. The oozing began again, the skin broke down, and his shorts were stained. He came back from work with long bloodstains on his legs that ran into his socks. She washed everything at night as he slept "*como los muertos*," like the dead, and hung it to dry over the heater.

Octavio could not work anymore. The Italian family that owned the restaurant was very sympathetic and caring. The owners gave him two weeks' pay and replaced Octavio the same day with a Mexican worker from the neighboring state of Puebla. The Poblanos had colonized New York City thirty years ago. The pioneer families sent for their relatives and established an open pipeline throughout the greater metropolitan area. Entire towns were deserted in the region as people moved to New York City, leaving grandparents behind. Gaudily painted retirement houses with new satellite dishes hoisted like masts from rooftops pockmarked the empty streets of their hometowns, a widespread scene throughout the Americas.

The exodus from Puebla had been profound and unsettling. The rural Mexican economy did not offer a viable present, much less a future. Entire industries had collapsed in the early 1990s after NAFTA was signed. U.S. agricultural subsidies permitted price differentials that Mexico could not match. Communities packed up and left for the big cities or the United States. The treaty was a stacked deck, and the Mexican worker would pay the price.

Liliana asked me what the possibilities were at this point. I was very open with her. We went over her husband's cancer, the sheer improbability of it, the gratuitousness of it at his age without any reason. Liliana was fatalistic like most Mexicans. She did not search for reasons to explain death and illness. Bad things happen and will happen. She did not indulge in guilt or question why us or why me. She knew she would be a widow living in her in-laws' house, managing three children, in a few weeks. The immediate pressure of economic survival would not allow the time and energy to indulge in what-ifs. Her father had left her mother a widow, and now she would follow. The symmetry was too obvious. The pauses in her comments told me more than what she had to say.

She asked me how long he had to live. "About a month," I replied candidly.

"Can you help me get him home?" She was direct and determined. Her look was intense. "He needs to be with his family. His children. They need to see him to say good-bye." I started to think about the meaning of a good death. A good death for him, for them, and for all of us taking care of him. This wasn't about abstract immigrants stealthily crossing the border stealing jobs from real Americans. This was a man and his wife trying to gain a millimeter toehold on a brutal economic ladder that was created by political and economic forces beyond their control.

The goal, clearly, was to get them both home, surrounded by their family and friends, to make arrangements for his medical care. It was the best we could possibly hope for under these circumstances. I was not sure we would be able to do this, I told her, but I promised to try. When we finished we hugged each other and she started to cry. She sobbed into my shirt and tie and started to laugh nervously as she looked at me. "*No pasa nada*, it doesn't matter at all," I said. She pulled out her cell phone saying "*permítame*," and called the Salcedo family to tell them what was happening. "We're coming home," she told them. They talked two to three times a day, but this was one of the few good-news calls. I gave Liliana my card and scribbled my cell phone number on the back.

I hoped she was right about going home soon as I opened the door and looked at her before slowly and quietly closing it behind me. I really needed to be alone now to collect my thoughts and emotions and make sense of them. It is impossible to keep withdrawing from an emotional bank account without making occasional deposits. I had an email to send, to see if it would be even possible to pull off a trip to Mexico for an undocumented, bedridden cancer patient and his wife. It needed to be soon or not at all.

I walked through the central part of the floor and cut through the administrative office space. I knew I could find an empty place to sit for a few minutes and think. As soon as I entered my office downstairs, the day would be launched and out of control, my control. The emails, phone calls, meetings, drop-in visits, real and imagined crises would intervene and would not end for another twelve hours. Better not to go there, yet. A colleague's door was ajar, as always, and her papers were piled everywhere, floor, desk, and chairs. Her signature five pairs of sneakers were lined up in a row. I knew she wouldn't mind if I chilled out here for a few minutes. There were some lights on down the hall in other offices. I shut the door and sat down and turned off the light.

Medically, it was clear what had to happen. This was the easy part. Octavio was dying. He was in a vulnerable and unpredictable state that could erupt anytime. We could not control it. The failed surgeries, open abdominal wound, and amputated leg told us that. He might bleed out at any moment. I knew my friends at the Mexican consulate would move heaven and earth to help Octavio. If he could make it home, they would try to make it happen. I decided to ask them.

I called my wife and we spoke about repatriating Octavio. Diana took it in as a normal thing to do under the clinical circumstances—a logistical issue, not a moral one. She said she would come, too. By sheer coincidence, we knew the town, the context, the language, and the local rhythms of life.

The medical team would be relieved. I called Umut to tell her. She was ecstatic.

I thought about Octavio, his cancer, and, if all went well, his final trip back to Mexico. Octavio and I had the same type of cancer and had received identical treatments. Diana had taken me to Tepoztlán for several weeks to recover. It was at a sensitive time in my recovery. Through a stomach tube, I was feeding myself canned protein and calorie slurries five times a day. Cathy, my swallowing specialist, had given me a 5cc syringe to practice swallowing small amounts of water. My throat muscles had to relearn how to function in unison a drop at a time. I don't know whether it was the air, the altitude, the sun, the volcano Popocatépetl that looked over the town, the birds, or the *corridos* that played from our neighbors' radios, but by the second week I could swallow baby food and abandoned the plastic umbilical cord tethered to my stomach. Diana had taken me to Morelos to learn how to live again. We were taking Octavio home to Morelos to die. I sat in the darkened office for a few more minutes and let the feelings wash over me. I had changed a lot in a year. The deep dive into an automatic survival mode had cut nearly every invisible social tentacle. I now had choices to make. Taking a patient home to Mexico to die. The only one who acted as if this were the most normal thing in the world was Liliana, who expected that we would all come through for them.

It was five thirty in the morning. Diana and I pulled into the south parking lot before the night shift started pulling out. It was a short walk into the hospital and a quick ride to the tenth floor. The corner room across from the central nursing station was filled with activity, and everyone was glad to see us. The physicians went over the supplies that I would be taking on the trip—first on an Aeromexico flight from JFK to Mexico City and then in the ambulance to the hospital in Cuautla. I had sedatives, morphine, bandages. Everything had been carefully packed and labeled in a small suitcase. I greeted Liliana, who stood before seventeen pieces of motley thirdhand luggage and nylon gym bags, holding everything they owned in life, accumulated over the past six years. Octavio was alert and awake and living off bursts of adrenaline. He wore his Yankees cap and T-shirt. The ambulance crew arrived a few minutes later, and we made our final round of hugs and good-byes. The ambulance EMTs (emergency medical technicians) and I got Octavio safely in the ambulance while Diana and Liliana made sure the luggage made it into the hospital van that was taking them to the airport. The lot was deserted except for a lone agent in the check-in booth. As the medics closed the doors to the ambulance, Octavio waved good-bye, his dark blue cap pulled down low, hiding his eyes.

Alvaro Jimenez from the *protección* office of the Mexican consulate flagged us down as we pulled in front of the Aeromexico departure area at Kennedy. He would accompany us until Octavio was safely in the hands of the physicians at a *seguro popular*, public hospital, in Cuautla. Alvaro had all the papers and permits to ensure that the handoffs from immigration to customs all went smoothly and there would be no unnecessary delays. Time was everything on this trip.

Three rows of seats had been removed in the rear of the plane so that Octavio's stretcher could be secured adjacent to the windows. After he was carefully patted down by a security detail and his pillows and blankets checked for contraband, we rolled down the catwalk to the plane entrance and got ourselves securely ensconced in the rear of the plane before anyone else boarded. A bolus of morphine took the edge off the long haul down the plane for the two-hundred-pound deadweight passenger. Octavio dozed through most of the flight, and Liliana and I took turns sitting next to him. Diana and Alvaro were deep in conversation. Passengers needing to use the restroom tried not to stare, but there was no curtain to shield Octavio from their curious glances. It wasn't too many hours before the plane made a left turn over the Hotel de Mexico on Insurgentes in downtown Distrito Federal with the volcanoes of Mexico City dominating the skyline to the right. The gray smog cloud smothered the plane as we touched down.

The airport *bomberos*, fire department, managed to carry Octavio from the plane down the steep steps from the rear of the Boeing 727 to a waiting ambulance while a team of immigration officials stamped our passports and waved us through, bypassing the usual paperwork and inspections. Octavio's parents, Brigido and Elena, were waiting next to the boxy Cuautla ambulance that had pulled up beside the plane. We secured Octavio in the back as his mother stroked his sweaty matted hair, tears streaming down her face. His father, skinny and leathery, stood stiffly outside, not moving and hardly breathing, staring into the distance after a handshake and brief introductions.

A young woman in a white uniform and white physician's lab coat approached me from the airport entrance carrying a cardboard container with coffee and sandwiches. She introduced herself as Dr. Laura Lazaro-Perez, the physician in charge of Cuautla General Hospital. She had made the trip in the ambulance to greet Octavio and his family and to formally accept the patient from my care. She offered me a coffee and a sandwich as we chatted for a few minutes about Octavio's case. Arriving travelers and families pushing trolleys laden with luggage streamed out of the electronic doors. They glanced over their shoulders in our direction, not missing a step.

"Laura, Seguro Popular has a new hospital in Cuautla?" I heard from the consul.

"The Morelos government is rebuilding an old city hospital on the main street. The Mexican government developed Seguro Popular, like your Medicaid program, ten years ago, to make sure everyone had access to a basic package of health care. Nearly fifty million people, half of the country, had nothing." And she added quickly, "So what is happening in the States, Eric? Tell me, how come you are fighting over insuring the citizens of the United States as more are losing insurance? And the costs are astronomical. We are getting medical tourists in Mexico and not just for cosmetic surgery and dental work anymore or to buy a year's supply of medication. We simply don't get it here. It just doesn't make any sense. We have no money and are doing the opposite."

"The politics of health care are all about money," I said, "very big money. Almost three trillion dollars and counting. The key players in the health industry, from the hospitals to the insurers to Big Pharma and the physician groups, have gotten so powerful that they can distort and deform what happens in Washington."

"Harry and Louise?" she said as she sipped a macchiato and looked at me through her wire-rimmed glasses.

"Exactly, Laura. Exactly." She was referring to the ad campaign financed by the Small Business Council that undid the Clintons' efforts at comprehensive health care reform in the early 1990s.

"But seriously, health care?" she picked up. "We were an embarrassment on this continent. We still have a long way to go. Some people complain that our program is '*Ni Seguro, Ni Popular*'—neither safe nor popular. But embarrassment is a huge motivator. When we compared ourselves with other Latin American countries, we had to start doing something. Long live national humiliation." She smiled.

"Embarrassment evidently doesn't work in the States," I came back. "Imagine a tide of economic refugees from the north in their silver campers driving to Morelos and Cuautla?"

"We are already seeing them coming. Look at the growth of gated communities here." She was matter-of-fact. "This is the new normal, Eric." I thought of our house in Tepoztlán, the high stone walls, the giant twisted black *ciruela* trees, the electrical storms and pounding rains from June to October, the walks to the shops and the market. I kept silent.

An ancient large brown van cruised to a stop in front of us, the doors opened with Liliana and Diana inside surrounded by six years of baggage. Brigido reached inside the ambulance to touch his son and to say good-bye to his wife before he hopped up into a passenger seat in the van. We agreed upon the route to Cuautla and pulled into the never-ending rivers of traffic on the *periférico* heading south to the toll road. This would take us out of the Valley of Mexico and over the ten-thousand-foot pass between volcanoes into the state of Morelos. I sat in the back of the ambulance and looked out the windows at the taco stands, colored plastic awnings and chairs, flat-tire shops, hotels, restaurants, football stadiums, and endless miles of houses, cars, and people. Where incoming roads brought traffic to a near crawl, dozens of Mexicans in Nextel orange jumpsuits sold cell phone cards, candies, custards, windshield wipers, and plastic toys. There were no sword swallowers or jugglers with flaming batons today.

Looking at the smog and the traffic, I thought of the sheer improbability of twenty million souls fashioning a life on a dried-up lakebed. This entire area had once been Lake Texcoco; the island city Tenochtitlán was ruled by the Aztec emperor Moctezuma until his fatal welcome of Hernán Cortés. We drove past a turnoff for Coyoacan, once the lakefront suburb for Cortés and now a center of bohemian life, bookstores, and restaurants. It was a paradoxical token of life and peace and quiet in the throbbing city.

As we snaked our way south, I checked on Octavio and gave him morphine and another bag of saline solution since his catheter bag had only a small amount of urine. I talked to his mother about her grandchildren and to Laura about Cuautla, balancing her career and family, plus the inevitable dose of Mexican politics.

Elena wept silent tears as she smiled at her son. She tried to keep him steady as we drove over the speed bumps and took the tight curves from access road to the highway to the local streets, avoiding the dense congestion. I looked at Octavio's mother hunched over her son and looked away.

The Mexican idea of death had traditionally been framed around the festival of the Day of the Dead or Día de los Muertos. The annual holiday starts at the end of October and goes on until the fifth or so of November, overlapping with All Souls' Day on November 2. Mexicans go to the cemeteries where they've buried their dead. They tend and scrub the grave sites and then carefully arrange flowers and food plus sweets to share with the dead. It is a time of communion with relatives, parents, grandparents, and children in a spirit of caring, loving, and sharing. It is not filled with grief and sadness. The dead are very present and alive in this national holiday, which can be traced back many centuries before the Spanish Conquest and has merged into the Catholic calendar.

I could finally see the new Walmart in the outskirts of Cuautla with its acres of empty parking lots. The upraised, rifle-wielding arm of Emiliano Zapata, the revolutionary leader of the early twentieth century, indicated the main turnoff to the city's center a few kilometers ahead.

We swung around to the front of a makeshift entrance to a nondescript building ten minutes later. Dozens of people were sitting outside on colored plastic chairs; there was a small, open-faced pharmacy with a metal grille covering the space next door. The hospital was undergoing renovations and was at half capacity. Everything was catwalks, plastic tarps, stacks of adobe-colored bricks, and roped-off areas. A middle-aged guy in a white guayabera shirt sat in front of a small wooden school desk at the entrance with an official-looking cap. He called patients to the clinics and limited access for everyone else. Food vendors hovered everywhere, their stands close by, catering to the visitors who sat for hours waiting to be allowed in to see relatives. They cleared the area to let us in.

Octavio was settled into a three-bedded room on a medical surgical unit with post-op patients recovering from C-sections, angina, lobar pneumonias, and a pneumothorax from a knife wound. Plain vanilla, concrete, whitewash, linoleum, no AC, barely room to get from one place to another sideways. Trays of soup were handed out by the candy stripers amid the strong smell of disinfectant and bug spray, the hum of a distant generator, and mariachi music filtering in the wide-open breezeless windows. There were patients in the two other beds; patients in beds lined the corridors. Student nurses in scrubbed and pressed uniforms bobbed between the beds and the rooms. Guards stood at the entryways while families, doctors, and visitors all wove their way through the hospital. As an American doctor bringing a dying young Mexican patient by jet plane to his hometown in the sweltering heat of the plains of Morelos, I felt like a Martian from outer space. This was the entry point for Octavio into the Mexican health system.

Octavio's receiving doctor and I went through the case in detail at the nursing station in front of a bank of computers. He made it clear that they were not a hospice and had neither the familiarity with taking care of dying patients nor the narcotics and other medications to keep Octavio comfortable for more than twenty-four hours. A pain specialist was available once a week. This was a bread-and-butter community hospital. The young man on one side had a leg fracture from an automobile accident and had been waiting several days for OR time and a metal pin to realign his tibia. On the other side, an old man with a deeply crevassed face with emphysema and bronchitis was sitting bolt-upright, wheezing with an intermittent deep phlegmatic tubercular cough as intravenous medications dripped slowly into his arm. I offered to get narcotics from a private pharmacy if the doctor wrote me a prescription. We negotiated his medication regimen and went over what they had in stock and what I had remaining in my box from Bellevue. Enough for another twenty-four hours, we were in business.

When I got back to his room, Octavio was sitting up in bed smiling and appeared comfortable. He and his two hospital mates were propped up, eating ice cream from cups with small red plastic spoons. Diana, on the way to Cuautla, had bought and smuggled in a liter of ice cream from Tepoznieves, our favorite Morelos ice cream store. *Beso de Angel* was dribbling from everyone's chin as nods and slurping noises greeted me. For the first time, I relaxed and smiled and joked with the Salcedos, his mother, and the other patients in the room. We had made it back to Mexico intact, and with Octavio in one piece. Exhaustion hit Diana and me at the same time. We said our good-byes and took a cab to our house in Tepoztlán nestled in the Tepozteco thirty minutes away. Unbelievably, after the day's ordeal, Liliana left the hospital to go look for a job. Ever since I'd met her on the ICU floor, she had been obsessed with work and their vaporized savings. She had nothing to bring back to the family compound.

The drive back down the sinuous road into the valley of Morelos through a break in the vertiginous cliffs that guarded the entrance to Tepoztlán was always breathtaking. We passed the ruins of old sugar haciendas from two centuries earlier when Morelos had been one of the largest cane-sugar-producing areas in the world. Its underground water supplies in volcanic earth had managed to support this vast labor-consuming industry, bringing extraordinary wealth to a feudal planter class. The inequalities fueled the anger and rage that led to Zapata's uprising in 1910.

We had planned on one more day, one more visit with Octavio before flying back to New York City. The entire Salcedo clan materialized, hanging out at the bedside and spilling into an empty ophthalmology waiting room. Kat sat next to her father, holding his hand. She had his same large, luminous eyes. They had reconnected. The young boys played in the hall, finding alternatives to the reality playing itself out in the hospital room. Octavio's mother had slept on the floor at his side in her clothes. Octavio's sister and niece sat outside, available to run errands. They were unhappy with his care in a public setting, the lack of privacy, the 250-peso-a-day cost plus medications (another 750 pesos), the commotion and noise. It was clear they needed to have him at home. It was something I could not suggest; they needed to get to that point themselves.

The parents were trying to come up with some money to pay the hospital; only the completely indigent paid nothing. The Mexican team had assumed control, and it was clear they were going to work with the family to ensure his pain control and complete care at home. The phone calls and negotiations were in process; he would be moved later that day. Diana took Liliana aside and slipped her a hundred dollars. Again, Liliana accepted this as a matter of course. They needed help and would not turn it down. We then went back to say good-bye to Octavio. I took his hand in mine and promised to come back and visit in a month. His eyes filled with tears, but he agreed to believe that we would see each other again.

After our good-byes to Octavio and Kat, we took the other family members across the street for lunch. Patients' families were sitting on the side of the entrance eating tortillas off paper napkins while licking their fingers. Cars kicked up dust clouds in the desert air. We were deep into the dry season. There was a long row of bright-colored plastic tarps providing shade for a dozen taco food stands in a row on the other side. Elena's, Erika's, Rosa's, Eugenia's. We strolled across and walked the gauntlet until we found one with the right atmosphere of TV on low volume, red plastic tables and chairs, blue corn tortillas and quesadillas on the large circular *comal* heated with a gas burner, a gigantic *cazuela* filled with crispy pig skin and red broth, and—most important—a smiling *anfitriona* or hostess to greet us.

We sprawled out over a few tables and put in our orders. We were surrounded by women except for Octavio's father, Brigido. We made small talk until the orders came.

Octavio's sister Barbara started the conversation. She had been in Arizona with her husband and had been picked up by ICE (Immigration and Customs Enforcement) and immediately put into detention. "*¿Tiene una hija?* Do you have a daughter?" they had asked. "If you want to see her you have to leave and not come back to the States for five years. If you come before five years are up we will put you in prison for two full years." They threatened and bullied her. They were Latinos themselves, Chicanos from Texas, Latinos who had grown up in the States and had their U.S. citizenship. She had left without seeing her husband, who drifted to New York City to stay under the radar of the immigration services and the deteriorating vigilantism of the Southwest. The Sheriff Arpaios who were making a name for themselves in Phoenix were all known through the informal networks where information was transmitted rapidly via cell phones and word of mouth. He wasn't necessarily the worst, she said, only "he liked the publicity and the power."

Octavio's mother, Elena, told us that she had made an attempt to visit her son when he was in the hospital. She had been granted papers from the Mexican consulate in Mexico City and told to cross at Laredo, Texas. After a forty-eight-hour bus ride, she arrived at the border. The U.S. ICE officials called the New York hospital, which denied that Octavio was a patient in the facility. They put Elena in handcuffs until the Mexican consulate was contacted in New York City and was able to verify Octavio's existence and his medical status as an inpatient. They released her but refused her entry. She was too distraught to try again through official channels. The pain and humiliation of the experience left her anguished and defeated. She took the next bus back to Morelos. The family wrote a letter to the Mexican president asking for assistance. They never heard back.

Octavio's cousin Jessica had jet-black hair and was on and off her cell phone throughout the meal, getting up a few times to talk privately, her back to us. She was in her early thirties and looked much younger. Her husband and kids were in Waco, Texas. She had worked in the States for thirteen years maintaining a household with her husband and four children, all of them U.S. citizens. While commuting to her job at Wendy's in the standard checkout counter uniform and apron, she was picked up by the police on a stop-and-frisk protocol. She was immediately taken to an ICE intake center since she had no identification, then transferred to a remote detention center. Her location changed four times in eight months. Middle-of-the-night rousings, the gathering-up of belongings, and being bused to new locations with no stated reason was the routine for the hundreds of detainees in orange jumpsuits who lived in an expanding parallel universe to the U.S. prison system. They gave her a blanket and a prison uniform and food in the morning. At the end of her eight months in detention, ICE officials eventually released her at the U.S.-Mexican border. The guards, she said, called her a "bitch" and told her to stay the "fuck" out of their land.

"Why do they hate us so much?" she asked me.

She made it back to her family in Cuautla, where she continues to participate in the daily life of her husband and children via phone calls many times a day. A virtual mother to a virtual family. The children, preschoolers to adolescents, the wife and husband are in suspended animation, waiting for some kind of reunion, for the possibility of a life together that may not happen. With each year that passes the ties that bind are frayed.

Sitting around the table, Diana and I acknowledged the widespread community of pain. We also knew it is the deliberate policy of the U.S. immigration service to raise the bar for economic immigrants. The reduced risk-reward ratio will supposedly change the decision-making behaviors of young men and women who risk their lives to get into the States. The costs and risks are considerable: the costs of a coyote, the risks not only of ICE but also of criminals engaged in the increasingly lucrative business of extorting and kidnapping immigrants heading north from Central America and Mexico.

Brigido had another order of *tacos de carne*, cheese, and mushrooms on blue corn tortillas with an orange-flavored drink. He mopped up the salsa with extra tortillas, sprinkled on some salt, and dropped chopped onion and cilantro onto his last mouthful. He looked chronically tired. He wore the same clothes from the day before, a brown-checked shirt and brown pants. He was skinny and had short gray-flecked hair. I asked him if he had ever spent time in the United States. "I never wanted to immigrate," he said. "Too many stories of prison time from my friends and their children. Plus, the heat in Texas is worse than Cuautla. Who would want to suffer like that for nothing? The drugs and alcohol have ruined more lives than the *remesas* have helped."

He then started to talk about the upsurge in the narcotics trade in Morelos. "It isn't like Michoacan here with *La Familia* [the narco cartel in Michoacan state] in charge, extorting and kidnapping. The cartels don't control the entire state. The drugs get shipped through Cuernavaca up north or flown through the airport in the city center. I am more worried about unemployment and the young people, though. What will they do to support themselves? How will they live? I couldn't even support Octavio, my own son in my own business. It dried up in front of my eyes after twenty-plus years. The corruption is everywhere in government and could spread to the men who cannot support their families, who cannot afford a house or an apartment, a girlfriend. If

BESO DE ANGEL 105

you cannot afford to get married to have a family, you are creating a different kind of desperation." Brigido was animated and angry as he talked. I had not seen him this lively before—just quietly helpful in the background of the entourage of women he assisted in his steady way. I would not see Brigido again as this Brigido. He couldn't protect his family and could barely keep tortillas on the table. His shame was shrouded in rage that he contained in order to be of service to others and his work.

"I used to have my own car repair business," Brigido said matter-of-factly. "With the economy sputtering down a dozen more businesses opened on sidewalks, parking lots, and empty spaces everywhere. Prices dropped for repairs and I had to lay off my three employees whom I had worked with for many years. I was embarrassed. They had wives and families. I knew all of them like family. The price of parts doubled in the last two years. Electricity and gas go up 20 percent a year minimum year after year. The *gasolinazo* or Pemex price increases on gasoline every three months forced me to sell my car, a much-used Chevrolet. I cut out everything that was not totally essential and charged only what my customers could afford. At this point, I depend more on credit and bartering. I didn't have a cash business left. I now do everything myself and bring in Raul, my brother, for the occasional big job, an engine or transmission. I have to keep everything locked up all the time or my tools will get stolen. No one can afford tools. I also repair everything and anything, from refrigerators to air conditioners.

"But I am just one man, and there are many more in the neighborhood. I hate the narcos, but I can see where things are going. Where the pressure is. Without jobs or a future, what are you going to do? Just how do you survive? Maybe if I was a young guy like my son I would go to the States and take the risk. It is kind of like a prison staying here if you are a young man like Octavio. So what is the difference, really? I see my grandchildren and don't see what they will do, where they will live. Who will they marry and how will they bring up children? We can barely bring them up. I sleep on the couch to allow my children the dignity of privacy. They lost their spouses a long time ago to immigration. The U.S. news reviles us, makes fun of us, makes us into thieves and criminals. Who are the criminals exactly? If Mexico is a criminal state or at risk of becoming one, why sell us advanced military assault weapons at border depots? Why launder the narco money in the biggest U.S. banks? Why purchase billions of dollars' worth of drugs?" Brigido was almost done but had not quite run his course. This was the Mexican street speaking loud and clear. "We are a relatively poor country, but not an impoverished country. We are a deep country with a profound wisdom. The United States is risking its own heart and soul by hating us, hating others." Brigido sipped his soft drink and looked at all of us and then turned toward a distant spot and lost himself into infinity.

I looked at Brigido with some surprise. He had been so taciturn and private. I knew he felt a great pain for his son. His wife was the emotional member of the family who looked after the grandchildren and kept an eye on the house. He tried to bring in some pesos and keep the lights on. He had a very realistic sense of the Mexican government, U.S. policy, what it meant, and where it was headed. Was this a look into the future for the United States, its own future foretold?

We paid the bill and all piled into our small VW for a short drive to the Salcedo house through the center of town and over the dried bed of the Cuautla River. Middle-class gated communities fell away as we slalomed our way into a working-class neighborhood where the work had evaporated. We pulled into a nondescript barrio of rectangular cement houses and cement sidewalks. There was barely a tree in sight. A few ancient dust-covered cars parked on the street. Brigido opened the door and welcomed us into his home. Octavio's two young children were playing on the floor; both had baby bottles filled with milk in their mouths, lying on their backs in front of a large color television screen. They squirmed and moved by pushing their legs against the ground, sliding across the floor. They were too old for baby bottles. This was a case of elderly grandparents taking the path of least resistance under enormously stressful circumstances, caring for another generation they were not mentally or emotionally prepared to manage.

There were no alternatives. The family was tapped out in every direction. Both children had obvious severe developmental delays in language and skills from benign neglect. They were never abused; they had food and decent clothes, and a loving household. The energy required to read to them, talk with them, and participate in meaningful activities for their age did not exist. The time, effort, and money required if they were to socialize with their peers, or take part in activities that might engage them both mentally and physically, were unavailable. The barrio had changed in recent years. It was not safe for kids to play in the streets and hang out without supervision. Every family was locked into its concrete bunker of a home. The family showed us pictures of Octavio as a young man and the marriage portraits of his parents thirty-five years earlier, a handsome couple. The Virgin of Guadalupe looked over the room from her altar surrounded by candles over the door.

As we drove away, retracing our steps through central Cuautla and back toward the giant Walmart leading us to Tepoztlán, we couldn't help but think about the Salcedo family. We were leaving a community shaken by seismic economic forces way beyond its borders. Mothers and fathers, brothers and sisters trying to make some sense of a world that had changed so much over the last few decades and was putting more and more pressure on them to keep a step ahead of a game they could barely make sense of. It was like a gravitational field from a black hole that pulled away at industries and livelihoods, added great wealth to a small class, and created a huge demand for illegal drugs. This new parallel economy was as big as the traditional one but spawned a level of violence and civil unrest that even defied the state "ownership" of lethal violence. We were bringing a young man home to be with his family during his final weeks. Yet we had become witnesses to the intimate violence that was part of economic immigration as it tore through communities and families.

The flight back was unremarkable, leaving at one p.m. and landing at Liberty Airport in Newark, New Jersey, that evening. Diana and I hardly spoke on the flight. Once we landed, we took a cab to our apartment, checked in with our family, ran through the pile of mail, ordered some takeout, and crawled into bed. We both knew the next morning would bring on the routines, emails, and phone calls that would begin to erase the physical and emotional drama we had been a part of.

Over the next few weeks, everyone who had cared for Octavio asked about him and Liliana. Octavio had made it home and was under the medical care of a daily visiting nurse and a physician several days a week. His pain was well controlled with a combination of narcotics and medications for anxiety in liquid form titrated to his changing needs. He played with his kids, talked with his family and friends as his strength allowed. According to his sister via a poor phone connection to my New York line, he was enjoying his mother's tortillas, hot to the touch, with coarse salt and green mangoes the day before he died.

Over the month Octavio lived with his family, through the phone calls and email messages and the conversations with his caretakers at Bellevue, I thought often about what it meant to so many people to have him make it back to his home. Octavio had threaded the needle in this brave new world. He had survived the human traffickers, the desert, terrible loneliness, and extreme working conditions to send a few dollars home to his family. His hope was to someday have his own concrete-bunker-like home with a couple of rooms on the empty lot next to his parents' house. A rogue cell had not obeyed molecular signals to stop unbridled DNA replication. Everyone had been moved by the spectacle of a young man made totally vulnerable. He had become dependent on the kindness of strangers.

From our perch in the inpatient building at 27th Street and First Avenue, recessed down a long walk toward the East River, on the high floors of Bellevue you can see for miles in a 360-degree arc that covers the lives of nearly twenty million people. As many people as in Mexico City. Within a few generations everyone within this broad radius has come from someplace else. Everyone has stories of leaving a homeland because of political persecution, economic collapse, civil wars, or the need to break out of the social grip of a traditional society that is too tight or too restrictive. In his attempt to create a modest better life, Octavio risked the little that he had. Reconnecting him with his home and family was a reaffirmation of life at its most elemental. In a world that is increasingly stressful and less predictable, more economically challenging and politically less governable, medicine is still about looking after the individual who seeks care.

The return to Mexico for a dying young man and his young wife was our opportunity to take the caring as far as we could. How people die and how we participate in their deaths is as much about us as about them. Our own humanity is at stake. In a society that is increasingly mesmerized by efficiency, measurement by numbers and a bottom-line mentality that extols profit and wealth over any other human value, the risk is clear to everyone I work with. When health care is now measured by a "medical loss ratio," and the percentage of spending on health care is considered a "loss," then we are really lost.

CHAPTER 5

The Qualification

The email was not exceptional. *Can you come to my next AA meeting tomorrow night. It is my 4th Step qualification. Would like you to be there. Sorry for short notice.—Arnie ps St Lukes in the Field West Village 7pm.* That was it, cryptic but crystal clear.

The invitation opened wide an entire emotional strongbox that had been dormant for at least four years. I was not the only one to witness Arnie skidding into the ditch. Watching a person slide into a deep hole and not knowing where it would end was slightly pornographic or schadenfreudesque as the bodies piled up. Deep wells of anger and sadness, families on fire, kids in crisis, broken marriages, and broken lives would pour out over a long time. The outcomes were prewritten; only the small print still needed to be filled in.

And now this email.

I was running late at work the next day, so I decided to take a cab to the AA meeting on Jane Street in the West Village. There was no time to decompress from a long day of listening to the *drip-drip* of cuts to funding health care for the most vulnerable. I asked the turbaned black-bearded Sikh cabdriver to let me off a few blocks from Hudson Street to walk the final ten minutes west along Christopher Street. The street was filled with cafés and bakeries, pet stores ("$300 Dollars Off All Puppies"), and trendy hipster bars and restaurants. Every other person on the street seemed to have a shih tzu, no matter how big and tattooed the guy. The evening was hot and steamy; by the time I came within sight of the Hudson River, my shirt was stuck to my back, with blotches of sweat everywhere. An electric storm was coming. A taxi was stopped at the red light when I got to the curb, all four windows wide open. A Pakistani cabbie nodded ever so slightly to the relent-less syncopated sound of Qawwali music rolling out over the street onto the sidewalk. He looked at me, still nodding, and did not miss a beat as he swished north through the thick damp air. I wished he had stayed there until the end of the song. It brought me back to Peshawar and another time in my life for a few brief seconds. The music was soothing and pulsated at the same rate as an internal pacemaker in my primitive limbic brain.

I was just on time, two minutes before seven. People were walking through the two gates to the grounds and filtering into the lovely brick building on the idyllic urban grounds of the Episcopal church. The large room was two-thirds full and I found a metal chair in a far corner between a bird-like woman in a white dress whose leg bobbed through the entire meeting and a middle-aged man with a short buzz cut and neat goatee dressed completely in gray from shoes to necktie. A thin woman of thirty-five to forty with frizzy brown hair was clutching the lectern while repeatedly looking at her watch, ready to begin the ses-sion on time. Precisely at seven p.m. she hushed the group, then asked for volunteers to man the clock when she started running through the AA mantra of mutual respect and asked for the 12 Steps and 12 Tra-ditions to be read by the membership. A plastic-coated white sheet of paper was passed from person to person, each reading aloud one step and handing the sheet to the next person. It was "step night," the third Thursday of every month. Members who had reached an important milestone in their progress "celebrated" the occasion with a meeting in which they could share their journey; they received a coin with the number of their years in AA. One day at a time.

Arnie was in the front row, three seats down from the evening's leader. After collecting the paper when the traditions had been read, she had some announcements about upcoming meetings, holidays, donations, and the need to be on time to respect the church's con-tribution of the building. She announced that Arnie was celebrating his fourth step and would be qualifying tonight. She beckoned him to join her at the lectern, smiled, and took a seat as the group applauded enthusiastically. He was clearly a regular and known to the group.

He had seen me come in and nodded a greeting, expecting nothing in return. A small smile acknowledging that I had come at his request. Nothing more would be said between us.

My name is Arnie. I have just completed four years in AA. One year for every step so far. It has been a hard, long journey. I have not made a qualification before. I have had my two and three minutes sharing things with this group and the other groups I have attended over almost five years. They have all been fragments, bits and pieces from my life that were all responses to things other people had qualified or said about their lives and their personal experiences. It has taken me a long time to be able to stand here in front of you and tell you what I can about my shipwrecked life and my many attempts to put it back together.

He paused and sipped some water.

Arnie was a man in his early sixties, comfortably dressed in a blue linen blazer with matching buttondown cobalt-blue shirt and freshly pressed slacks with gray New Balance racing sneakers. His hair was thinning, and he had lost a good thirty pounds since the last time I'd seen him four years ago. He was trim and clean-shaven with an almost imperceptible hesitation in his presentation. You would only notice it if you knew him. The old aggressiveness was tempered, held in check, as if on a leash, without any strain. I sat back into my chair, crossed my legs, and blocked out the rustling in the room, the overhead fan giving a faint respite to the humidity and the heat from the other bodies. People idly fanned their faces with paper, books, a stray ancient *People* magazine, and 12 Step literature.

My story is not a pretty one. It is no better and no worse than the hundreds of stories I have heard over the years in several thousand AA and Al-Anon meetings here and wherever I have traveled. I am one of those guys who had to destroy everything I had. My sponsor first used the term with me auto-da-fé, a burning at the stake. They used to do that to Jews during the Spanish Inquisition, but I lit my own fire. I had to

almost die to get a life, any kind of life. In fact I did kill myself
in some way. I mean, I destroyed myself, or the remaining part
of myself that had not been destroyed already by my addictions
and bad judgments. My deceptions and lying were all that I had
left by the time I nearly died in Bellevue Hospital. But to finally
come around, to make it, to be here tonight, I had to go down
a lot farther than I ever thought possible. I mean I had to let go
of any remaining hidden pretenses that I was holding on to, or
that held me in their grasp. Was the addiction mine to choose
or was I in thrall of the addiction? It doesn't matter really, two
ways of looking at the same thing.

Listening to Arnie, I remembered the call a few years back about
him from the Bellevue emergency room. "Eric. He's back. He's hallucinating and acting psychotic. I sent off a drug screen. There is a
lot more going on here than you can imagine." I got it right away and
headed for the hospital.

Arnie relaxed some as he got into his story.

I was one of those guys who they make movies about.
Wall Street *with all of the lifestyle that went with it. Michael*
Douglas as the evil monster without values who used other
people. When I first saw it I denied it to myself and to everyone
around me as a fantasy and bad image of a profession that had
a job to do in society even if we didn't like how it was done.
Like a garbageman, I said to myself. Not everything smelled
good but it was necessary work. Capitalism wasn't pretty up
close but it was better than anything else that had come along.
Creative destruction. You blow up businesses and lives and
then get to crow as you pick up the pieces, scrape the pension
funds into your balance sheet, and go on the prowl for other
objects of your desire.

It first started with a back injury. I don't even know what
caused it and it's immaterial, it does not matter now. My doctor
saw me and did some X-rays and gave me some prescriptions

for pain medications. Vicodin tablets. Though it is blurry, the beginning steps I mean, since by the time I was finished it was ten different kinds of prescription medication and hundreds of tablets every couple of days plus anything else I could get my hands on.

So Vicodin, little white tablets. Not the mother's little helpers from the songs of the 1960s. Valium for stay-at-home moms who couldn't bear the stress and boredom of being locked in their houses with two kids, the dog, and no one to talk to. Just some white tablets for pain. I was a regular heavy drinker at that time. Always had a bottle of wine with dinner and a drink or two over lunch. In fact, I had bought a wine cellar at an auction from Sotheby's. I mean the entire wine cellar of a longtime collector who died with thousands of bottles in several carefully monitored and air-conditioned warehouses plus a thousand bottles in another apartment next to his filled with cases and racks of wines from France, Argentina, Chile, South Africa, and a huge bedroom filled with single-malt Scotches, collectibles, the best, most esoteric and delicious. There wasn't a day I did not drink; it lubricated my work and helped me deal with the stress of the brinksmanship and the deal making. There was nothing unusual about it. We all did it and then went to private gyms and men's clubs for a sauna and massage. Part of the executive compensation package.

The white pills took away an edge of anxiety, stress, and some other dimension I hadn't even fathomed at the time. My life was becoming unwound, though I didn't see that, either. I had been through several marriages, failed relationships, extramarital affairs, and the latest trophy marriage was coming apart slowly but surely. I treated her like my other acquisitions. The cost, the benefit. A wife as an ROI, a return on investment. My life was like the morning after, the feeling of desultory emptiness that slowly lifts and then you get on with things. But it never lifted; I was living in a perpetual, terminal phase of the morning after. That is, until the white pills took it away. I was

free now of that nagging feeling of incompleteness and a deeper
fear that I didn't want to approach at all. That would come
much later, when things fell apart.

I sat there listening to Arnie tell his story to seventy-plus people in
a room on a hot humid New York night with lightning flashes coming in the windows like spasms from another universe, but the air still
heavy and dead. The thunder would arrive later. His chauffeur had
steered toward Bellevue four years earlier, when he turned ashen and
complained of nausea. When I got to the emergency room, he had been
thrashing about and hallucinating about hearing voices that wanted to
kill him. He was drenched in sweat, and a nurse was wiping him down
with a wet towel. He was now heavily sedated with morphine for his
chest pain and tranquilizers plus a shot of Seroquel, an anti-psychotic
medication for the hallucinations and agitation. The attending in our
psychiatric emergency room had come down the hall to advise on the
situation. The patient's initial EKG showed an inferior myocardial
infarct in progress and a tachycardia at a steady 120, his pulse racing
under the stress and need to keep up his cardiac output. Now with his
agitation and delirium/hallucinations, it was clear that his heart would
be at much greater risk—and that there was something else going on.
He had no previous psychiatric history. One of our doctors had Arnie's
wife on the line, and we were getting phone numbers of his family doctor, specialists, and key contacts to put the puzzle together.

There was something about the narcotics that gave me a
release from a distress I hadn't even identified to myself until
it was gone. But I went back to my doctor a few times and got
new prescriptions since the pain was not better. I went through
the usual CT scan and MRI scan rituals plus the obligatory
referrals to multiple specialists who couldn't find anything
but bone spurs and degenerative spine disease. Half the docs
offered surgery and half prescriptions and half said, "Do noth-
ing." An enlightened non-interventionist even recommended
rest, acupuncture, tai chi, the finest spas and massage therapists

*available, and of course to cut down my schedule, relax, and
take a vacation. She cautioned about the medications. I did
all of that except the rest and relaxation and cutting down of
meds. The opposite. I accumulated at least fifteen more doctors
that year, who all prescribed not only the Vicodin but Oxy-
Contin in increasing dosages plus benzodiazepines like Valium,
Ativan, Xanax, and Klonopin. I had an elaborate schedule to
see them in rotation. At work I made up fake appointments
every week that looked like I was busy going to meetings
around the city. I took the prescriptions to different pharma-
cies and paid cash every time to avoid the insurance company
inquiries and computer-driven letters to my physicians. Within
a year's time I was a regular user. A regular Dr. House or Nurse
Jackie on Wall Street. I took my pills every few hours, had them
hoarded away, and had my dealer doctors scattered around
the city all cleverly hidden from one another. I arranged it like
I was planning a merger or acquisition with military precision
and took care of all the details. Nothing was left to chance.
Except I forgot one thing. The alcohol and the medications
interacted. I had memory losses. Minutes were gone. Then
hours. Then entire days were gone. They weren't blackouts in
a drunken stupor. They were chemically induced erasures of
parts of my memory banks in my brain. Everyone noticed it
and discreetly wrote it off or covered for me and assumed it was
too much work, stress, pushing myself too hard, maybe a little
aging thrown in. I was like that guy in* Memento *who had to
write down his life on his skin.*

*By this time I had branched out to other drugs, other medi-
cations. Since I was who I was, the doctors gave me samples
and other prescriptions for tranquilizers, benzos, sleeping
pills, anti-epileptic medications, and anti-depressants. I had so
many prescription medications, I couldn't keep track of them
or remember what they were for. I had bags of prescription
medications stashed in my apartment, my office, my weekend
house, and suitcases I used on trips. I couldn't keep track of the*

drugs. During a business trip to Europe, I ran out of Oxy and got into real trouble for the first time. I got sweaty, very anxious, and had a craving that was burning a hole in my head and my insides. I faked a kidney stone and got some narcotics in the emergency room and a prescription. That was Paris, France. I was an international drug operator by this time in my new "career." By day an international financier and by night desperate to make sure I had my supply of drugs. I was increasingly doing stupid things, more careless. Lying became a habit. Then it became a normal way of living. It became living.

Arnie's description brought the memory of a young radiologist to mind. He was a new attending, smart and capable, with a lovely wife and two adorable children. He came to see me after an emergency room visit for the abdominal pain of recurrent pancreatitis where he had received intramuscular narcotics and a prescription. The problem with the entire story was that the pancreatic enzyme amylase level in his blood never was elevated, although the amylase was high in his urine. One night after a couple dozen visits to the emergency room and similar follow-ups with different doctors, I realized what was happening. The next time he came in, we ordered a urine culture along with a urine amylase enzyme. The amylase was elevated in the urine, and the culture of his urine grew out bacteria that colonize the mouth. Our salivary glands also make the digestive enzyme amylase, and he had been spitting in his urine to raise the amylase level, giving a falsely positive test. When I confronted him with these findings and his obvious drug addiction, he was remorseful and talked about an old injury and inadvertent narcotic addiction. He looked sadly pathetic. There was no answer to my phone calls the next day. Overnight he had packed his house and left town with his wife and children, never to be seen or heard from again. Addictions ruled his universe. Drug-seeking behavior no matter the cost.

I started lying to my wife, who found stashes of medication. My medical problems became more elaborate, and the

*specialists I went to and the treatments multiplied. Each one
was plausible by itself, but together they made no sense. There
was no one pulling them together except myself—I was the
impresario of my illness or addiction. I would tell my ex-wife
medical stories my friends and colleagues told me. I collected
them and hoarded them as my own. But it was really my
mood swings that affected her the most. She couldn't put them
together with the alcohol and drugs. I forgot huge amounts
of time. I had nightmares from Klonopin for almost a year.
Nightly horrors dredged up from my childhood that were
played out in Technicolor as I kicked my way through the blankets and avoided death by gang and Mafia members out for my
blood. By this time our marriage was a mess; she was living in
another bedroom and moved a lot of her belongings to another
apartment we owned in Tribeca. My libido had shriveled up
along with the rest of me. I blamed her immaturity, her superficiality, her criticisms, her lack of criticisms. I blamed her being
there and her not being there. I worked at undermining her
self-esteem with a watchmaker's precision. I knew exactly what
I was doing and could not control it or did not want to control
it. We had a more formal relationship that got colder over time.
Have you heard of zero degrees Kelvin? It is the coldest temperature there is. It is the temperature of interplanetary space. It
was the temperature of my relationships. Zero degrees. I didn't
notice and I didn't care. Little did I know.*

*My work became a substitute for my family and friends,
and everyone understood or seemed to make excuses that supported the high-flying lifestyle of an arbitrageur, deal maker
extraordinaire, at the top of his game and packing in a couple
of lives where there was only room for one. I wasn't aware of it
at the time but I recruited people to aid in my personal deceptions. Dropping a few comments here, an indiscretion there. A
few too many drinks, trips, meetings, late nights, pressure from
deadlines, financial reports, mergers and acquisitions. I was so*

successful by day—how could that not be the real me, the real deal? The issues had to lie elsewhere. Perhaps not enough home support, lack of understanding, caring, selfishness, and superficiality. Not mine but my wife, my family, everyone else. And the money. It stunned people into a complicit silence. Lifetime security for family and friends alike. Silence was purchasable from everyone around me. I looked down on all of them as sycophants for hire. Just tell me the price, sir.

Arnie, back in the Bellevue ER, was too physically labile to go to the cath lab even though he was heavily sedated. There was something strange about the hallucinations. We got the alcohol level test back; it was moderately elevated, but this was too early for withdrawal and the DTs or delirium tremens, probably the most lethal withdrawal syndrome from alcohol. There were times we had to give hundreds of milligrams of Valium intravenously to patients who were seeing bugs crawling over themselves and the walls. Their hearts racing, blood pressures sky-high, and adrenaline levels off the chart. It took a lot to break through the entire body's hyper-alert nervous system as alcohol leached out of the system.

Arnie's liver enzymes were elevated, there was a mild anemia—and otherwise nothing was remarkable except for a cardiac enzyme bump indicating early injury to the heart muscle. The toxicology urine screen would be back shortly. Plan B was to bring him to the coronary care unit with one-on-one nursing and keep a close eye as his condition evolved. By then his wife had arrived. A stunning blonde half his age was waiting in the family room with two adult children from earlier marriages. They were all about the same age. I entered with some trepidation. There were deep histories hidden in plain sight, and we as physicians not infrequently became the receptacles for the rage and anguish that hadn't been touched. The wife was clearly in charge and was going to direct traffic. Facts, names, phone numbers, prognoses, percentages, options…She let the children have their say respectfully, but treated them as emotionally unstable and incompetent to handle the real issues.

*My addiction to everything I got my hands on was my prob-
lem and had become my family's problem. But I didn't realize
that until later. I rationalized and denied everything as work
and stress and lack of understanding of the key people in my
life. All of the doctors I saw except one just kept ordering more
tests. They played me and I played them for prescriptions so
the game would keep going round and round. It was legal and
I didn't have to steal anything or do anything that wasn't prescribed by New York's elite medical professionals. There was
one psychiatrist I had been referred to for possible depression
from chronic pain who listened to my pressured speech and
hyped-up diagnosis and treatments who said to me one day,
"You are an addict." I never saw him again and went about
my business. There was no system. There is no system. No one
connected the dots. The privacy laws gave the doctors plausible
deniability to not talk to one another or my family so the game
could go on. It was an inconvenient diagnosis and I could pick
and chose at will by this time any other diagnosis I wanted.
I channeled migraines, slipped disks, kidney stones, recurrent abdominal pain, spinal stenosis, sciatica, and neuralgias
I couldn't pronounce. And others I read about, heard about,
dreamed up, and then acted out. The world started to come
apart a bit when something happened in my family. It was the
first time something got through the heavily fortified tissue of
fabrications and falsifications I had built around me. But only
briefly.*

He took a pause and took a long drink from a plastic bottle of
designer water. People were quiet in the room. Many had been there
before, and many had done a lot of things that would never be revealed
in a qualification, or with their sponsor. Nothing was off-limits. He
slipped off his jacket and slung it over an empty chair. Beads of sweat
glistened on his forehead. His shirt was blotched with irregular dark
spots and stuck to his chest. He wiped his neck with some paper towels
a willowy twenty-plus-year-old female member handed to him. Step

13? Where you fuck the new and emotionally vulnerable AA members. I couldn't help but wonder. The New Balance sneakers squeaked on the freshly waxed wooden floor as Arnie moved around the lectern.

My eldest son tried to kill himself. An overdose. The entire family including my ex-wives rallied around him. He was found by his law school roommate, barely arousable, with a bottle of pills and a note to his family. Prior to his suicide attempt, he had become more reclusive. He had stopped attending his classes. From being a top student the first year, Martin had gradually slipped off the grid by the middle of his second year. He was hospitalized at the best institutions and received top care by the best doctors and psychiatrists, social workers and psychologists money could buy, literally. But the point of the story is not just my son's near-death experience and depression. The emergency room overnight doctor showed me the pills he had taken. They were in a ziplock plastic bag. I took them out. Every single one of the orange bottles with white screw tops had my name on it. Every single one was from a different physician, nurse practitioner, or physician assistant. They had all been my prescriptions, filled in my name, that I had squirreled away in some dark corner I hadn't even remembered. My son had discovered my stash sometime earlier and made them his own. My addiction had become his addiction. His addiction had led to his inability to function. He slipped where he never had before and the sheer absurdity of it, the panic of it had left him needing more medication to control the anxiety and the despair—and ultimately to the feeling that there were no solutions. Every road was a dead end was how he put it. The entire episode was covered up without asking anyone to cover it up. He was weak and had a problem. Me. The stress of growing up with too much of everything and an overpowering father. Overachieving father and a son who couldn't cope. The only thing missing was an absent mother to make it complete. I didn't lift a finger then to change that story. It would have been too much to ask

*of myself. A bit of honesty was in a very short supply. I just
accelerated my own pill taking and alcohol consumption. It
smoothed things out. The sharp edges were smoothed over as I
chewed some bitter white tablets and washed them down with
GlenWhatever, golden liquid in finely cut glass. I glowed and
life went on. A mere speed bump. I wouldn't be derailed yet.*

The room was completely quiet. You couldn't hear anyone breathe.
A father had just sacrificed his son. *Oh, God said to Abraham, "Kill
me a son."* Everyone in this room knew that the deepest and dark-
est secrets were never shared. You go public with what is pretty safe
and sanitized. In a case like Arnie's, there were always more skeletons
dumped into killing fields. This family was a breeder reactor for psychic injury and pain. It would demand more human sacrifice. More
lambs to the slaughter. Who would be next? Would it be by drugs,
alcohol, cutting, food, emotional distancing, promiscuity, or the intergalactic emptiness that lives at the bottom of lovelessness?

I remember how complicated that family meeting proved. *Were we,
the physician team at a public hospital, competent enough to care for
a leader of the free world?* A reasonable question from the blond young
wife. This was clarified when wife number four made some calls on
her cell phone outside the room. She asked me to talk to Arnie's international TV celebrity cardiologist at a prestigious medical center several miles to the north of Bellevue. The professor was down-to-earth
and apologetic. I believe he knew implicitly this had nothing to do
with heart valves, clogged vessels, or pacemaker malfunction. "Is
there anything I can do?" I summarized the case and asked him to
fax me Arnie's records. He didn't have much to add except the pain
syndromes, the normal stress tests, some specialty referrals, and to
keep him posted please; he gave me his cell phone number. We stressed
the unknown nature of what we were dealing with since a myocardial infarction was one thing...but a myocardial infarct complicated
with drug withdrawal and a mystery syndrome causing hallucinations
and aggressive behavior requiring chemical and physical restraints was
another.

I remember my nursing colleagues from the former St. Vincent's hospital telling me about the alcohol prescribed to the hospitalized priests and nuns to prevent their withdrawal symptoms. Perhaps we were seeing a pure and simple withdrawal from a pharmacopoeia of possibilities all interacting to make his brain's hippocampal neuronal synapses fire wildly or not at all. I called my colleagues at the poison center that was staffed in a city laboratory building across First Avenue from Bellevue. "Man, sounds like PCP to me," said my colleague on the phone, matter-of-factly. "Forget the free-world-leader stuff. You soak some PCP in marijuana and he may not come down for a few weeks." A few hours later, the tox screen came back positive for alcohol, benzos, OxyContin, marijuana—and PCP. This was the sort of OD we normally see rolling in from the ghetto or with pimply teenagers from New Jersey suburbs in their parents' black Benz SUV. Not from a guy who owned a floor in the Dakota. We had a dual diagnosis ("double trouble") ward, 20 East, full of patients hearing voices, seeing things that weren't there, and at the same time detoxing from heroin, cocaine, alcohol, benzos, methadone, and everything else you could grind, liquefy, inject, snort, pop, inhale. Most didn't have a chauffeur, air-conditioned wine cellars, or tricked-out personal 747s with truffles and gold foil grated on your mac-and-cheese. The symptoms were identical, and treatment and recovery were going to be complex no matter how much money you had in your personal piggy bank.

I had entered a bizarre world that I wasn't even aware of at the time. Despite the fact that I was acting bizarrely and had memory outages like New York City blackouts in the 1970s, the company was making big money and my immediate colleagues covered for me without missing a beat. I caught a few comments like "Take some time off, long weekends," but nothing more substantial. My family world had contracted. By intimidation and a bullying style, I managed to keep everyone in line. Huge doses of buying stuff for everyone seemed to keep people happy and allowed me to dose my guilt with something besides pills and alcohol. In a funny way I considered myself a pusher or dealer, controlling my family and colleagues with money, apartments, trips, jewelry, cars, and special favors called in regularly for mediocre performance, indifferent effort. Pusher father, a husband creating a smokescreen that hid the real problem as I was driving off a cliff with black smoke coming out of the exhaust pipe.

The beginning of my turning point happened during my hospitalization. I don't remember anything of the first few weeks. I came to the hospital with a heart attack. The doctors told me they brought me to the intensive care unit and sedated me and were unable to treat me more aggressively with balloons, stents, or surgery because I was in an agitated state. They told me I was psychotic. I have no memory of this at all. They evidently sedated me and then had to restrain me. In fact my heart disease, or the heart attack, went from a small one to a medium-size one because of all of the stress I put on my system from the drugs I had taken. This part was all information that my doctors, the whole team of them, told me weeks after I was admitted.

In fact Arnie did take three full weeks to stabilize from the psychotic symptoms. He was kept under heavy sedation to make sure his heart was protected from an internal hormonal storm.

Evidently when I was stable enough from my heart attack they transferred me off the intensive care unit floor directly to a psychiatric unit. The one they call "double trouble." It is for patients who both have psychiatric problems and are withdrawing from drugs. You see, I had started to use marijuana along with all of the other medications I was addicted to. I know it sounds ridiculous since I was already taking so many drugs and alcohol, but it relaxed me. I got into the marijuana and had a 1-800 cell phone "delivery service" drop off an assortment of marijuana selections, like Ben & Jerry's, in sandwich bags when I went to pick up prescriptions from the pharmacy. The deliveryman, a grad student in plasma physics with a ponytail, said he had something special for me and gave me some freebie joints along with my regular supply from his breast pocket. I didn't know what they were. A few days later I smoked two joints in my bathroom at work. I'd had a long day and too many meetings and was off to another benefit uptown where I am on the board of directors. I got indigestion in my car and some chest tightness and told my driver to take me to the nearest hospital. Bellevue was a few blocks away. I found out a few weeks later when I returned to consciousness that the joints were laced with PCP.

Phencyclidine was legendary in emergency rooms around the country and in psychiatry. It was a bear and invariably left a mess in its wake. Also known as PCP or angel dust, hog, Chuck Norris, Hulk Hogan, and fry sticks, it was originally made by the pharmaceutical company Parke-Davis as an anesthetic fifty years ago. It produced a post-operative psychosis and was abandoned but rediscovered as a drug of abuse, since it's easy to make with a home chemistry set, and is usually combined with marijuana or LSD. It is sprayed on the leaves of cannabis, oregano, or mint and then smoked. The intoxication phase begins with euphoria, confusion and delirium, psychosis, agitation, rapid heart rate, and high blood pressure with increased salivation. This leads to a stupor with wide-open eyes that beat rhythmically in different directions and is followed with grand mal seizures. The final stage is lethal, with coma, strokes, heart failure, and muscle breakdown causing kidney failure. The stages are mutable and patients move among them. Sedation and isolation in a quiet room with careful observation is the cornerstone of treatment. The psychosis can be transient or prolonged depending on prior psychiatric illness and or exposure to multiple drugs. As Steve Ross, our chief of addictive diseases, always reminded his staff, take a careful, detailed longitudinal history. "The Devil, God, and the Diagnosis is in the details."

I was locked up, a free pass to psych. That means that two physicians signed an order to lock me in an inpatient psychiatric ward for up to ninety days. There is a buzzer at the door to get in or out unless you have a key. You need privileges to even go for a test off the unit. To exercise on the roof, catch a breeze, or smell the city air in the metal cage has got to be earned. I was so sedated on injections of Seroquel—a medicine for psychosis— plus Ativan, a benzo, that I don't remember the first couple of weeks on the unit. They said I was zombie-like and better for it since the PCP-induced hallucinations and agitation fluctuate until it fully wears off. There was a one-on-one aide with me all of the time. They call the aides BHTs or behavioral health technicians. The BHTs who looked after me were in their twen-ties and thirties, young men and women who didn't let me out of their sight—not to go piss or shit, to the shower, to my Spar-tan bedroom, or to the dining room or treatment area. They quickly got to know what I liked, my favorite sports teams, skiing in the deep powder snow of Alta, Utah, smoking Cohiba Puros from Cuba, and listening to Mozart operas and old Nat King Cole records. Pretty soon I had The Marriage of Figaro *on a small tape player and magazines my family brought in of the special things from the parts of my life I had abandoned little by little years earlier. From* Popular Mechanics *to* Forbes *to the* Financial Times. *They would talk to me for hours and ask me questions about my interests. It's funny, but over a few weeks I came to depend on them and learned about their families, their special interests, places they wanted to visit. It was like a weird Scheherazade. Trading tales from different kingdoms. Each one a foreign language to the other person. I knew more about them and they knew more about me than my own family. I cared more about them than my own family. Just their presence, sit-ting next to me in a yellow plastic chair, calmed me down. I got weaned off the zombie medications. I was only on methadone for my promiscuous narcotic addiction—if it was a white tablet I swallowed it—and they tapered away everything except for an occasional dose of a tranquilizer and something to help me sleep. Sleep, precious sleep, had been destroyed a year earlier from the marijuana.*

We had a unit meeting every day around nine thirty. The staff came on the unit and all of the patients sat in a big circle in the large open day room.

They were a motley crew. Actually, we were a motley crew. I was one of them. I lost all pretensions about who I was. The odd thing was that I felt safe for the first time in years. Safe in a mental hospital.

I was just another patient with a combined psychiatric problem and drug abuse. Period. It was nice to be anonymous. The locked unit, the presence of the staff, the nurses, doctors, psychologists, social workers, activity therapists, peer counselors, yoga teachers, students—it all felt okay. I had tried to pretend and hold myself together for so long, it felt good to be in a place where I was looked after, where there was no more room for lying, deception, cheating, judgments, fears of falling and failure. I could relax talking to my morning BHT, a twenty-eight-year-old Dominicana, Melissa, in charge of my mornings, about her marriage and my failed four marriages plus countless infidelities leaking out to everyone, myself included. Infidelity was my life's theme. That occurred to me when I was speaking to her. In the middle of a sentence about another interesting thing I had seen or done or visited, I started listening to myself. I shut up and had nothing else to say for a couple of days. I started to listen to the other patients really for the first time.

There was a jumper on the unit when I was there. He had been on drugs and depressed and hanging from a bridge where he had been hauled off by pedestrians and the police. The staff called them jumpers. We had half a dozen admitted when I was on the unit. They jumped in front of trains, from bridges, off apartment houses. They were chased by their demons. There was a young Latino guy who came in with satanic designs on his clothes. He talked to me about Jesus and the planets he had visited. A young black man was beside himself with the idea he might have to go back to prison for a parole violation. He had been abused and re-abused repeatedly in prison. Sexual merchandise was what he was. Small, pretty, and defenseless. He paid for his protection by sucking cocks. He was unpredictable, and we were all afraid of him on the one hand and terrified for him possibly having to go back to jail on the other hand. There was a schizophrenic graduate student from CUNY hearing voices. She looked like my daughter, almost identical. I hadn't paid attention to my daughter, my own daughter in any meaningful way in years. I had no idea who she was or what she was interested in. I knew more about the BHTs and the other patients on the unit than about my own wife and my children. I could plan a complex hostile takeover and the percentage points on shorting the currency of a sovereign country but I could not have a cup of coffee with my wife and sit still and hear what she had to say about her day, her friends, her fears, her desires.

There was a pause in the room. Arnie sipped some water, wiped his neck and forehead, and the group coughed and rustled in their seats. As I sat in the back row, I felt his wife's desire for vengeance in the room. She was a full partner and a well-known litigator in a blue-blood New York law firm. She had a career and was more complicated than your average TV-special blond young trophy wife. There was something she said, or rather didn't say, that made me uneasy—something about how she looked at me. Arnie was looking for redemption and rebirth. Humiliation had a way of being the gift that kept on giving, a lifetime of payback, but of a different kind.

We knew, back in the Bellevue moment, that the hardest part would be post-discharge. It wasn't clear at first what was alive in Arnie's life and what wasn't. It might not be clear for some time. The bridges with ex-wives had been torched and burned to the ground. The current wife, or "merger and acquisition" as one of the counselors murmured, was distant and disconnected. Jean, I remembered. "I want the best treatment for my husband. No expense will be spared," she declared a dozen times. "He has to be transferred to the finest institution in the United States for these medical issues." She never could name them. This was refrain number two in the first forty-eight hours of his transfer upstairs to the locked world of inpatient psychiatry. Her cell phone was glued to her head as she repeatedly called in consultations with his distinguished New York physicians, who all told her the same thing: *Keep him where he is. Leave him alone. He is getting the best care possible.* Mixing economic class is hard for most people to swallow, especially when it comes in so many colors and accents.

Finally Jean acceded to the reality that he'd be treated at Bellevue. She set up a virtual mobile command center and insisted that he be under a John Doe alias; no information could be shared with anyone, under any circumstances, without her express written permission. She made it clear that there would be severe legal and financial repercussions if this demand were not accepted 100 percent. Two of her lawyers arrived in their thousand-dollar Italian suits and met with our senior staff, legal team, and security under her written authorization. Arnie essentially ceased to exist except as incognito patient X with a Latino name. We usually reserved this privilege for mob leaders and drug dealers who had been shot, stabbed, or beaten within an inch of their lives. That kind of alias. But Arnie was not at risk. How would the market factor in a hospitalization on the psych unit at Bellevue? What would the herd do led by computerized algorithms? Hundreds of millions of dollars were at play. For a hospital that defined itself by caring for patients where social risk factors often overshadowed the medical issues, the problem of too much money was not in our differential diagnosis. Too little played a role in most of our patients' lives. The irony, of course, was that Arnie's problems with drug addiction and its rippling effects were no different from the problems of any of our regular patients.

I caught up with Jean one day by chance sitting alone in a tiny empty office we offered her. She came every afternoon, was buzzed into the narrow warren of offices with her black leather briefcase, computer, and phone, and waited for visiting hours. I'd heard that Arnie was being evaluated for discharge, so I stopped to talk to her. "So, good recovery," I said. "He should be discharged soon." She looked at me perplexed.

"I want him here for the full ninety days."

"I don't understand. Arnie will be here until he is ready to be discharged with a safe follow-up plan. His case is reviewed in detail every day by the entire team. Everyone has input."

"The transfer was written by two psychiatrists and is legally binding for ninety days." She spoke to me as if I were a child. Something was different now. There was no emotion. Pure calculation.

"Ninety days is the maximum we can keep anyone here without getting another judge to sign on for an additional period in special circumstances. If people are better and able to leave, the ninety-day issue is moot." I said it slowly and clearly.

"I don't agree with your evaluation. He will need the full ninety days and perhaps more time under supervision and evaluation." I was getting it now.

"He will be declared competent and able to leave at a certain point. It is a physician judgment call." Why did she want him here longer? She didn't have to live with him, she could divorce him, move out, have another life, move on. What didn't I know about human motivation?

"My lawyers will want to review his records and we will appeal any decision this hospital makes to a judge. I know you have a court in the building."

"What's going on?" I asked her straight-up.

"I want him to suffer. It's hard to say, Doctor. I don't even know what to call it. It's not hate exactly." She dropped her force shield just this once; I never saw it again during the entire time I knew her. "He slapped me in front of a roomful of people. Important people in my life, my career, my future. He thought I was some piece-of-shit floozy he could abuse and ignore at his whim, his indulgence? He never even remembered what he did. He was so far gone on the Klonopin, Oxy, and his whiskey. He thinks he can get therapy here or anywhere, then ask for forgiveness and be fucking redeemed. No fucking way, Doctor. He buried himself. He will stay that way. We are not tadpoles, even though his kids act like them sometimes. He can't cut off our arms and legs and they just grow back.

"When he was in the ICU there was a family meeting. He was calling everyone names, cursing and being, well, just himself, I guess. I didn't even hear it, so pathetic really. One of your nurses, a tiny brown woman from India or Bangladesh, I don't remember, interrupted the meeting. She said loudly and clearly, looking directly at me, 'No one tells me to get fucked. Not even your husband.' Then she was quiet again and didn't say another word. That was the moment for me. I needed to hear it from one of your nurses, who had never used those words in her entire life, who never let herself be humiliated or spoken to like shit. I had eaten it for so long I couldn't recognize the taste or smell."

There was nothing to say. I heard her loud and clear.

Arnie's children came by, but there wasn't much they could add to the conversation. The oldest daughter broke down and sobbed through her tears about the "death of my father." Martin came in and out of the picture, always alone. He would appear to see his father and then abruptly leave. He had taken time off after his overdose, and Arnie had a trust fund at the ready. The One-Strike Law did not apply in this universe. He wasn't black. Stop-and-frisk was not ruling his time on the street. He could have as many strikes as he could afford. The youngest daughter, Raquel, lived in the city by herself and came to see her father dutifully. She hardly ever said anything. Hiding in plain sight was her disguise, allowing the rest of the family to speak for her. She volunteered no opinion and offered nothing to the treatment team. She had a secretarial job with an NGO. We wondered where her anger had been hidden.

The discharge process ended in our court on the nineteenth floor, the prison floor. Arnie was sitting next to his lawyer at a small wooden table. The wife sat at the back of the room with her two lawyers. Demetre, the tall, thin, laconic "seen it all" psychiatrist who ran double trouble, was in the dock with a stack of charts piled next to him. "This is highly irregular," Judge Geffen said to no one in particular.

"The patient has been cleared by his psychiatrists for discharge citing no clear and present danger to himself or anyone else. He has no evidence of cognitive impairment to preclude discharge, and plans have been arranged. I don't know why you are wasting my time." He looked up at the Italian suits in the back of the room, apparently unimpressed. The judge's annual salary was what these guys made every two weeks, not counting end-of-the-year bonuses. He wasn't going to be moved by any verbal artistry. But I soon realized that the point was not to win this one round. It was a declaration of war by another means.

"Judge Geffen, sir, if I may approach the bench. There are many inconsistencies in the record, days of missing documentation, lack of agreement by the team caring for the patient—"

At that point, Judge Geffen cut him off. He was angry and sat up in his chair. "Just what do you think this is? We are not in criminal court. You are not playing with a jury's sympathies and manipulating a mistrial for your client." He turned to the psychiatrist, who watched unblinkingly the show of humanity alternate between farce and tragedy.

"Doctor, in your opinion is the patient of sound enough mind to be discharged?" the judge asked directly to Demetre and then looked at Arnie. The room was silent. The guards had stopped dozing a long time ago.

"Yes, Judge. He is ready to be discharged."

"Case dismissed." The judge hammered his gavel with extra force.

They were calling the next case as we filed out of the room. A disheveled Chinese woman, tiny, talking to herself in whispers of Fukienese, was helped into the room by her Americanized teenage daughter in a short skirt and short asymmetric haircut with a hint of purple streaks. The legal team and wife had left by the first elevators. We retreated to the eighteenth floor without much to say. We knew from what we had just seen that there'd be more to come.

The discharge day was difficult. I mean on the one hand I wanted to leave and get back to my life. On the other hand I had destroyed so much of my life that I didn't know what I was

*going back to. I knew I couldn't pick up where I had left off.
That part of my life was finished. I had taken care of that. I was
a shattered human being. My wife sued for divorce immediately
after I was discharged. She had moved out when I was in the
hospital. The board of my company made it clear it wanted my
resignation, for health reasons. My office was taken over by the
acting director. If it had just been alcohol, I might have been
able to stay. Alcohol was fashionable. We have presidents who
do that, and it almost makes them more fit or electable. Hallu-
cinogenic chemicals and psychotic breakdowns were something
else, I guess. As far as my children went, I had to ask them for
forgiveness. Then accept their anger, their rage, and endure it
as part of who I am and what I had done to them. I hurt them.
I put them at risk. What does forgiveness even mean? As someone said, it's impossible to forgive because even by saying the
word we bring back into focus all the harm we've done.*

He stopped and paused for a few moments in front of the group.

*After I was discharged, I had a really good therapist I saw
several days a week in Midtown. At first I was on methadone
for the narcotic addiction and had to come to Bellevue six days
a week to pick up my liquid medicine, swallow it, and come
back the next day. After a few months of stabilization, they
switched me over to buprenorphine, the pill form—a narcotic
substitute you put under your tongue once a day. Now I can go
once a month and pick up thirty tablets from my doctor after I
pee into a cup for a tox screen.*

Methadone had been tried on addict volunteers in Lexington, Ken-
tucky. A synthetic narcotic invented in Germany during World War
II when opium and morphine were unavailable, methadone was long
acting, and the highs and withdrawals of opiate use were eliminated.
The Narco Farm—which took over a prison in the bucolic countryside
from the mid-1930s to the mid-1970s—became a treatment center for

thousands of narcotic addicts over four decades. It was shuttered as the country moved into a more confrontational and prohibitionist attitude toward drug usage in the 1970s. There was a fear that large numbers of Vietnam vets were addicted to the heroin widely available in Southeast Asia. The War on Drugs had been declared by Nixon on June 17, 1971, in a calculated attempt to attract Southern white voters to vote Republican. It was part of the pushback from the Lyndon Johnson civil rights era ending Jim Crow segregation. The push to build prisons and incarcerate blacks and Hispanics for small drug offenses was building momentum. The prison population would swell from under a half a million to five times that number plus tens of millions more under state surveillance as ex-felons. The politics of drugs trumped any meaningful treatment approach. Arnie had skittered through a corner of a gulag warehouse for the underclass. I wondered if he knew that the larger story in which he was a bit player was every bit as tragic as his personal story. I wondered.

I was sitting in my therapist's office a little over four years ago in one of our usual sessions. He was a seventy-five-year-old white-haired frail man who wore frayed white buttondown shirts, no tie, and faded tan chino pants and scuffed black Rockport shoes. He had stacks of books in his office everywhere. Sometimes you had to clear off your chair since he wrote all morning and saw patients in the afternoons in the same office, a ground-floor room in his house on Jane Street in the West Village. We had two chairs in the room sitting ten feet apart looking at each other when he said to me "Arnie, you are an alcoholic and a drug addict." For a year we had talked psychobabble. I felt good—I had seduced my therapist and he was in my corner, another acquisition and attestation to my getting better. I had continued drinking like nothing had changed, since according to my world I did not have any problem with alcohol—just drugs. My shrink called me on my hypocrisy and made it clear he was neither seduced nor enchanted with my storytelling. The scab hurt when he pulled it off like that. He called one evening a few days later and told me to join him at Sixth Avenue and 12th Street the next day at eleven thirty a.m. I met him and he walked me to an AA meeting at St. Vincent's hospital. He told me to go inside and keep going every day for at least three months. He agreed to continue to see me on that condition. Non-negotiable. He turned around and walked off.

I went inside and never left. The first year I ended up going to five meetings a day. I couldn't do anything else and desperately needed the meetings and the phone calls from my sponsor every morning at eight thirty. I am here today to celebrate my fourth year in AA. Really the completion of my fourth step.

Arnie had left out large parts of his "journey" into his heart of darkness. This was an edited version for a semi-public audience. He had started using cocaine years earlier than he let on with a mistress twenty years younger on business trips he took regularly to Europe. We never got to the exact bottom of how much Ecstasy, Viagra, cocaine, benzos, alcohol, and PCP went into the mix to fuel a grueling work and clandestine social schedule. By the time he had gone to his doctor for back pain and received his narcotic prescription, his drug habits had been well established and he was deep into the 1-800 universe of drugs delivered on Vespa scooters like pizza. His kids were a mess—far more than he let on. The oldest daughter had severe eating disorders and had been hospitalized repeatedly (though not at Bellevue). Martin had been arrested for attempted rape, but somehow, miraculously, he got off and the charges were dropped. But hey, the story was close enough. Like all stories, this one was fungible. There are certain things we cannot say, not even to ourselves.

I looked around the room slowly. The overhead fan turned without making any noise. There was the barest hint of a breeze of warm air coming through the windows. The coffee machine hissed and popped. A stack of AA literature was sitting on a windowsill. The 12 Steps and 12 Traditions were curling up in the heat from their perches facing the main room. I looked at individuals and wondered about their stories and their secret lives. The pain in the room was palpable. How many

there were still incapable of speaking out loud to a group of strangers brought together by the same misery and affliction? But they had
crossed the doorway and had made some preliminary commitment
to doing something. How many had been there for twenty-plus years
and had made the meetings their life, a necessary construct around an
inner chaos? A person could begin the process of reconstituting a life
with the group's norms and rules and rituals. The serenity prayer was
a lifeline—it allowed people to distinguish between the things they
could and could not change. It allowed a modicum of hope, of self-
acceptance. There was a lot going on in the room that was unsaid, but
the very fact that people came back to the same place to hear and talk
to one another week after week was something. The room offered a
space to try things out without coercion in the privacy of one's own
head.

Arnie thanked the group for their time as they applauded him. The
meeting leader in her pink sweater and blue plaid dress, her electric hair
now damp and stuck to her neck from the heat and moisture, came up
and gave him his four-year coin and shook his hand. They hugged, and
he found his seat near the front of the room. Arnie was asked to choose
the members present with their hands up to respond for only three
minutes to his qualification. He chose a dark-haired Asian woman sitting across from him to start the comments. She thanked him for his
qualification and noted how very difficult it is to forgive oneself. I only
half listened to the comments as the room rustled and people got up to
use the bathroom, stretch, find some water, and readjust themselves. I
knew we wouldn't talk after the meeting or likely see each other again.
He was on a journey he had chosen to let me witness out of respect for
our dozen conversations and interactions. It was a way of telling me he
was now in a different place, on his own and self-sufficient, capable of
managing his affairs without intermediaries and special interlocutors.
A graduate from our chemical dependency and recovery program both
inpatient and outpatient to a private life. The message was received. It
was both creation and reinvention.

As people were stacking the chairs against the walls and gathered in
clumps to talk, I walked out the front door into the hot West Village

night. Heat rose from the hoods of the cars; air conditioners exhaled heat down Grove Street. I found a French wine bar with a few empty seats by the window. I pulled open the door to escape the heat and sat in a corner with a glass of red wine and a few small plates of tapas facing the bar and the street. The buzz of the conversations of couples hunched over tiny tables, hands clasped, hung over the room, the waiters dressed in black hovering lightly in the background. I opened my black notebook, looked out the window, and pondered the nature of forgiveness.

CHAPTER 6

A Heart for Rabinal

Sometimes you choose to be involved with patients and sometimes you don't. It just happens.

Checking my email early on a Wednesday morning, I spotted a message from a cardiology fellow. He wanted to meet with me with—as he put it delicately—"some urgency" about a patient who was on the telemetry, or heart monitoring unit. "Complex medical case, Guatemalteca with end-stage heart disease." I texted back that I could meet him in an hour in the coffee shop, my de facto second office. My own coffee was better, but I liked the change of scenery.

I found Dr. Lenny Perham in a booth in his white coat, stethoscope dangling around his neck. It was now late afternoon; the place was nearly empty except the take-out lines. Danny, the Greek waiter, wearing a baseball hat and carrying a pad with his hieroglyphic scrawl, saw me and brought me a cup of coffee and a seltzer water. The effervescence soothed my radiation-scarred esophagus and scoured away the remnants of the pasty saliva.

"Dr. Manheimer, we have a tough case and need your help on this one." I nodded and he kept on going. "She is undocumented." I knew where this was going.

The story was long and had many inflections and unknowns. Lenny knew the medical issues with great precision and presented the case to me as if he were on visiting professor rounds, not missing a beat. "This thirty-nine-year-old single mother of two children was transferred to Bellevue five years ago. Soraya Molino walked into Woodhull's emergency room with a complaint of progressive weakness over six months and a new symptom of breathlessness simply walking a couple of blocks or up the flight of stairs to her first-floor apartment."

"Lenny, you don't have to make it so official, just tell me the story. Eat your burned bagel and cream cheese and chill." He smiled, relaxed, added a thick smear, and ate and talked at the same time.

"She worked the night shift in a dry-cleaning factory in an illegal warehouse in a desolate part of what little non-gentrified Brooklyn remains. She liked the work with a dozen other women from all over Latin America. They commiserated together, shared family stories, gave advice, and formed a makeshift support group. Like the cigar factories I've heard about in Cuba, the women took turns reading to one another out loud during their breaks, and the news let them share stories from their homelands." This was a story.

"At her neighborhood hospital, Woodhull in North Brooklyn, she was evaluated and admitted to the coronary care unit. The signs and symptoms of congestive heart failure were straightforward. On a routine chest X-ray, her heart was twice its normal size, the veins were distended, small amounts of fluid collected in the 'gutters' at the angles between her diaphragm and her chest wall, and the thin puffy white streaks over her diaphragm were typical of atelectasis or lung collapse. She didn't have TB, and her bones were normal. In fact, in all other respects she was a normal thirty-nine-year-old attractive black-haired woman with an angelic face and a quiet disposition who answered every question with *Díos te bendiga*, or *Gracias por todo, Doctor*, almost like a tic." Our patients seduced us many times with their modesty and simple graciousness in a sea of suffering.

There was one deviation from the usual heart failure issues. In fact, two. One was of immediate concern. The other would involve many health care and legal professionals for years. The immediate one showed up on the EKG, or electrocardiogram: lots of extra heartbeats. Wide loops from diseased ventricular muscle instead of the tightly angled normal electronic traces from the normal atrial pacemaker. The ventricular beats activated by the stress on her heart were multifocal, coming from many latent pacemakers. They came in rapid runs.

Ominous, they gave her doctors tachycardia. Like a map of the electro-magnetic noise from the Big Bang, her EKG was too interesting!

After observing Soraya overnight, Woodhull faxed over the EKG. This was slow V-tach, or ventricular tachycardia. A cardiac rhythm that was a killer, a "widowmaker." Random events we have all heard about, a collapse on a sidewalk, standing in an elevator, walking to buy some milk. We had an unknown window of time to get her over to Bellevue and put in a defibrillator, an electronic device the size of a pack of cigarettes, slipped in a "pouch" under her skin that could both receive the electric cardiac signals and send an electric shock if the internal software program detected a malignant rhythm. Her own heart had become a ticking time bomb. The killer was not the short-ness of breath that left her panting and stopping halfway as she crossed Brooklyn's Broadway under the ancient elevated subway train tracks to the overflowing emergency room. It was the ominous electrical sig-nals of latent pacemakers stirred into existence by a heart running on empty. Why did Soraya have a failing heart?

We got Soraya Molino in the afternoon by ambulance with copies of her medical records. Our cardiac care unit, or CCU, is on the tenth floor. It is part of a continuous circle of intensive care unit beds for the sickest patients in the hospital. The views from the rooms are airplane vistas of all of the boroughs of New York City and New Jersey. It is like a 360-degree control tower for the city's airports. I would find out later that Soraya had not arrived by plane—it had taken her months to walk to Brownsville, Texas. Sixty-six days, in fact.

Soraya was greeted by the cardiac team after she had been settled into her bed, an IV slipped into her arm and hooked up to our moni-tors. The ominous rapid ventricular beats were on the screen in spasms of three, ten, seven with normal beats in between. The lethality of V-tach is speed. The heart beats so fast, there is not enough time for the ventricle to fill with blood; the cardiac output plummets and the blood pressure falls to zero. Nothing in, nothing out. The patient col-lapses immediately. If a normal rhythm is not restored and the brain is not supplied with oxygen, the patient is brain-dead in six minutes.

The cardiologist called the cardiac cath lab and activated a room and an entire team within minutes. They wheeled Soraya to the interventional laboratory for the multi-hour procedure. Her sister Clara held her hand in the industrial elevator bank as the team moved. Neither of them spoke English aside from a smattering of phrases and *please* and *thank you*. Her sister had been a highly trained nurse in a Guatemala City general hospital and was hardwired for trauma and decision making on the fly. Like many immigrants who were lawyers, doctors, PhDs, and accountants in their native lands, but here drove taxicabs or worked in homes and back offices.

The Filipina cath lab nurses were there to greet her in Spanish. She was somehow made at home in their high-tech work space, a space-lab-type room filled with electronics, video monitors, a cold metal table, bright fluorescent lights. Everyone dressed in scrubs and covered with lead aprons. Two cardiologists were totally focused on the monitors as they slipped the metal wire leads into place while half their brains watched the electrical squiggles of Soraya's beating heart. They knew the risk of triggering her heart rhythm into a sudden death spiral with their manipulations. No one wanted to provoke the cardiac arrest they were working to prevent. There was a constant stream of "*¿Qué tal, chica?*" "*Ahora vamos a moverla aquí a su derecha.*" "*¿Hiciste pipi, mi amor?*" Her sister came in for a few minutes to kiss her and stroke her hand; then she went to sit in the waiting room just outside of the lab door, where the family's anguish could be monitored by the staff just as they were monitoring the V-tach of the patient separated by ten feet and lead-lined walls. Our dual monitoring system worked well, the heart of the patient on the table hooked up to ultra-high technology in a five-million-dollar lab, and the heart of the family member sitting on a two-hundred-dollar bench outside. The procedure went smoothly over a few hours. Soraya was watched for a couple of hours and then brought back to the CCU. She would spend five more days there while the extra water in her lungs was squeezed out with diuretics.

Soraya had Chagas' disease, caused by a bug bite—the "kissing bug," it's called. The reduviid, assassin, or kissing bug lives in thatched roofs in Mexico, Central America, and South America and bites a sleeper's face, usually near the mouth or eyes, leaving a small red mark. It's attracted by the blood flow to the face. The parasites then travel to different organs with an affinity for the heart and the intestines. This is a very slow and progressive disease, measured in decades. Carlos Chagas, a Brazilian epidemiologist, looking to solve some of the mysteries of malaria and its devastating effects on the Brazilian workforce, had come across a "new" disease in 1909 and traced its transmission, its insect source, and its clinical manifestations. Now blood transfusions transmit the disease throughout the Americas. The initial symptoms of Chagas' disease are usually trivial and brushed off. If the disease is recognized early it can be treated, though the current medications are toxic and require several-months-long treatment regimens. After it spreads to the heart over decades, the scarification process leaves it like a balloon filled with water, no propulsive force.

My black notebook in hand, I scribbled, wrote, and diagrammed the evolving events as Lenny walked me through the case. A year after her first hospitalization at Bellevue, Soraya needed a new heart. That was the essence of the conversation. I had drawn a big heart with a question mark through it in the notebook. My mind was moving quickly now. She was under forty years old and had an end-stage heart that had been carefully evaluated for any treatable disease. When a heart is functioning at only a few percentage points above zero, the options narrow drastically. They wouldn't have knocked on my door if there were other options.

I paid the bill, left Danny a big tip, walked down the F-Link to the main hospital building, and pushed 17 on the express elevators.

There were two women in the single room facing north. The older woman sitting in a chair was about fifty-two, with a harder face than her sister, lined and without eyebrows; no tufts of hair sneaked from under the blue cloth cap covering her head. She got up, smiled, and said, "*Buenas tardes, Doctor*," when I came in. Soraya was lying in bed, with her black hair on the pillow, a slight smile on her face. In a soft voice she said, "*¿Qué tal, Doctor?* How are you?" They had been expecting me thanks to Lenny and the cardiology team. I pulled up a chair and positioned us in a small semicircle so Soraya could be propped up comfortably watching and listening to us.

Indira, her nurse from Kerala, the southernmost state in India, with long black braided hair to her waist and a magnetic soft smile, brought in Soraya's dinner from the gunmetal-gray incubator double-parked outside the room. Clara poked around the tray and tried to find something for her sister. Finally Soraya said, "I can't touch the food. I will get sick again." She was clear, better nothing, but with a nuanced apology. "It is my fault, I am so sorry." Everything was being done to help her. The physicians had been frustrated with her nausea and immediate vomiting. She had lost muscles and strength. Following her weight was useless since she retained water from the heart failure. Simply seeing her skinny white arms and the perfect outlines of her bones through increasingly translucent skin was sufficient. I was thinking about Dr. Karnofsky again and his infamous score.

The diagnostic evaluation had been complex and involved additional heart catheterizations looking for atrial enlargement pressing on her esophagus, an endoscopy hoping for a treatable stomach ulcer or reflux and inflammation, and a psychiatric consultation. Tiredness, lack of enjoyment, and her appetite changes registered a tentative depression. A trial of the latest-generation anti-depressant was suggested and added to her increasingly complex multi-medication regimen for heart failure, anti-coagulation, dyspepsia, and heart rhythm control. We were pushing ten medications at last count. I wondered if we weren't poisoning her inadvertently with combinations of interactive toxicities. Under their breath the physicians' discussion had been about cardiac cachexia, a wasting illness like anorexia or starvation. When the heart is so large and dysfunctional, it can consume oxygen and calories like a gigantic sinkhole, leaving crumbs for the metabolism of daily life.

"Look," I said, "it's dinnertime. I have an idea. It has been a long day and, Clara, I'm certain you haven't had anything since coffee this morning. And I missed lunch."

She nodded and threw in, "I am fine, Doctor, don't worry about me."

"There is a place across the street. In five minutes I can bring up some home cooking Latino-style. Okay, Dominican, but maybe it'll pass inspection with two Guatemaltecas?" They were smiling now and gave the go-ahead. "What is your order?" I pretended to be a waiter and wrote down their simple requests.

"Rice and beans, *por favor. Moros y Cristianos.*"

"*Moros y Cristianos,*" I answered. "*Por supuesto. ¿Nada más? ¿Carne, pollo, salsa, res, pan, dulce, nada de eso?* That's it, nothing more, meat, sweets, sauces?"

"*Moros y Cristianos únicamente, Doctor, por favor y gracias,*" they finished together in a chorus.

I got up, gave them *El Diario*, and went out to First Avenue. I breathed in the exhaust fumes from the triple starting lineup of double-decker tourist buses and waited for the traffic to stop at the red light. At the corner of 28th Street, large boxcar-style steel food carts, all different sizes and shapes, sell an assortment of food, from falafel to *shawarma* to hot dogs and halal. A line snaked out to the traffic light on the corner. A balding young man, around thirty, wearing a white apron covering his large belly and a smile manned the enormous grill like a conductor at the Philharmonic.

"Hey, Doc, the usual?" I said no thanks, just plain rice and beans, nothing else. I got two sodas as well and a seltzer water for myself. He packed the white plastic container with warm sweet-smelling black beans and rice, added a few falafel "for the road, Doc," and packed everything in a plastic bag with napkins and plastic forks.

I handed him a five-dollar bill and thanked him profusely. "I'm on delivery service, Miquelito!"

He waved and laughed as I zigzagged back across the street in between cars. "If you ever need a job…" was the last thing I heard him shout.

Clara opened the plastic white container overflowing with *Moros y Cristianos*. She divided the food into three portions and handed them out picnic-style. Soraya ate slowly but with gusto. She took small bites, mixing the black beans in their sauce with the white Mexican-style rice and sucking on the morsels before swallowing them. We talked for the next three hours without a break. I forgot about her eating issue until her sister picked up her clean plate and put everything neatly back in the plastic bag. So much for our standard differential diagnosis. I would have to add rice and beans. I made a mental note.

"Tell me, where are you from in Guatemala? How did you end up in Brooklyn?" Such New York questions; it was almost impertinent. But we were sharing a meal together. No candles and no bottle of wine, but the evening was quiet. There were sighs from both sisters. Soraya lay quietly but attentively as Clara began the tale.

"We are from a small town in the Highlands of Guatemala, San Juan, a tiny *pueblito* a few kilometers from Salamá in the state of Baja Verapaz. It is near the central commercial town of Rabinal. Many hours' drive north of the capital, Guatemala City. Our parents were very poor farmers. They are still alive and living in the area they grew up in"—Mayan country heading toward the Chiapas border with Mexico.

Clara continued, "There was barely enough to eat when we were kids. Once a week, meat was the treat, a chicken, some goat meat, maybe pork. The kids went to a local school, and I, the oldest daughter, made it to Guatemala City and stayed with a cousin. I studied very hard, living like a hermit on vapor alone, and was accepted into nursing school. It gave me a profession with a decent standard of living, a regular income, not much but enough." Clara talked openly and clearly. She had a story to tell and an audience who was not going to judge her.

"My *pecado*, sin, was to marry a man who suffered from '*mamitis*'—a mama's boy. The first offer. He never left me alone for a moment. What I thought was love was really hatred. He was jealous of everything I did and gradually restricted my movements from the house, my visits with friends and even neighbors. Over a couple of years I went to work and returned home, to cook and clean for him and satisfy him sexually. At his whim, like whistling for a dog. That was it. My life contracted." She made a sphere with her hands the size of a basketball and then crushed them down to a clenched fist.

"I often woke being beaten on the face and head. My alarm clock, a brutal drunk *cabrón*. He fractured my arm and I spent three weeks in the hospital having it pinned and getting rehab therapy. You know, it was the best thing he gave me. I finally had time to think. I planned my escape from his attacks and his infantile attachment to his mother, who lived next door. Most important, it gave me time to examine my life and the imbecility of marrying the first man who asked me. A poor stupid naive girl from the Highlands. We were a dime a dozen, many sold themselves for a few quetzales to buy food." The recounting was matter-of-fact. It happened, these are the facts.

"I walked to the hospital where I worked from the bus stop every day and passed a deep *barranca*, ravine, that ran through the city. Barranca Guayama. There were frequently bodies at the bottom of the *barranca*, thrown there the night before from passing cars. Tossed out like garbage. Many of the bodies were *descuartizado*, quartered, with heads missing and signs carved into their chests or foreheads. You learned to walk by quickly, trying not to look, covered with a shawl. You didn't talk about it. It was normal." She took a breath and looked at her sister, who was listening intently and nodding in agreement. "I took my boss's kids to the Cloisters last weekend. I work as a nanny. Imagine you found bodies cut up and stuffed just off the walkways under leaves and brush. A foot sticking out. New ones every day.

"At the General Hospital in Guatemala City the rate of alcoholism and violence, beatings and rapes increased every month, as predictable as the sun coming up. The police did nothing. You avoided the police at all costs. They dragged around Las Zonas, the neighborhoods, on high-powered motorcycles, covered in black Kevlar, with machine guns over their shoulders. They swaggered and demanded. The violence once limited to gangs over turf, drugs, and petty theft had changed. It penetrated everyday life. From buying milk at the store to walking your dog. Random assaults and beatings, kidnappings, murders, gang rapes or young women sold into sexual slavery where they had to live and adapt. And homes themselves, I mean inside your own house, your own apartment was no longer safe. It was contagious and spread. The temperature rose and kept rising."

"When did you decide to leave?" I asked when she paused to take a bite.

"It was unbearable to watch it and it was unbearable to be a part of it any longer. I planned my escape with a coyote to the United States. I would leave my two nearly grown children with a relative to finish school and then send for them. My only other move was to kill my husband, but then he would be with me forever, as a nightmare. That's how contaminated my thoughts had become. My only way to preserve my humanity was to leave." Clara was calm, and her voice did not change its inflection. It was the humiliation that stung her so deeply. More painful than his fist.

Clara took a minute to drink her soda. We were all quiet together. Soraya broke the silence. "Clara, tell the doctor my story. I have no *animo*, no spirit, to talk now." Her sister gave an almost imperceptible nod.

"My sister had no education except the most minimum grade school level available in Salamá. Barely reading and writing. Good for bearing children and cleaning a house. She met an older man at a community dance in San Juan who courted her for six months with flowers and cheap sweets. She agreed to marry him, a virgin in body and in mind. The violence in our home area was terrible. Rabinal had been a massacre zone. Soraya was too young to know what was happening and had never left the town. Our parents never breathed a word. I think they had seen too much in their lives of suffering. It was all about survival. Nothing else.

"My sister's marriage was not a happy one, but it ended more tragically. They had a son, Tomás. Her husband ignored her and left her on her own for months at a time. One time he didn't come back. He 'disappeared.' In fact the town was disappearing. All of the towns were emptying out. Ghost towns with elderly men and women left tending small plots of cornfields on steep hillsides. There was emigration to Mexico and to the United States. There was something new on the streets. Narco violence. Young men on *motocicletas*, motorcycles, or small pickup trucks carrying heavy weapons high on drugs controlled the neighborhoods and violated women randomly and regularly." Clara knew that her sister's story was more than a personal story. It told of the destruction of a society. "One day," Clara continued, "her husband's right hand was left outside her doorstep."

She knew she and Tomás, then six, had to leave. She saved and borrowed three thousand dollars from family and friends to join a group of sixteen men and women leaving from the Mexican border town Tapachula to Brownsville, Texas. "The journey would take two months and be very hard and dangerous. My sister had no idea." Things can always get worse. Beware of false sentimentality, my mother warned me. Many years in the medical profession had taught me firsthand.

Guatemala was both the Beauty and the Beast. I was familiar with the areas Clara was talking about. I thought back on the trips that Diana and I have taken there, once on a crazy journey to Tikal in the Petén via the Usumacinta River in a dugout canoe at the height of the civil war. A young Mexican man rowed the canoe. What were we thinking? Another more recently to see an ancient performance of pre-Conquest origins in Rabinal that Diana was writing about. It was a magnificently gorgeous country. But also a ravaged one on so many levels.

The terror had started with the fall of newly elected President Arbenz in the 1950s in a CIA-backed coup blessed by President Eisenhower in a Cold War frisson, requested by the United Fruit Company. The destabilization established a pattern for Latin America and made it the "Empire's Workshop"—felicitously named by the Latin American historian Greg Grandin. What followed were repeated changes in government, coups, countercoups, and the increasingly heavy hand of the CIA. Advanced military training in Vietnam-style counterinsurgency warfare has been provided for generations of military leaders in Latin America by the U.S. military at the School of the Americas in the Panama Canal Zone and later in Georgia.

By the early 1980s, Ríos Montt, a fervently evangelical general formerly out of favor, exiled to Franco Spain briefly and trained in the School of the Americas, became president of Guatemala. The uprisings that occurred sporadically around the country, the strikes by schoolteachers and workers, were seen as the work of communism, which in the U.S. lexicon meant unlimited logistical, military, and financial support. Ríos Montt understood the Yankee mentality well, along with the trip wire that opened their pocketbooks and trumped any minimalist congressional oversight. Ronald Reagan called him a great friend of the United States while he devised a scorched-earth program, Victoria 82. He lifted his tactics from the playbooks of the failed war in Vietnam, the village pacification programs. He amplified the role of Los Kaibiles, the counterterrorism black-ops group that was headquartered in the Petén, in northern Guatemala in the Yucatán, in special camps along the Usumacinta River. We happened to have been their guests at their training camp for five hours on that ill-conceived trip as they cross-examined our Mexican rower. These young recruits were carefully chosen and carefully brainwashed to be unsentimental killers.

Victoria 82 was a campaign to eliminate villages in the Highlands, in Rabinal, in Salamá and its surrounding areas. The idea was to "drain the sea"—to exterminate men of recruitment age for the insurgents and terrify the remaining population into submission. The fish in the sea were the Mayans and Ladinos or mixed-race Guatemalans living in their towns. Terror became a critical strategy, one might argue the essential one. As Mayan groups turned against each other, and Ladinos turned against Mayans, the links of trust, kinship, mutual assistance were dissolved in the blood of forced murder, picking apart the jealousies and animosities that are latent in all communities. The leaders were deliberately marked for execution or exile.

Father Ricardo Alemán, a Catholic priest who lived for nearly thirty years in the Verapaz districts and knew the Molino sisters and their families intimately, had come to see Soraya. Clara had emailed him from her boss's apartment when her sister had become ill, apologizing for not going to speak with him directly. He visited often, and was always animated when he joined the conversation. He had witnessed the Red Handkerchiefs. Young men, wearing red scarves around their necks, would come into the center of Rabinal and shoot young men at point-blank range. They would shoot any women coming to their aid and anyone else who looked or acted suspicious. They left one man alive to pile the corpses on a truck and drive it to Salamá. The driver would stop short of the forensics building, get out, and stand by the back of the truck, where he would be shot, stacked with the rest of the corpses, and driven into the stockade. The head of the red *pañuelos*, handkerchiefs, who rode on a motorcycle outside Rabinal, was himself shot to death by the son of one of his victims. He asked not to be tortured, as he had tortured so many by his own hands. They put a bullet in his brain and threw his body down a *barranco*.

Clara and Soraya recounted many stories of their lives in and around Rabinal and Salamá and the isolated village of San José. They were remarkable survivors, lovely human beings, with integrity and deep humanitarian values. What category of naturalization and immigration could the Immigration Customs and Enforcement arm of the U.S. government put them in?

Soraya's personal story continued to evolve over a series of more frequent hospitalizations. The fluid built up more rapidly in her legs, her abdomen, and her lungs as her cardiac function dropped another percentage point. Her weakness progressed with less tolerance for walking and doing any household activities. Our social services arranged a van to take her to her office visits. She was months behind in rent, but the neighborly and kind landlord was not going to put her out on the street. We had a little time to pull together some additional community resources. The clock was ticking, however, and we could all hear it. Soraya would make it to cardiology clinic on a Wednesday afternoon. I would get an email that she was in the CCU later that day.

As I sat on the edge of her bed or pulled up a chair close by her side, she and I would talk, her voice barely a whisper. Sometimes Clara was there, and occasionally Father Alemán would come to chat and say some prayers in his white short-sleeved guayabera no matter the temperature outside. Soraya sighed. Her life's good days had been measured on one hand. She suffered and then she suffered some more.

One day Clara told me about her sister's trip from Tapachula to Brownsville. We came up on the elevator together, and I asked her to join me for a few minutes. I was drawn to her directness and clarity. She was always completely present and focused. She was never sentimental and did not burn with pity or anger. I borrowed the head nurse's office. Leslie was wise and emotionally connected. She knew the issues were more complex than what showed up on a monitor and was comfortable looking after the medical issues and being on call for anything else that was needed. She cleared off some space for us to sit. "Here, guys, it's all yours. Let me know if you need anything. The coffee is fresh, help yourself." She pointed to a Mr. Coffee machine and quietly closed the door, taping a "Do Not Disturb" sign to the outside.

"Clara, I am not only concerned about your sister Soraya. You have your own medical problems." It was clear she was getting chemotherapy. How she could help her sister and keep functioning was a real question, at least for me.

"Doctor, I will be truthful with you. I have learned not to complain in my life. It doesn't pay and doesn't make anything better. It is what it is." She settled into the chair and, as always, was direct and forthcoming.

"I had some spotting six months ago, and delayed because of my sister and her health issues and my own denial. Being in the business like you, I thought it might be fibroids or something similar. Finally, the lady I work for took her kids on a trip and I made an appointment to be seen here."

"And?"

"The doctor found a mass in my uterus. The ultrasound and CT scans confirmed a cancer. A couple of weeks later I was in the operating room for a hysterectomy and lymph node dissection. Everything was removed."

"Clara, I don't understand how you managed to look after yourself and your sister. Who looked after you?" I was incapacitated beyond comprehension by my own cancer treatments.

"After I recovered from the surgery, the oncologist put me on a chemotherapy regimen every month for six months. I am just about finished. I won't tell you it has not been hard. I focus on my sister, which keeps my own fears and private demons at a distance. I also don't have a choice." She was very emotional at this point. I hadn't seen her go there in the dozen visits we shared together. "I honestly don't care about myself at this point. It isn't about me and perhaps not about Soraya, either. We may follow each other into the ground. She has two children. One by her husband from Salamá. The other child,

Laura, is from a common-law husband she had a relationship with when she arrived in New York City alone and without a cent." The children were a big concern of ours also. We didn't know what would happen to them if Soraya died. The archipelago of relationships in her life was fragile, in and out, very poor, floating from job to job and state to state, wherever something could be found.

"Roberto tries to help out, a couple of dollars here and there for his daughter. He is not a bad man. Just struggling to function, and he has another family in Florida."

"Is there anyone in Guatemala who could take the children? Your parents? Your kids? I am sure we could get the embassy to fly them home." We did this all the time with other countries.

"It is not possible under any circumstances, Doctor." She was emphatic and clear. I heard *No way.* "There is no one who can care for the children. My parents are old and need help. My own kids are struggling and barely keep their heads above water. But even more important, I will not send them to Guatemala. There is simply no future for them there except more of what we went through. They are much better off here as orphans of the state. I'm not sure if I am more afraid for the boy or the girl. That may be a cruel and strange thing to say." Better to live an undocumented life scratching a living without daily violence.

"Soraya barely survived the trip from Tapachula. You need to know a little of what happened. Maybe you will understand why I need for her to survive. To see a little more of life than what she has seen. If it is possible.

"Tapachula has turned into an *infierno*, a hellhole for immigrants from Central America," Clara continued after a pause. "She signed up with a trafficker from Rabinal who arranges passage with known coyotes. He had a good reputation from neighbors and other families we trusted. He delivers the immigrants to his partners in Mexico at the border. This was a trusted network." She wanted to make sure that I knew they'd gone into this seriously and carefully.

"What we didn't know was how bad it had gotten on the Mexican side. The coyotes had sold out or been killed by Las Maras. The gang extorted existing networks for half of their profits and then kidnapped half of their clientele to extort more money from their families in Central America or the United States—and even then sometimes sold them to brothels or to other cartels.

"Soraya did not stand a chance. She and Tomás got to Tapachula a few miles over the border with the Mexican coyote. They went to a safe house for transfer to vehicles to take them up north. At the safe house the entire group of sixteen was handed over to Las Maras. My sister was the pretty young woman, innocent, not capable of escaping or even killing herself. They took her north all right. They pimped her the entire two months it took to get to Brownsville. They said it was a 'tax' she had to pay since her family was too poor to send more money to free her. That she was in fact lucky. The other alternatives were far worse. Tomás was sold, she didn't know to whom or where he was." Clara stopped, and we both sat and looked at each other for a moment. I was entering a zone I didn't want to go into particularly. We saw a lot of pain and suffering, but of a different kind.

"For sixty-six days she was raped by a dozen men. They took her at night, they took her in the back of the van, the truck, the side of the road, the bathrooms. She was nothing, a rag, meaningless. It was a miracle she was still alive when they dumped her at the end of the nightmare ride. I think they let her live because she had simply survived. It was insane, a perversion of respect. From a gangster's perspective if you survive humiliation, shame, there was a weird respect that accompanied the degradations. They got what they wanted. She paid in full. They honored their promise from Tapachula, Chiapas." Clara was trying to find the words so I could understand the logic of the illogical. The randomness of survival. Honor among killers and torturers?

"How did she recover? How did she manage to keep going?" Suffering had an infinite number of pathways into the future. From lives destroyed, lives deformed, to lives re-created in part or in whole and everything in between.

"The thing that most people see with my sister is a young woman, with soft white skin and her black hair. One part of her is very vulnerable. It is because she is too trusting. Despite all the things in her life she still trusts people. That has not been taken from her. I don't trust anyone except her. Spiritually we are not sisters. I am alone, totally alone, except for her. But trust is her great strength. She has never been alone. She always has some people working with her and for her no matter the circumstances. She spent two years looking for Tomás. He finally showed up in the U.S. detention system. A Catholic group helped Soraya free him. But you cannot imagine the shape he was in, emotionally and physically. Still is, actually. Some scars never heal—especially when you are young, as he was." Clara paused again and let it sink in before she continued. "Anyway, her trust helps her. Even her landlord had begun to protect her and her kids." I remembered meeting him when he brought her to the hospital the last time.

"Tell me about him."

"He's nice. A good man. A Cuban who was six or so when Castro took over and his family left the island. He's a widower who has lived in Brooklyn forever. He speaks English, which also helps her arrange her treatments. And like all immigrant Cubans, he got citizenship right away. The one-year rule." She knew something was wrong with the picture.

The other side of the anti-communism story, I thought, but didn't say.

A few days later, I spoke to Soraya in earnest about her heart disease. I needed to make sure she understood what was at stake and what we might or might not be able to do. The focus of her team of cardiologists had been obsessively on her ejection fraction: the ability of her heart to pump blood. When she first shuffled across Broadway into the emergency room at Woodhull hospital, the echocardiogram showed diffuse impairment of her heart function. While it normally could squeeze out 60 percent of the blood in the left ventricle, it had dropped at that time to half the normal amount. She had now reached the point on the curve where things accelerated rapidly downhill. A 50 percent drop from normal to 30 percent was one thing. A 50 percent drop from 30 percent to 15 was another entirely. Fifteen percent was at the lower limits of survivability. The barest functioning with no margin for further loss. At 30 percent you couldn't play tennis but you

could look after yourself, bathe, dress, walk the dog, do some shopping, and travel around town pacing yourself.

"*Soraya, tenemos que hablar de tu corazón.* The inflammation has
taken its toll and is progressive. At this point your doctors do not have
more medications. We are in a corner *sin salida,* without an exit." I
had been very careful to let her doctors do all of the explaining and
pacing the discussions. We were in constant communication.

"I understand, Doctor. My heart is failing and there is not much
time left. How much do you think?" Time is all relative. Prediction of
death in medicine is notoriously difficult. On the other hand, it would
be a copout to not answer her question. She had to make arrangements. And she wanted to live. Despite the difficulties in her life, the
few pleasures it had offered her, she had been happy listening to stories
in the middle of the night at the laundry, seeing her sister, watching
her son and daughter grow up. She was thankful for the kindnesses of
people who were taking care of her.

I sat on her bed and held her hand. "At the rate your heart disease
is progressing, Soraya, you will need a new heart, a transplant. You
will need it within a few months. Your disease is progressing more rapidly now. You cannot do the things now that you did even six months
ago—even three months ago."

"How can I get a heart if I don't have papers?" She got to the central issue directly. A lot quicker than I had planned. "Maria my social
worker says that is not an option without a green card. The doctors
talked about a machine hooked up to my blood plugged in all the time
to keep me going, but they said that a heart is not possible." For Class
IV heart failure, there were not a lot of options. New technologies had
pushed an artificial pump or LVAD, a left ventricular assist device,
into the market at some of the transplant centers. It was used to keep
patients alive while they waited for a transplant, or used as a mini
pump hooked into the arterial blood system in and of itself. It was
complicated and required a support network; it was not free of its own
risks and complications. One of my patients rejected it outright as an
option since even bathing was an issue. For some it was not a life; for
others it was life itself.

I left when Indira came to take Soraya to the bathroom and give her a bath.

Two weeks later all of us involved in Soraya's care held a meeting to clarify our strategy. The social work department had a large conference room with beat-up wooden furniture and long cracks in the walls from the pile drivers smashing huge metal posts into the landfill, putting in the foundation for the post-9/11 Office of the Medical Examiner's DNA lab that clipped both our light and the views south, exactly where the Trade Center towers had billowed smoke a decade earlier.

The door was wide open and I could hear laughter and voices in Spanish and English. Soraya had been released a week earlier, but we all knew it was just a matter of time. Renee, who ran the social work department, was trying to figure out what could be done to help Soraya's kids. The boy, especially, was difficult and had all sorts of behavioral issues. Could he be placed? She was blunt and on point. "Worst-case scenario planning."

I decided to focus on what needed to happen so the end-of-times scenario didn't kick in. "We are clinically at a very vulnerable point. Soraya could have a cardiac arrest at any moment; her congestive heart failure could advance with another organ tanking or ten other complications. You guys are old hands at this and know the consequences as well as I do." I didn't realize that the Soraya Molino team had not permitted themselves to really believe that this was the end of the line. Protective mechanisms allowed people to do their work with the idea that she had more time. When you approach the speed of light, time slows down. In this case, time was speeding up.

"Clinically we are going to act as if we can get her listed for a heart. That means a battery of tests, a complete psychiatric evaluation, detailed notes from the heart failure team. I will own that piece. We will try to make it happen." The group was clearly in agreement. She was too young, she had suffered too much, the kids were half in limbo now. "I will need all the help we can get from legal services and social work to keep pushing her paperwork. Let me know who to call." Time to pull out all the stops. At least we would go down trying to pull this off. If Soraya died, we would know we did what we could within the system's constraints. It was as much for us as for her at this point.

The group spent the next hour outlining the social issues, from schools to food stamps, rental assistance to grief counseling, transportation to homemakers, and donated clothing to adoption services.

I was physically in the room but mentally in another zone as Renee ran her meeting. I drifted back to my first conversation with Lenny. I was pissed off and tried not to show it. Why shouldn't she get a heart? The undocumented could donate organs. And did at appallingly regular intervals as young, undocumented workers accepted high-risk jobs. But they couldn't receive organs, even when donors (like siblings) were ready to donate and physicians were willing to operate for free. What was going on?

Organ donation was not a simple matter. You did not fill out a form, mail it in, and then find out by return receipt that you had been accepted and that a warm pulsating organ was waiting for you in an operating room a ten-minute walk from your apartment. It was more like a giant lottery, a national lottery with local decision making, but a lottery nevertheless.

By federal law all five thousand–plus hospitals in the United States participate in organ donor identification and inquiry with families. An organization has regionalized the country into networks and has close ties to physicians, hospital communities, transplant centers, and a national group that uses a computer database to connect organs with people in need based on blood type, other medical factors, the changing clinical status of patients, and availability. These groups meet regularly, are professionally administered, and are dedicated to the simple proposition that to donate organs is to save lives.

I made phone calls to my colleagues at transplant centers around the city and to my friends who were heart failure specialists. This was a bread-and-butter case. They dealt with end-stage heart disease every day, using all the tricks of the trade: the drug combinations, intravenous medications, diets, complicating factors, miscommunications, instructions, visiting nurses, daily weights, and at the end of the journey LVADs or heart transplants.

I knew we had to get past the psychiatric evaluation. Drug addictions and incapacitating mental illnesses precluded receiving an organ. Soraya's depression was reactive, formed out of the chronicity of her illness and its debilitating humiliations. She was not a depressed person. The opposite was true. She had an anti-depressive personality.

But I knew it would be harder to negotiate the legal issues. It was almost impossible to get an organ for an undocumented immigrant. I spoke to my colleagues in the heart failure community and went over the case in detail. They agreed to help in any way they could. Bellevue does not do transplants, but it is a major donor hospital. We have a very close working relationship. They would make her case known to the transplant group. They would forgo the thorough evaluation and accept ours. But there was nothing they could do about the legal issues.

I knew it, of course. It seemed unfair and unethical to accept organs from undocumented immigrants and not allow them to receive. I looked out the window before turning to my email. And there it was. An email from Clara. It had been in my inbox since the morning. Soraya was marrying her mild-mannered, soft-spoken Cuban American landlord. Could I join them for a toast at five that afternoon near city hall?

The heart for Soraya came shortly after she was accepted into a transplant program in New York City. The evaluation team at the transplant center adopted her immediately. They fell for her graciousness, her smile, her "*gracias a Dios.*" They fell for her life from Salamá to Tapachula, the coyote transfer to a gang of human traffickers. The night laundry work and the catch in her breath several years ago. I think they fell for the fact that in her entire life she'd had only a few weeks, maybe a few months, of happiness. Sometimes one person stood for all of the others who didn't make it. That, plus her ejection fraction was now in single digits. She needed the next compatible heart.

A gypsy cab careening around Grand Army Plaza broadsided a twenty-two-year-old bicycle rider on a bright Wednesday morning. He was brain-dead immediately from massive brain injury. The organ donor team met with his family at the local hospital. They agreed that the best that could happen from this tragedy beyond imagination was to allow other people to live. His organs went to save many lives.

We all did not know what to say after such a long journey with Soraya. We had held her hand and listened to her stories. We had adjusted her medications and moved heaven and earth to get her a heart so she could have some years that were joyful and lived without fear and the threat of death, rape, or harm to her children. We had given her a heart for Rabinal. A partial payment for the chaos and suffering that didn't have a voice. She had never thought she would have any time of enjoyment in her life. She never entertained a fantasy of happiness, satisfaction, or relationships; she never thought that anything was owed to her. Everything was God's will.

When we found out from the transplant team that she had died, a bit of all of us died at the same time. We know we cannot predict who will survive and who will not after a heart transplant. There are too many moving parts, too many variables, from technical complications to rejection, blood clots, and infections. But the futility of what we'd done overwhelmed us. The vast emptiness laughed at us.

CHAPTER 7

Four Generations

The morning was a dense haze. It was the fifth day of a warm-weather inversion that encased the city in a thick gunmetal-gray shield. The air did not move, keeping ozone and car exhaust gridlocked over the city. People were edgy; the hospital was packed and the emergency rooms, overflowing. Special shelters were opened around the city to protect the weak and the aged. I stopped by my office briefly to drop off my sweat-soaked sport coat and slip on a clean white lab coat. I had a visitor waiting in my office anteroom. She had thoughtfully bought me a coffee and a cream-filled Italian pastry spilling from the napkins.

"Hi, Yolanda." A big smile appeared from under her signature large dark Dolce and Gabbana glasses, and then the invariable hug. She showed me a quick picture of her newborn son and her fifteen-year-old wannabe-doctor daughter on her BlackBerry to catch me up on family matters as she followed me into the inner office. I took a couple of bites and a sip of the coffee as she brought me up to date on half a dozen of our recent patients in common. Yolanda Valera was the NYC Organ Donor Network's Bellevue representative. More part of the family than an "official," her business was always fraught and bordered on the outer limit of emotional tolerances. Hearts breaking all the time was too heavy a load for me.

"Hey, you emailed me about coming to the labor floor. That's not your usual hangout," I intoned anxiously. I sensed this could be a disaster with repercussions that would spin endlessly. The smile and a hug were no indicators, no matter the circumstances, and the circumstances on labor and delivery were a worst-case starting point. "Give me two minutes and let's head upstairs."

"I got a call from the head nurse, Anne. She'll be here any second. She is with the family now explaining about a C-section with Dr. Girardi." She took over now. "Anne gave me a heads-up call. The first brain-death study has just been completed and they have the C-section team ready to go."

"You got a call about what exactly?" I didn't have the time or energy to let this drag on.

Yolanda heard the edge in my voice and got very professional and technical very quickly. "A young woman, twenty-nine years old, was pregnant with her second child, in her third trimester, due in a few days at most, at home working in the kitchen, watching TV, on the phone, the usual stuff when she had a sudden severe headache and vomited over everything and everybody. Her mother was with her and had her lie on the couch and put a cold wet towel around her forehead. She came back within minutes from cleaning up the mess and she couldn't wake her daughter up. An ICH." *Jesus*, I said to myself. Intracerebral or brain hemorrhage. In a twenty-nine-year-old woman. What was going on? We strode down the labor and delivery suite and parked ourselves in the head nurse's empty office.

At that moment Anne opened the door to her office and saw me; we nodded at each other. A thin attractive middle-aged Filipina with a ready smile and a pageboy haircut, she eschewed melodrama and focused on the business of taking care of patients. We had been colleagues for years and gone through many challenging battles over everything from late-term abortions to midwife-obstetrical-nursing turf wars that reminded me of the Thirty Years' War. Not all hospital politics was benign and ended with a handshake. The thing that bound Anne and me together, more than anything, was only known to five other people and our respective spouses. We were members of the Platinum Club.

For several years we met with three to seven other staff members over a monthly lunch at the Greek diner across First Avenue at a corner table away from the crowds and noise. All of us had been diagnosed with cancer within a year of one another, and all of us had platinum chemotherapy. We christened ourselves the Platinum Club. Lifetime memberships were all that were offered. There were no dues and no elections, no mailings, and none of the annoying mealtime fund-raising phone calls.

"Anne, what is happening now?" She was agitated; her face was always a dead giveaway to her feelings. It was one of the things I liked about her. She was professional but not an automaton.

"The family is devastated. They are crying and inconsolable at this point. It turns out the Sahagún family matriarch, the grandmother, is in our rehab unit now recovering from another round of surgery. She has been here on and off for over six months." She paused for a couple of seconds to let it sink in.

"We got consent from the mother, Marta Sahagún, legally the next of kin, for the C-section to try to save the baby. No husband in the picture or significant other. That was our first priority. The baby's life is giving them a focus and Dr. Roman is with them as my nurses are setting up the room for an elective C-section. Peds is already here to assist. Should be under way in ten minutes, no more." The mother was like an incubator for the baby at this point. Her blood pressure and blood tests were normal. The fetus was getting what it needed from the placenta to stay alive for the time being. Anne was efficient and ran a tight unit, but she was stressed and I knew she was working on auto-pilot now. The radiation had taken its toll on her. The exhaustion was impossible to describe and it went on and on, month after month.

"Hey, Anne, you said Sahagún?" I said. This was not a common Spanish name.

"Yes, you know them, Eric. They asked about you already. I thought you had seen them by now when Yolanda told me you were texted. Marta and her crew are all in the doctors' lounge. We gave it over to them. She may be a single mother who just lost her daughter, but she has worked at Bellevue for over twenty-five years. We had to set up limits on which staff could stop by. Everyone loves her. She is like the queen here. It is too much." She was pretty depleted herself emotionally.

Marta was a *limpiadora* or housekeeper for the hospital way before I arrived. I had gotten to know her when she would sneak out the parking lot entrance for a Lucky Strike in the Sobriety Garden, the space created by recovering drug and alcohol abusers in treatment at Bellevue. The handmade garden paths and artwork, Gaudiesque in their strangeness and munificence, were wedged between an exit ramp and the medical examiner's new glass sarcophagus. I recognized her one day as I waited for a ride to take me to the city council. She had a lovely way of greeting everyone with the Caribbean "*mi amor.*" "Have a great day, *mi amor...*" How could anyone resist? So we started to talk and gradually got to know each other over several years with bits and pieces of conversations stitched together from waits for elevators, in line for coffee, in the medical library when she came to clean and I was holed up writing a paper, the errant cigarette in the Alice in Wonderland garden, and two years ago about her own health concerns.

Dr. Roman, the attending obstetrician, poked her head in the room. "C-section in five minutes." We looked at each other and had nothing to say. She shook her head slightly and that was it. Many years of working together had given us an ability to communicate telepathically when necessary. This was one of those times. Anne reached into her desk and without asking handed me some fresh green scrubs. While she and Yolanda went out to sit with the family, I changed in her office and walked the fifteen yards down the main corridor of labor and delivery to the entrance to the operating rooms.

Perry was the senior OB anesthesiologist. He wore wire-rimmed glasses and was tall and lean; he never aged. He was already checking the lines and numbers on his brand-new Dräger anesthesia machine with a young female resident in scrubs and a heavy teal sweatshirt he was supervising. On the operating room table covered with several blue paper sheets was an enormous mound of a person. A quick guess put Irene Sahagún at close to 250 pounds. A huge round ball of a human being with an enormous panniculus (belly) that moved with the force of gravity, sliding and hanging from her small frame. It was impossible for the surgeons to lean over the patient and proceed safely. This was not going to be a three-minute slash-and-burn emergency C-section with an infant's heart decelerating and the time ticking mercilessly.

Dr. Roman asked one of the general surgeons who specialized in bariatric surgery to join her. Manish Parikh came in the room gowned and ready to operate. "Let's try this bariatric-style," he said after a quick glance at the patient and the room. He organized everyone to slide the leg pieces on the table apart and cushioned Irene's legs in extra sheets and soft blankets.

During the procedure "time-out," all of the patient's identifiers are read out and signed off by the treating team. Parikh started, "Holy...Sahagún. I operated on her mother a year and a half ago. I know this woman." He backed out for a few minutes, went outside, rescrubbed, and came back in. "Okay, sorry about that, ready now. Let's do the time-out again." His voice was controlled, but the humor and banter with the staff were gone. It was going to be all by the book. You could only hear the circulating nurse's booties scuff the linoleum floor as she walked around the room and some rustling and muffled single-word comments from anesthesia.

Parikh knew they had time. The baby was well oxygenated. Its heartbeat could be heard and seen on another monitor looking at the fetal heart strip. They divided up the tasks quietly and efficiently. After a careful dissection through a foot of white and pink fat tissue with tiny red pinpoint bleeders cauterized on the way down, they reached the dusky red-blue uterus. Dr. Roman took over and quickly had a little girl by her feet and then in her arms. Brenda swooped in from peds and took over with suctioning the mouth and handling the baby. She was pink and breathing and squawking.

It was time for me to go and see Marta and her friends. The baby would be fine, in the neonatal intensive care unit (NICU) for a couple of days and then to the nursery. Who would be looking after the baby was another matter. Marta had a million issues to deal with. Now a million and one.

I pushed open the door to the doctors' lounge across from the nursing station. Marta was seated near the window overlooking FDR Drive snaking southward toward the Brooklyn Bridge. Techs, supervisors, hospital police, messengers, transport, nurses, translators, social workers were all in their uniforms filling the rest of the large conference room. I recognized most of them, and the room fell silent. My eyes locked on Marta, and I went over and hugged her tight. Her tears said it all.

"Marta, your new grandchild is fine. A little girl. Does she have a name? She is with the pediatricians and on her way to the NICU, we can go there a little later and you can hold her."

"Dr. Eric, I don't know what to say. *Mi amorcita* was fine. She had a headache, I mean a really bad headache, she was pale and cold. I put her down to rest and three minutes later she was lifeless. *Mi amor...*" I held her hand and rubbed her back. The friends stood back a little and let us be together while they talked in the background.

"Isabela. Isabela is what Irene wanted to call her. Her great-grandmother's name, a *partera*, a midwife from another time completely." She dried her tears and looked around the room for a moment. "*Yolanda, por favor.*"

Yolanda and Anne slid their chairs closer. "Marta has agreed to donate her daughter's organs, Eric. We talked about what Irene would have wanted." Yolanda had Marta's other hand in hers, and her arm was around her shoulders. The two came from similar impoverished backgrounds in the *campo*, the countryside, in two different countries. They had both struggled to make it through hard work. One had an extended social network through hundreds of daily encounters over the years at a big public hospital. The other through hundreds of visits with complete strangers at the most difficult times of their lives in the same big public hospital. In the end it was all about "*mi amor*" one way or the other.

Six months earlier, I had found an envelope in my inbox with my name written in block letters: "Doctor Eric." Inside there was a note on paper ripped from a grade school notebook in Spanglish. *Por favor, Doctor, mi mama is in hospital, Cuarto 1024. Can you see her. Olimpia Gutierrez.* Signed *Marta Sahagún, the cleaning lady.*

I took it into my office and tried to remember Marta Sahagún. And then an image came back of a smiling, very large woman with a big laugh and husky voice and a cigarette cough who pushed her heavy yellow-and-black plastic cleaning cart quietly through the halls. Though invisible to most people, Marta had enormous dignity and goodwill that added a comforting feeling to the medicine floors. She was middle-aged with jet-black short hair and bright red lipstick on her lips permanently in a half smile. She felt proud to have a job at Bellevue Hospital. "*Dios mío*," she would say, "with all of the great doctors and patients from around the world." I hadn't seen her in some years.

After dealing with my office stuff, I went up to check on Marta's mother. Omar Bholat waved me over to join rounds with his team as they were wrapping up a case discussion with a family whose young adult daughter had a close call with an extreme case of ulcerative colitis. When the discussion of what to do next closed, the group moved amoeba-like fifteen feet down the corridor, parking in front of Olimpia Gutierrez's room number 1024.

Through the sliding glass doors I could see an overweight elderly woman on a respirator. A technician was changing some tubing and settings on the ventilator while a nurse was finishing recording her vital signs and changing a dressing on a clear plastic tube that snaked from four different clear solutions in plastic bags, feeding medications slowly via computerized pumps hanging from a single pole like postmodern stoplights in a futuristic Gotham out of a Batman movie. A heavyset woman with jet-black hair was tidying up two chairs in the corner covered in sheets and blankets where she had clearly spent the night. I recognized Marta when she turned and spotted me through the glass doors.

The chief resident, a sturdy Chinese woman around thirty in scrubs and black clogs, who had been up all night in the OR, began her summary, "This is day number seventeen in the unit for Mrs. G, a seventy-two-year-old woman who presented by ambulance to the Bellevue emergency room in severe congestive heart failure. She felt nauseous and was slightly uncomfortable and had gone to the bathroom. Within minutes she was finding it difficult to breathe. Her banging brought her daughter to her side, and a 911 call brought an FDNY ambulance to their apartment. The family lives on the edge of Greenpoint in Brooklyn, and there are two hospitals within minutes nearby. The family insisted on Bellevue. All of the family's doctors are here, and her daughter is an employee here." She looked into the darkened room at Marta. The group's eyes moved with her.

What had brought her to the hospital in the middle of the night were the effects of long-standing coronary artery disease, the accumulation of fatty deposits in the blood vessels supplying her heart muscle. The rupture of a cholesterol-filled "plaque" triggered a cascade that clotted off the vessel. A heart attack was in progress. She was sitting bolt-upright in the ambulance while hacking up frothy white pulmonary edema fluid. Her heart was barely squeezing, and the backup pressures in her lungs were literally pushing fluid from the vessels into her air spaces. The EMT crew radioed in that she was within minutes of a cardiac arrest.

It took only a few seconds to give her some morphine when the gurney came to a halt in the treatment room. Her wild-eyed look calmed down. The anesthesiologist rubbed her arm and told her he was going to put in a breathing tube as he pushed in another intravenous medication. The lines on the EKG electrically sampling different parts of the heart muscle showed an evolving heart attack. A trip to the cath lab, five minutes away, would have to be delayed until she was hooked up to a dialysis machine to filter her blood and to get some fluid out of her system. She was in a no-win situation. With kidneys that had failed two years earlier, there was no room to maneuver.

Several hours later, the cardiologist came out of a heavy metal side door directly from the cath lab into the side corridor where Marta, her daughter Irene, and friends were seated on a wooden bench. Dr. Pamuk was all business but quickly recognized the family's distress. "Mrs. Gutierrez did well with the procedure. There were no complications." She got the most important news out right away and then settled into the decisions that had to be made. These would be hard ones for everyone involved.

"Your mom," she continued, "has several blockages in her coronary arteries. We can't get to them with our catheters. All we could do safely was get in, make a diagnosis, and get out quickly." At this point she was joined by Denise Collachio, a young heart surgeon, who introduced herself and stood quietly while Dr. Pamuk finished. "There is too much disease, and the locations of the blockages make it impossible to treat her in the cath lab. Plus, she needs to settle down from her heart failure and get another dialysis treatment." The cath lab had sophisticated radiology equipment that would assist the cardiologist in threading in tiny plastic tubes to investigate the integrity of the most important blood vessels supplying the heart itself—and many times to treat blockages with small balloons at the same time.

"So there is nothing that you can do for my mother?"

Dr. Pamuk looked at Denise Collachio, who continued, "I have looked at the pictures, and it is clear that surgery is the only approach for the disease she has. However, this is a very high-risk situation. Given her weight, diabetes, dialysis, diffuse vascular disease, and poor heart function, her risk of dying from the surgery is 50 percent. Plus, there is a high rate of complications from infections to strokes." Denise was direct and unflinching in her assessment, but she then spent a long time with the family drawing diagrams of the surgery until she was sure they understood what was at stake. Bypass surgery meant taking some veins from her legs and arteries from her chest wall to "jump" or bypass the diseased ones supplying her heart. "A lot of people would choose to do nothing. It is an okay decision. Sometimes doing nothing is the harder decision to make." *True enough*, I thought.

"And if we do nothing?" Marta looked at Denise. The question said it all. This was always the hardest question to answer.

"Marta, this is a really tough question. Why don't you talk with your mother? We can operate. Once you have all of the information and feel comfortable we have answered your questions, it is your decision. Different people will answer differently. We will go with your decision." I was impressed with her neutrality, how she presented the case. I had seen so many misrepresentations of the odds and options to families. Physicians would buckle under the pressure, the guilt of not offering some treatment or hope. Genuine informed consent was harder and less common than most people assumed.

I remembered a high-volume altercation between our internists and surgeons over a patient who was an intravenous heroin addict with a recurrent infection of a heart valve from shooting up with dirty needles. "But you have to operate on him, it is his only chance. He will die otherwise." The internists were adamant. The surgeon responded just as adamantly: "We operated on him for a valve infection and heart abscess and put in a brand-new plastic valve eight months ago. He chose to inject himself again and reinfect his valve. Not me, I didn't choose to reinfect him. He will die from the surgery. That is a near certainty. I don't want to be his undertaker. I am just a surgeon."

The 1 percent "solution" prevailed. I had seen it in action before. Any-chance philosophy meant an intervention. I had seen more than one woman with metastatic breast cancer in an ICU on another round of *let's try this chemotherapy*. The impetus for that procedure came from the seemingly well-meaning oncologist who couldn't accept the death of his patient. Who exactly was being treated in this situation?

The surgical team operated on the addict with the infected valve. The patient had a stroke and died a slow death in a nursing home. The surgeon never again let sentiment overwhelm his hard-earned experience. The internists learned that not everything could be fixed. A patient's death is often experienced as a total failure or a narcissistic injury by most physicians. Better to keep treating or hand off to a waiting squadron of consultants.

Marta sat with her mother in the cath lab recovery room. The decision was a given. We could all see it coming. "*Mi mama* would like the surgery." The surgeon went in to talk to Olimpia with Marta, and they reviewed everything again. The old, nearly blind woman was exhausted. "*Hija*, you decide. I am too tired. I trust the doctors. But you decide." Marta stroked her mother's hands gently and patted back a strand of her gray hair. She was not about to let her go.

The six-hour operation was a success—four bypasses and daily dialysis kept her alive and her lab numbers in order. The fact that Olimpia was obese, however, confounded her treatment and recovery by another order of magnitude. The team was indefatigable and kept pushing her to do more for herself. A special mechanical lift got her into a chair. A family member was always at her side. She was slathered in cocoa butter, her hair was washed and combed, she was exercised gently and fed with food brought from home. The ship slowly turned around while the team held its breath.

When the team left, I stayed behind to talk to Marta. Despite everything that had happened with her mother, she was totally composed. She had gained a considerable amount of weight. The rhythm of illness, hospitalizations, surgery, complications, more treatments, testing, and conferences was to her part of the natural course of events. My secretary had graciously brought up some breakfast for the two of us as we used a small family conference room to talk about her letter. Marta Sahagún was effusive in her greeting. It had been at least three years since I had seen her.

"Dr. Eric—" She paused. "I wrote not about my mother, but about myself. I need your advice on what to do about my own health. I know my mother is getting the best care possible." Despite two weeks sleeping on chairs in the ICU, she was animated and shrugged off the fatigue.

The fact that her mother was not the main event caught me by surprise. I'd been sure there had been some miscommunication between the physicians and her family that needed intervention. Those were the usual calls from family or from frantic social workers brokering angry families who were living the horror of imminent losses.

We went on a few more minutes about her mother. Olimpia's weight, her massiveness on a tiny frame, made everything more difficult, including her breathing. She was five foot four and weighed 270 pounds. She was enormous by any measure, and her inability to move around since she'd lost her eyesight a number of years ago, complicated by her dialysis regimen, resulted in another jump in weight and her diabetes ricocheting out of control—despite the steady attendance of visiting nurses and meticulous monitoring by her family. She had been progressively more depressed. She barely left her bedroom during non-dialysis days and expressed a lack of a will to live. She was ready to join her husband, who had died in an accident involving alcohol and stairs a decade earlier.

"Marta, it sounds like your mother has had every known complication

from diabetes related to her *obesidad*, obesity." The Olimpias were filling our clinics and the hospitals around the city and country.

"*Sí, Doctor.* She has had every complication, and pitifully so have
I." She looked at me, embarrassed, and sat still. There was a fading
resemblance to her mother as a young beautiful woman from the pictures in the intensive care unit room.

"Marta, tell me what I can do to help you. You know I will do what
I can."

"Doctor, I have some papers here outlining my medical problems
and was hoping you would go through them and help me understand
what is happening to my body and what direction or options I have. I
am scared of all of it and do not want to end up like my poor mother,
suffering for years at the end of her life, a lifeless life. Totally dependent. Like a child now." She pushed across a manila folder with her
name in Magic Marker, filled with twenty pages of computer printouts
and a CD in a plastic case marked "CT scan Sra. Sahagún / Alfonso
Reyes, MD."

I pushed back in my chair and took out the papers, putting the CD to
the side. They were a mix of office notes, a biopsy report, X-rays, and
laboratory tests covering the last eighteen months. I read them carefully and made some notes on the manila folder, then took a moment
to leave with the CD and review the scan on a computer down the hall.

"This is pretty heavy stuff, Marta," I said to start the conversation.
We spoke half in English and half in Spanish, as she always had in the
hospital. The handful of medical information that she had given me
had dire implications for her. "I will be totally honest with you. You
came to me for a second opinion. But I cannot do that unless I can talk
to you honestly and openly."

"Doctor, that is all I want at this point. No time for fooling around.
I fooled around for too long and now I want to see if I still have a
chance at a life. I can see clearly with my own two eyes where I could
end up."

"Well," I said, "the good news is that you have medical conditions
that are still reversible. The bad news: What you have is in many ways
as serious as cancer and in many ways as bad or worse." I had Marta's

attention completely. "Let's start off with the simple stuff. You have inflammation in your esophagus, from acid reflux. There is a change in the cells lining your esophagus called Barrett's. That will keep your GI doctor in business for a few more years." I smiled to see if she had her old sense of humor. She did not.

I continued from Dr. Reyes's records. "The biopsy shows a fatty liver with early cirrhosis. The inflammation from your weight has caused a reaction by the liver's cells. This reaction causes micro-scars to form, like a million tiny cuts that heal with tiny scars. What your father, Andreas, did to his liver with alcohol is happening to your liver with fatty deposits that don't belong there." I could not have put it more graphically or directly to Marta. She had such ambivalence toward her long-deceased father. The shame from his drinking was only over-whelmed by the time he hit Irene, his granddaughter. Neither Irene nor Marta ever forgave him. He was dead to them before he died.

"It is like a giant map of New York City with all of the streets laid out—then little by little, a few here and there are blocked off, and over many years more tiny blockages appear. Then after a while there is no place for the traffic to go. There is huge congestion for miles and miles until people can't even pull out of their driveways."

I flipped over a page of paper and sketched out a cartoon liver, half of it a normal liver, half cirrhotic. "Your blood tests show that there is inflammation, the liver enzymes are elevated. It is like what you would see with a viral infection. But the good news is that your liver is able to make all the key proteins to prevent bleeding. It's like a factory, and so far it is continuing to do its work. You have not crossed a point of no return." I paused and she interrupted.

"Andreas had cirrhosis from drinking. Can I get that from my weight?" She put it straight on the table. She'd refused to call her father anything but Andreas after he hit Irene.

"Yes, it can cause cirrhosis." I pushed back from the table.

"I don't even sip a beer on a *quinceañera* and I could have the same thing as my alcoholic father, who broke his neck under the influence of Coke and rum in my own building." She spoke softly and to herself more than me. A rhetorical commentary on the absurdity of life.

"Marta, you have other problems from obesity that are not trivial. I see that you have seen a specialist in breathing problems. You have severe sleep apnea. It is also associated with hypertension and heart problems."

"My daughter Irene thought I was dying. I stop breathing for long periods at night and she rushes in to wake me up. I would snort like a horse, she told me after she waited for what seemed like fifteen minutes to her. She called me *la potrilla*, the filly. For many years at work here, I was exhausted all the time. I was going home, cooking, and going to bed earlier, but I never felt rested. One of my neighborhood doctors heard my daughter call me *potrilla* and she asked more questions about snoring and tiredness. That's how they stumbled on the diagnosis.

"I thought it was stress, family issues, money problems, Andreas's drunkenness—life, you know! So I have a breathing machine at home. I hook myself up at night with a plastic mask and strap. Between my mother's equipment and my machine, our apartment resembles a car mechanic's shop—or a Stephen King movie," she added, smiling finally.

"Yes, Marta, that plus hypertension, high fat levels in your blood, arthritis in your knees that makes it hard for you to walk, you are on six different medications, and you see four different doctors routinely plus at least half a dozen specialists in the last couple of years, from endocrinology to pulmonary to orthopedics to a liver guy." I let the facts hang there for a few seconds. Obesity is the new scourge—an epidemic of diseases, all interconnected, beginning in early childhood. How ironic that the disease of affluence begins early and hits the poorest classes the hardest.

"What bothers me the most of all is the page on family history." I pulled out a sheet with some indecipherable physician scribble on a barely legible Xerox. "It says here that your daughter has diabetes. We haven't talked about the elephant in the room, have we?" I didn't speak this with any irony.

"You mean that I have diabetes and that I have been on different medications for diabetes and have started insulin two years ago?" she said to the table.

"No, not about you, Marta." She looked at me.

"Your daughter, Irene, has diabetes and is on metformin. And your daughter's son, Jaime, who is seeing Dr. Nguyen here at Bellevue, has a metabolic syndrome. Meaning his system is diabetic in all senses except the high blood sugar." Talking about her daughter and grandson brought Marta's gaze right into mine.

"Your family through four generations is a disaster zone of medical diseases and all of their complications." I added, not for effect, but just to speak out loud what I was thinking: "No more than twenty feet from us, your mother is being kept barely alive, a miracle of modern technology. And from her point of view and yours, from what you just said, it's not much of a life. You have just shown me your own reports, which say exactly where you are headed. Marta, you are a very smart woman. Let's figure out a solution." I didn't want to rely on Wizard of Oz technology to treat organs in extremis.

There was a parallel track running in my head as I was reading Marta's medical record. Were the members of this multigenerational family victims of their own irresponsible behavior, an inability to make the "right" health decisions for themselves and their kids? No one forced them into White Castle or Wendy's. No one else loaded up baskets with high-fat salty snacks in the neighborhood bodegas or carts in C Town supermarkets.

But, I thought, that does not explain the epidemic nature of this disease. What about the trillion-dollar industry that overproduces food in gargantuan quantities and fights for every square inch of the attention of every consumer around the world? It targets young consumers using social media experts who test colors and songs and pay off sports figures and media stars to hawk their wares. There's no gun to anyone's head, but there is a brain trust of über-advertisers, marketers, psychologists, sociologists, anthropologists, food scientists, and brain researchers unlocking the secrets to taste and pleasure. They study brain-based neurohormonal control and the environment to create vast demands for their products. What's the difference between this kind of addiction and the cultivated addictions to nicotine, cocaine, crystal meth, or heroin, for that matter? This is real translational research, from the National Institutes of Health bench laboratories to the corporate marketing strategists to your neighborhood food store.

I pulled my focus back to the here and now. "Marta, first things first." I held up the manila folder. "The health issues you have now are not going to get better on their own. No amount of wishful thinking will change the outcome. And the Virgin of Guadalupe is silent on this issue. You know that." The corners of her mouth hinted at a smile. I didn't play the Virgin card very often, and hope was not a plan.

"I can see from Dr. Reyes's notes that you have been through virtually every diet and group without success."

She nodded. Clearly she knew a lot better than I did about diets and dieting. "So what, Dr. Eric. Is there nothing to do? Did I really miss *el barco*? I need to be careful, *la vida no es un sueño*, life is not a dream"—one of her favorite expressions. It was exactly the right question to ask. I looked at Marta and thought about her mother having heart surgery to squeeze out some more earthly existence, if luck cooperated.

"Have you discussed surgery for obesity? Bariatric surgery?" I didn't hesitate to bring up the subject any longer. After extreme skepticism about a surgical "solution" for serious obesity, I had become a convert of sorts. At least for Marta, as an individual. Surgery would do nothing to combat the epidemic of global obesity. It would take political will on the scale of the surgeon general's report on cancer and smoking to change the rules of the game even slightly. Smoking was still the biggest single killer in our society, over four hundred thousand deaths a year. Every generation of physicians has a prototypical disease, the one that wreaks havoc with almost all the organs. Learned professors of medicine would say, "You can learn all of medicine by studying disease X." For my father's generation it was syphilis. For my generation it was alcoholism. For the current generation it would be obesity, hands down. It affected every organ.

"Dr. Reyes looked into it, and I simply cannot afford it. It is over fifteen thousand dollars. We barely make it from rent check to rent check. And you have to pay cash in advance." This was the biggest-growth surgical business in this country. Hundreds of thousands of operations were being done every year. It was surgery in a high-risk population and not something you fooled around with unless you really knew what you were doing. Fatalities from elective surgery were the stuff of the *New York Post*. No one wanted to end up between those covers.

"Look, Marta, we have a program here for weight surgery that I would like you to look at and judge for yourself. The payment is not an issue."

She looked up in disbelief. But she quickly looked down again. "I know there are many types of surgery, and it can be dangerous. Particularly with the medical issues I have. I have to look after my family, you know." She was right on the button and better that way. If she proceeded it would be with full knowledge aforethought.

"Okay," I said. "Think it through. Go to the Wednesday conference open to the public; you can meet Dr. Parikh and decide for yourself. The surgical part is over my head. The reports from Reyes are in black and white. Your mother is three doors down the hall. My job is to get you to the right doctors. The rest is up to you. But you have to do something. This is not a situation where you can do nothing."

"I will think about it," she assured me. "I will come up with a plan."

That was the last time I saw her before Irene's death. I still could not believe it. Marta's aged mother had gone home, against all odds. And now the joy of Marta's life, her real *amor*, was gone. Thinking back on our earlier conversation, I realized how much higher the stakes were than either of us could imagine.

I, and half the hospital it seemed, went to Irene's funeral. A cortege of vans, school buses, official cars, Dial 7 limousines, and private vehicles snaked its way down Manhattan's spine past the Essex Street Market and over the Williamsburg Bridge. Magnificent views south onto the gentrifying warehouses and tugboats pushing their huge loads against the rapid East River current sprawled out beneath a gray sky melting into the infinity of Brooklyn. The car was silent except for the regular clicks like a railroad car from the metal braces slicing across the asphalted road. We were all lost in our own thoughts about the senselessness of so much of what we saw every day. The carnage of wasted lives from violence, bad decisions, carelessness, drugs, alcohol created a mobile shell that we carried with us through the days and years of work. It was a semi-permeable membrane that allowed small doses of the raw pain and suffering to penetrate but effectively kept most of it out. When a senseless death occurred within the protective force field, we were all vulnerable. We were very exposed. The pain of our own immediate losses, a spouse's life-threatening illness, a drug overdose of a beloved cousin, the jealous rage that took a life ruffled the silence with a barely suppressed scream. Irene's death had spread a low-lying cloud of agitation and vulnerability through everyone.

We turned off in the heart of the Orthodox Jewish barrio. Storefront synagogues and matzoh bakeries, shuls, and hundreds of new red-brick apartments with metal grilles covering the windows and tiny porches were salted through the neighborhoods for the rapidly expanding community and their large families. A clot of young women gathered on the front steps surrounded by dozens of kids jumping rope and playing tag. We wound our way deep into East New York. We passed chicken wings, Pedro's Pollo and Pollo Campero, "the best" pizza shops, mofongo Dominican takeout, Jose's Churritos, Hamburger Heaven, Hamburger Paradise, Hamburger Joe's, and every national chain plus an infinite assortment of tiny bodegas selling lottery tickets and baloney. Thousands of small shops eking out a precarious existence in no-man's-land.

A huge granite Catholic church loomed into view when we turned down Myrtle Avenue. Hundreds of our colleagues and friends and relatives from the Sahagún neighborhood network were lined up around a corner slowly feeding into the building. The women wore black dresses and large floppy hats that they held on to as a gust of wind kicked up. The men were in suits of different colors with shiny black shoes. Pockets of people stood in the street, between triple-parked cars, chatting and hugging. Traffic was backed up; a couple of cop cars were pulled onto the sidewalk, and cars were diverted through the red lights. No one honked.

The ceremony helped to heal the wounds. The priest had known the family through four generations. Given the mixed nature of the masses entering the church—Muslims in hijabs, Jews wearing yarmul-kes, Methodists, Lutherans, Evangelicals and Pentecostals and even a few Catholics—Father Martí, a Cuban refugee from the 1980 Mariel boatlift, quickly took stock of the flotsam of humanity that rode the tide to the base of his pulpit.

"We are devastated by the loss of Irene Sahagún. Each and every one of us will carry this loss for our lives. It touches us and reminds us of how fragile life can be, how the flicker can go out with a tiny gust of a breeze. How do we find any meaning in this death, the loss of this young woman?" There was no answer. And he left Jesus aside for the moment. He left the question hanging in the air unanswered and allowed all of us to try to answer it from whatever view we had that might make sense of the senseless tragedy.

It took a long time for everyone to walk past the family, say two words, give a hug, and return into the sunlight. I took a gypsy cab lined with dangling crucifixes and saints back to the hospital, alone. In my hand I had the clear plastic bookmark-size reminder of Irene with her picture, the dates of her life, and her mother's expression at the bottom, "*La vida no es un sueño.*" Life is not a dream.

What would become of them? What were their options? How could I, or any doctor, treat a medical disease that was essentially a public health catastrophe? We did not have sleuths like John Snow—the man who removed a pump handle on Broad Street in nineteenth-century London to end an epidemic of cholera. How do we put a stop to the obesity epidemic that is killing patients globally in massive numbers? Just talk to your neighborhood pediatrician. My peds colleagues were becoming internists as obesity and its medical "side effects" became ubiquitous. Obesity and its Siamese twin Type II diabetes were obvi-ous correlates of calorie-dense foods, from Agent Orange–colored chips to the vast dead sea of colas. "Pouring rights" put sodas within the reach of every school kid and hospital patient, all in exchange for the pathetic amount of bribe money that went to school districts and municipal budgets starved for tax dollars. These predatory practices of focused advertising consciously, purposefully, put populations at risk.

For twenty years, as a young physician fresh from a big-city hospital

training ground, until middle-aged maturity and experience had satu-
rated me with clinical and hospital-based medicine, I sat in office/exam
rooms with patients and their better halves and listened and discussed
weight reduction and diet changes plus exercise ad infinitum as the
solution to the most common medical ailments that brought patients
through clinic doors: hypertension, hypercholesterolemia, reflux
esophagitis, heart disease, and strokes.

This experience in my office was repeated in millions of office visits
by millions of patients with similar efficacy. The zero-effect dilemma.
The magnitude of the obesity epidemic and the failure of medical
weight reduction interventions has outsourced the "problem" of dieting and weight management to the innumerable diet "authorities." It
has spawned a multibillion-dollar industry that is ballooning as fast as
the obesity epidemic itself. With depressing and predictable regularity,
studies have replicated the irrefutable facts. Dieting has a very limited
effect on weight loss that is at best modest and transient. The traumas
and stresses of everyday modern life can be assuaged by instantaneous food gratification. For anyone experiencing a bad day at the office,
domestic tension, parenting challenges, and financial downturns, food
is one of the sure ways we can get some relief no matter how transient.
Then we push Repeat a few hours later.

Months passed and then the insistent buzz of a text message cryptically reminded me, *coffee marta lobby don't forget!!!!* I sat stuck in
traffic in Lower Manhattan as half of the streets were barricaded off
for either a presidential visit or the relocation of a high-security prisoner. The ubiquitous black police helicopters reverberated loudly overhead. I wondered when domestic drones would provide surveillance.

Marta waved me over to a corner seat as I walked across the
polished granite floor. "*Hola, mi amor...*" We smiled. "I'm going to
check out the surgery," Marta said. "I can't afford not to, not with my
three babies—you know, including Mama."

"They need you," I said, taken aback by the starkness of her situation.

"Ha," she laughed, though it was not her old, open laughter.
"Before I couldn't afford the operation and now I can't afford not to

try the operation." The doors to the auditorium where the bariatric surgery session was starting had just opened. "I'll go with you for the first part," I said as we walked toward the doors.

There were a hundred people milling, all oversize, two-thirds female, young folks in their early twenties and middle-aged men and women and partners. The English/Spanish buzz continued as people moved to fill the seats and lined the walls around the room. The community needed lots of room to spread out. Oversize arms hung over the backs of chairs as the slim young surgeon in a crisp white jacket took the microphone and welcomed everyone to the bariatric surgical open house.

There was simultaneous Spanish translation. This was no accident, and not only because a large part of our population was native Spanish speaking. The Latino or Hispanic health paradox suggests that first-generation immigrants have healthier children—despite relatively lower socioeconomic status and lower educational attainment—than comparable white populations in the United States, probably due to breast-feeding and stronger social networks or other "mechanisms," but second-generation immigrants lose the advantages of the first. The data showed that Latinos had obesity rates second to none in New York City. The Mexican immigrant group was at the top of the list. The issues were as varied as the Latino populations themselves but seemed to suggest that cultural norms optimized chubbiness and size as desirable in young children. Throughout Latin America, obesity was looming as an enormous public health issue. Fast foods, high-fructose snacks at a four-year-old's eye level in every conceivable store across the continent had created in a generation a nightmare health debacle.

Dr. Parikh spent half an hour running through a series of slides that spoke directly to obesity and its effects on health. I glanced over to get a sense of whether Marta recognized him from when Irene's baby was delivered, but she showed no signs of it.

"There are several types of operations for obesity now. We operate using special techniques that make only small punch-like incisions in the abdomen. We insert instruments and operate using a movie camera on a big screen. There is no need for a big incision, and the healing time is much shorter. You are in one day and home that night, or at the latest the next morning." He showed some real slides of actual surgeries being done, with the instruments alternating with colorful cartoons. "But the most important thing to show you are the different kinds of procedures and why you might choose one or another. I will help guide you to the right one for you but ultimately it is a personal decision. We have three guests here today who have had the three types of surgery, and they will explain to us why they chose a particular type of procedure."

Two women and a man came out to the front of the room and sat in chairs facing the audience. "Mr. Clark had the band two years ago," the surgeon said by way of introduction. "Can you tell us about why you chose it and a little about yourself before and after the surgery, Isaiah?"

A black man in his midforties stood in front of the room. He wore a dark chocolate-brown suit, brown shirt, and tie. His head was shaved and shiny under the lights. He carried himself with dignity and looked fit. His deep voice resonated off the four walls. He didn't need a microphone. We all wondered where the patient was.

"I was a bus driver for New York City in Queens and Brooklyn for nearly twenty years and loved my work. I am a big man, over six feet as you can see, but I weighed more than three hundred pounds and had to go on disability over five years ago. Back pain, arthritis in my knees, hypertension, and diabetes. No smoking and no drinking. But I aged twice as fast as anyone else, like I was in a movie at double speed." He smiled and the audience laughed with him.

"Not working got me pretty depressed. It affected my marriage and my relationship with my kids and grandchildren. I was totally useless. The more sedentary I became, the more weight I put on. No job, nothing to do but watch television and sit. My only satisfaction was cooking and eating. I was worthless in my own eyes. My doctors treated me well. They had visiting nurses in to check on me and I had the latest medications, all six of them, computerized instructions and phone calls from a case manager twice a week. My life was all about medicines, doctors, nurses, and the constant threats and fears about strokes, heart attacks, and cancer. The first took my mother and the heart attack my father when he was my age. His first of four heart attacks. Until he was on oxygen and his legs were the size and appearance of a fireman's legs with the pants on." The eyes of everyone in the room were glued to Isaiah. He was speaking to and for all of them.

"I read about surgery for obesity in a magazine and didn't think anything of it. An interesting article, but it sounded like an experimental treatment. Surgery for obesity? Not for me. I was not going to be a guinea pig. Then one day coming here for a routine checkup—my monthly therapy session, as my wife called them, because it got me out of the house and out of her hair—I saw this flyer, the one you have in your hands about this meeting. We came together and we listened and I set up an appointment to meet the surgical team two weeks after that meeting. I saw them many times over six or eight months before they put me on the surgical schedule. They made it clear this was serious surgery and it would not work unless I was dead serious about it myself." He looked at Dr. Parikh, who was sitting off to the side listening as if it were the first time he'd heard the story.

"It took me a little time to get used to the idea since I was a full-time patient by then. I mean a professional patient, my new job. No pay and no benefits but full-time job. With high blood pressure. With diabetes. With high cholesterol. With arthritis. Even with depression and anxiety. The whole shooting match. 'What don't you have, Isaiah?' Minerva my sister asked one day as I was going through my medication list and blood test results. That did it." He paused a minute and sipped some water from a Poland Spring bottle.

"During the time of coming to see the surgeons and their team, I met a lot of patients who were coming back for checkups after their surgery. They were getting checkups, adjustments, having their weight monitored. They were all losing weight, some faster than others, and some were struggling. But what got me was when I talked to several who were a year out already. One gal, she was my daughter Mona's age, had lost a lot of weight and then was off her medications by twelve months. She was working again as a secretary, looking after her kids, and wearing her wedding dress around the house, because she could.

And you will hear from Adriana in a minute." He pointed to a lovely dark-haired woman sitting two chairs to his left. She nodded and smiled to the audience. Isaiah had the group in his hands.

He turned to the screen, and the projector flipped on. Isaiah showed the group on some cartoon slides how the band worked. The deceptively simple idea involved putting an adjustable plastic ring, like a small dog's collar, around the top of the stomach, creating a much smaller pouch for food. Saltwater solution would be injected by a syringe into a reservoir every four weeks, through the skin in the abdomen, tightening the ring and making the stomach pouch smaller and smaller while still allowing food to pass through into the intestine to be digested. It usually took about eight months to get to the right size for a particular patient.

"So after half a dozen adjustments, which were done at home by a visiting nurse, my meal sizes dropped drastically and I was feeling full. The weight came off regularly, and with it the pills I was taking came off as well. First the meds for depression and anxiety. I was doing something for myself and didn't feel dependent and useless. Then my blood pressure was normal. My cholesterol came way down and I only needed a small amount of the Lipitor—and even that is being negotiated with my internist. But the most important is, I don't need the meds for diabetes. I mean I don't have diabetes now. Talk about free at last!" He was a natural preacher and enjoying sharing his success with the group.

The other speakers covered the other procedures in the same personal way. The question period took a long time. Dr. Parikh spent as much time as was needed going over the complications and how the team customized the procedure for each person. "It takes time to figure this out, and people change their minds at the beginning. That is normal and part of the process. There is no rush. The day you are wheeled into the operating room, you need to know it is right for you. That is the test. Just like the folks here did this morning. I won't operate on anyone who is not ready. It is not fair to them or to my team."

He finished more somberly than I had remembered. "You have heard the success stories here today. There are complications. We have done well, but there will be problems. That is why we take our time and don't rush anyone ever."

While Marta Sahagún cornered Dr. Parikh, a line behind her rapidly accumulated oversize patients clutching their handouts, medical records, and X-ray files, stretching toward the exit.

After Marta's surgery and recovery, I met her again for coffee. Months had passed. Isabela, her granddaughter, was starting to walk. A photo on Marta's phone showed a smiling and thriving little person. "She's my little girl," Marta said, bittersweet. Doña Olimpia was doing well, she told me, and Jaime was okay, though he still had weight issues. Marta had slimmed down somewhat. She looked younger, nicely dressed, and oddly optimistic, considering everything she had been through. "I stopped smoking, Doctor," she said proudly. *How do people survive?* I wondered. Resilience. We would prescribe it, if only we knew what it was and how to get it.

"You know, Doctor, Irene took Jaime to the WIC program, the Women, Infants and Children program, until he was five years old. She'd wanted to breast-feed but they gave us free cans of infant formula from Carnation. What can you do when you have to work and you have the cans sitting there? You get hooked on convenience. And your baby is hooked on Carnation!" The Carnation "wars" were international, playing out in Africa as well as the kitchens of middle America. WIC's forty-year mandate was to provide calories for poor people. Ten years ago it was waging a battle with the food lobby to provide fewer calories for a large percentage of its mothers and kids as the "first responders" of an obesity epidemic sat in WIC's waiting rooms.

Marta looked up and around. "You have Pepsi here at the hospital, Doctor. Exclusive contract?" I nodded and rolled my eyes. She added: "Just like in the public schools. I heard the mayor signed with Snapple an exclusive contract for the city of New York. A way to bring in money to pay for education. Snapple and education? Our neighborhood hospital has a Burger King sitting in the lobby. You can smell the fries when you go through the revolving doors." The near-vegan, thin to anorexic, jogging, calorie-counting physician workforce promoted prevention and über-nutrition in the small outpatient cubicles, took care of the heart attacks, kidney failure, and foot infections on the inpatient units. And we contracted for a few bucks with the omnivorous industry that was the problem on the ground floor.

I looked at Marta. This was not the typical *mi amor* stance. This was a different woman, not just because she'd lost some fifty pounds. There was a new look to her—not determination. She had always been determined, determined to survive, to care for those she loved, to connect affectively with the world around her. This was different—a new focus maybe, a new intensity.

"How much did the hospital make?" she asked directly. I was taken aback.

"Hm," I said, thinking back. "The public hospital system signed a multimillion-dollar ten-year contract with PepsiCo in 2002."

"How much do you guys get?"

I did the mental math. "In a six-plus-billion-dollar corporation, this would amount to less than two hundred thousand per year for each hospital."

"How much does it cost to treat diabetes?" She was not going to let it go. I smiled at her—I could see now what was different.

"Well, let's see. Two hundred thousand dollars would cover the cost of one laser in our clinic for diabetic eye disease, the number one cause of blindness. Each treatment costs nearly a thousand dollars in a private doctor's office. And you need a lot of treatments to prevent the blood vessels from oozing and blinding the patient." I got her point.

The medical industry had been breached by corporate interests, from drugmakers, to orthopedic implants, to cardiac stents, among a host of others. The relentless focus on the individual patient ignored the social determinants of health that brought patients into the hospitals and offices to begin with. The social gradient of obesity was superimposable on a zip code map of the United States by income. The poorer the zip code zone, the higher the rates of obesity and the darker the color. At ten-year intervals, the rates were rising astronomically. The Southern United States lit up as the epicenter. A Rand McNally of a public health epidemic playing out daily in hospitals near you.

"I used to go with my parents to Puerto Rico when I was a child,"

Marta said. "Their parents still lived there in the 1970s. We would go deep into the rain forests, way away from any town. And there'd be a Coke stand. A rutted road four hours from nowhere and the red Coke truck would be tipping its way along the godforsaken path to drop off the bottles and pick up the empties. This poison is sold everywhere. Everywhere."

She took a sip of her coffee. "I finally feel that it's not my fault," she said, looking up at me. I was confused. "I mean my fault that Irene died."

I was stunned. "How could that be your fault?"

"I keep hearing it. My fault that I smoked. My fault that I ate too much junk food. My fault that Irene ate too much junk food. My fat, my fault. It's not my fault," she concluded, softly.

"I know, Marta," I said. "Look at the patients in this hospital. It's an epidemic. An epidemic is not one person's fault."

"I'm not going to let my babies grow up like this," she promised, though the words seemed directed more toward herself than to me.

The debate of debates over obesity in our society, like many others, has boiled down to personal responsibility. It is as old as American pie and hauled out periodically and dusted off to engender political support for a business-friendly agenda that promotes a citizen's natural right to buy what she wants when she wants in the quantities she wants.

The key strategy of the food industry has been taken from the legal, legislative, marketing, and risk-adjusted playbook of the tobacco wars. Many of the protagonists are one and the same, RJR Nabisco the most notable. The overarching narrative blames the irresponsibility of individuals as the root cause of obesity. "Why aren't parents paying more attention to their children?" say the letters to the editors. Consolidated corporate media receives its largest advertising budgets from the industry and gives it a pass. Corporations are providing their markets with choice. Government regulation, the mantra plays out, stifles the great American job machine and its innovation engine. Its most recent iteration has been the self-serving preemptive laws called collectively the

Personal Responsibility in Food Consumption Act. These laws have been adopted by half of the states and ban lawsuits against the fast-food industry. A tactic the tobacco industry wished it had in place before it paid out billions in settlements. Call it second-generation tactical maturation. The strategists from one decades-long engagement are older and a lot wiser when it comes to limiting liability, Congress, the Supreme Court, and the consuming public.

"Tell me about Doña Olimpia," I said, in part to change the topic.

"She's good, Doctor." Marta smiled. "She gets up, bathes, fixes herself up—her clothes, her hair. She can't see much, but she can feel—and she wants to feel nice. Jaime reads to her; she holds our baby. It's good for all of us. She'll be seventy next week."

It was remarkable the skill and teamwork that we could put into taking care of a septuagenarian diabetic with advanced vascular disease on dialysis and blind, with a 99 percent blocked left main artery to her heart, and bring her to the point where she could function modestly back home. We did the best we could with each patient in our hands. And yet I wondered what we could do to prevent our patients from getting these preventable diseases. We always said our job was not to solve world hunger, just take care of the patient in front of us. Where exactly did our responsibility start and where did it end?

Marta got up to go back to work. She promised to stay in touch.

The tachycardia of the hospital never seemed to slow down. In fact we all remarked that modern life was characterized by the loss of the ebb and flow or the sine wave of events. Everything now was about efficiency. Multitasking had become malignant, and all of the social media had an intrusive quality despite having a rationale for every "convenience" they offered.

I saw Marta's invitation to the "Runway" party one evening as I was finally getting to my mail. The flyer announced that the surgery department and Bellevue were sponsoring an event for bariatric patients a year after their surgeries. It was coming up in two weeks. She had scrawled on the bottom: "I have something to tell you."

I could feel the music pulsating and hear the shouts and laughter coming from inside the huge rectangular conference room on the top floor of the old TB building, with views to die for. The annual Runway was well under way.

I stood in the back row against the western windows with the late-afternoon sun streaming in and heating my back. Dr. Manish Parikh came over and shook hands. We smiled. He was soon engulfed by his patients and their families. A familiar face flashed on the screen. Marta had chosen a picture after she had gotten married and Irene was five years old. In a corner, an elderly woman sat in a wheelchair. She wore wraparound dark sunglasses and a pristine white linen blouse. Her hair was tightly coiled and her nails were painted. Doña Olimpia had made it out of Brooklyn to her daughter's celebratory walk. Jaime sat holding Isabela, who was now an active tot. It had been two years since her daughter's death. They had survived.

Marta came up beside me—I hadn't seen her. "So guess what," she said, excited.

"Your family is all here," I guessed, cheating.

"Yes, but not that."

"You've lost all the weight. Your diabetes is gone."

"Yes," she agreed quickly, "but not that."

"I can't guess. Tell me."

"I was voted onto the board of Healthy New York City. The local organization that fights the fast-food industry. I'm going to work there."

"Wow." I congratulated her. "That's fabulous!"

"They're going to pay to fight the *cabrones*, the bastards!"

"Wow." I really was speechless. "You're leaving Bellevue?"

"Yes. I mean no. I'll be back. But not as a patient. I'll be tormenting you till you get those Pepsi machines out of here!"

"Fair enough! Torment away."

Just then her name was called. "Now we have M A R T A, folks…" The emcee went into her medication regime before and after. "Only one pill now, folks, only one pill, do you hear that: one pill!" Marta had started to walk down the runway in her wedding dress in high heels with a confident swagger that had her audience whistling and chortling with enjoyment and good humor for her and for themselves. She reached the end, a few feet from where I was standing, looked me in the face, and blew me a kiss. Then she turned on her heel and walked slowly away as pictures flashed on the screen of the new Marta Sahagún. The crowd erupted in applause.

CHAPTER 8

The Singularity

Jeffrey had been brought in by the Port Authority police, found at the bus station in central Manhattan curled up in a fetal position under a makeshift cardboard roof between garbage cans. The cul-de-sac where he had been found was used by some of the city's hard-core homeless in bad weather when an icy wind spiraled up the avenues from Battery Park at the southern tip of Manhattan. The cops were pretty tolerant of the regulars in desperate times, regardless of the broken-window theory that related crime reduction to the arrest of squeegee men, jaywalkers, and unlicensed street vendors. Jeffrey had been a regular in our emergency room for a few years now. I'd known him since his schizophrenic break fourteen years ago, although I had not seen him for at least two. His delusion was that he was a Jain, a practicing member of an Indian religious sect. Mahendra, the physician in charge of our psychiatric emergency room, called my office and left his name and extension.

After attacking the metastasizing cloud of phone calls, emails, voice mails, text messages, tweets, beeps, and teetering piles of snail mail plus a show of force by the trauma surgeons about operating room delays for acutely inflamed gallbladders, gaping colostomies overdue for closure, and knife and gun club wounds that needed second-look surgery, I dropped downstairs and headed toward the adult psychiatric emergency room (CPEP) one long corridor due east of the main emergency room. Finally some midafternoon peace and quiet.

I nodded to the middle-aged black hospital guard. She wore her long hair Rasta-style, tied up in a single long ropy tail. She sat behind her ancient brown Formica-and-metal desk and was alert to everyone in the room. As I walked into the waiting room, full

of policemen and patients to be evaluated, I found myself looking through the Plexiglas walls directly into the coed CPEP holding
area. The staff were in civilian gear, pants and sneakers, and had their
IDs clipped to their shirts. They were idling around the room, heads
swiveling like compact radar units on destroyers, except for one stocky
red-haired woman on bathroom check. Every patient wore tissue-thin
pajamas washed ten thousand times. Many were lying on stretchers,
their feet poking out from the sheets and white blankets, heads covered with pillowcase turbans or limp forearms to block out the intense
fluorescent lights. The constant din of people moving about, talking, and shouting added to the hyperventilating atmosphere. Several
patients were lined up in front of the single bathroom, shifting from
one foot to the other, tapping on the door, their paper slippers half off
their feet. Another passel of patients sprawled out, using a long row of
blue plastic recliner chairs as small beds, like on the deck of the *Queen
Elizabeth 2* during another era through the lens of Fellini.

There he was—Jeffrey. He looked fifty years old, though I knew he
was really about thirty-five. He wore our standard faded hospital-issue
pajamas with a thin white blanket over his back like a Haredi prayer
shawl. He rocked gently back and forth as he spoke to the talking
heads on the flat-screen television secured behind a Plexiglas protective box. His beard had turned gray since I had last seen him. His hair
was biblical in length and gnarled in tangles. He looked like an Old
Testament prophet. Yellow cigarette-stained fingers with long curved
filthy fingernails jabbed at the carefully groomed and perpetually smiling faces on the TV. His teeth, where there were any left, were yellow-
ish brown rounded stumps. His eyes were sunken and had dark, deep
circles like makeup. He had a pale white paunch streaked with dirt or
shit visible through his half-unbuttoned pajama top. He looked in my
direction and scanned me for a moment, apparently without recognition. His eyes fixed on mine for a few seconds before he turned back
to the screen and continued lecturing the two mannequin-like news-
casters. They were twin sexless plastic Barbie dolls trapped in their
flat-screen world unable to respond to Jeffrey's jabbering on about
Christ, Muhammad, Yahweh, and the benefits of Jainism.

A middle-aged man in a crisp white attending physician's coat, stethoscope in the right pocket, without a wrinkle or hair out of place, opened the door to the interview room and welcomed me into his domain, Bellevue CPEP. Amartya Mahendra was a Pakistani psychiatrist who had a distinguished career in surgery and pathology before switching to the study and treatment of serious mental illness.

"It is more interesting than surgery and pathology put together, Eric. I couldn't resist it. Like an unseen seduction I got drawn into it after doing hundreds of autopsies and brain dissections. My first love. I know it sounds strange. Once the physical part of medicine was revealed, I became interested in the invisible part. The emotional life of man, the strangest, most unknowable, and most fascinating parts. Psychiatry, or whatever it is called, is pure mystery in an infinite regression of permutations no matter how many diagnostic labels are put on it. Medicine is my wife and family. Please don't tell Wendy!"

I had met his "real" American wife and gorgeous seven-year-old daughter, the true loves of his life. Over hamburger specials slathered with ketchup and mustard in the hospital coffee shop, he had told me about his training in London and later in the Bronx. We had also talked about his homeland, where I had spent some time in 1986 as a guest of the Karachi-based Aga Khan Medical Center. While in Pakistan, I had worked in the tribal areas in the Northwest Frontier Province, now the sanctuaries of the Taliban and Pashtun resistance to another empire's incursion into what became the Soviet Union's graveyard. Because I had once sat under tables when Russian helicopter gunships strafed the Pashtun refugee camps, I had some street cred with Mahendra and some primitive idea of where he was coming from.

"Mahendra, how is business today?" I asked him, knowing he enjoyed telling me the stories behind the stories of his patients' medical problems, as well as the fault lines of the intricate politically connected systems we relied on when it was time to send them out into the "real" world. Mahendra particularly loved to talk about what was real and what wasn't. He claimed it was his goal to figure it out by the time he was done. He figured one of his patients who appeared to have a delusion was really an all-knowing one with the truth embedded in the riddle of his delusion. "You never know, Eric. I have learned more from my patients than they have learned from me. I have been doing this for over twenty years—don't forget—and that is after two other medical careers. Plus both of my parents and my sister are physicians." He smiled. He clearly enjoyed keeping me alert and thinking.

"We are over census by fifteen patients, definitely in the red zone." He felt that getting over census by twenty-five patients created a hostile environment where an individual patient's personal space evaporated into thin air. Violent incidents were conjured into existence from an inadvertent touch, the wait for food, disrespect from a medication nurse, a gaze that lingered half a second too long. Pushing and shoving could escalate into a vicious assault. De-escalating acrimony and heading off tensions were mental martial arts. It meant accurately reading emotional language, decoding it in the moment, and having the tools to bring the tension down...with humor, a favorite sport, a candy bar, or a game of checkers. Mahendra and his team were all black belts. I loved to watch them in action.

"So why are things so tight, Mahendra? What's the deal?" My tone was neutral and matter-of-fact, though I thought I knew the reasons.

He looked into the waiting room behind my shoulder and said, "Just take a quick look around the waiting room and you have your answer. This is not magic, really. You can see there is not a chair available and we have three sets of cops here with new drop-offs." I could see the cops slouching against the walls, talking on their cell phones or to one another, sipping their bottomless paper coffee cups. The box of Dunkin' Donuts smeared with jelly and chocolate was sitting on the one empty chair in the room.

I swiveled around in my chair while he narrated, "The two patients across from us are old St. Vincent's regulars. We hired many of their nurses when they imploded into Chapter 11 bankruptcy and were picked up for multimillion-dollar condos. Or vice versa." Mahendra loved the total absurdity of the city, the madness, the dark matter and dark energy of the contact sport of politics, and the sheer—his favorite Yiddish word—chutzpah. He always had questions to ask in return when someone asked him to explain why Pakistan was so corrupt and how its intelligence agencies could be so inept. He knew everything contained its opposite. Contradictions were not what they appeared to be, and desire was not a four-letter word.

He continued without breaking a sweat, "So this was like a home-coming for everyone. We should put up a sign stolen from the land-mark Catholic hospital where you couldn't get a prescription for birth control pills but where there was top medical care for the gay and les-bian community of the West Village. 'Welcome to St. Vincent's. Wel-come to Reis Pavilion,' though I imagine it is part of the new condo deal, they get some of the memorabilia to add historical value so they don't have to pay taxes for ninety-nine years, or something like that.

"Some of the patients are here all the time. In fact one of them has been here over a hundred times in the last two months. His personality disorder, addiction to medications, and maybe a touch of something new from the street pushed him to come in, be discharged, and return in a few hours. We even started a special group to deal with 'frequent fliers.' Steve, our chief of addiction services, put together a new pro-gram with the emergency room and the Outreach Crisis Team to see if we can stem the tide. We get a thousand dollars a day for an admission and seventy dollars per outpatient visit and only a pittance of that if the patient has insurance. Go figure. I am just an ignorant guy from the city of Lahore in the Punjab. What do I know that the guys in Albany do not?" He was on a roll. Most people who worked in the medical system did not know how the system worked. He clearly did.

The simple explanation is that it is not a system. In no way shape or form. It is a congeries of interest groups that has carved up and distorted how health care is paid for and delivered into balkanized protected feu-dal states enlarged and serviced by armies of lawyers and K Street lobby-ists and ready-willing-and-able politicians. "Where I come from, people don't want to get vaccinated; it is a CIA plot. Here politicians warn peo-ple not to get vaccinated because it causes autism with the implication that it may be a CIA plot. Like the Rapture, Eric, the time hasn't come. We have to be patient." Mahendra smiled his enigmatic smile.

We spent the next forty minutes going through each of the fifteen cases in the waiting room that, because of the overcrowding, had become an extension of the CPEP proper. You could feel the body heat, the emotional intensity. At that moment an aide in a beige uniform wheeled in stacks of plastic food trays. Everyone looked up, and the temperature dropped a few degrees. Food always had a soothing effect regardless of the source. We had halal chicken for the Muslim patient in the corner, Chinese food for the young woman with the police, and plain ordinary cold greasy American grilled cheese sandwiches, iceberg salad, and solid bricks of apple brown Betty for everyone else. The cops were take-out specialists and used their smartphones to GPS local menus and order out. A couple of detectives went down to the Greek coffee shop to chill out on their break.

"Jeffrey, or Mr. Jain as he prefers to be called now, was brought in after midnight by the Port Authority police." Mahendra turned around to look into the unit sitting area, now converted into over-census sleeping quarters using the *Titanic*-like deck chairs. The middle-aged prophet was gesticulating to the wall and talking to a fellow male patient who was oblivious to his entreaties and fixated on a verbal altercation going on across the room being smoothed over by two tag-team behavioral health aides, one male and one female. I had seen them in action when an out-of-control psychotic patient was brought in handcuffed and bound to a stretcher. Bolshoi or James Bond, pure and simple. The patient would be stripped and searched, re-dressed, and put in the unit to chill out in a few minutes. Hardly a word would be spoken. Tie in place, not a wrinkle in the putty-colored Gap buttondown. Shaken, not stirred.

"You probably know him better than we do," Mahendra declared out loud to no one in particular. Just a statement. "Where are his parents now?" he asked me finally. He knew I had followed Mr. Jain, aka Jeffrey, for a long time. We all had patients we knew better than others, a few that got to us in some personal way. Most of the time we didn't take the time to figure out why. The why could ramify in deepening and widening circles. If you stayed on the surface all the time, dealing with the "facts" of the cases, you did not know very much at all. The treatment plan was a caricature, copy and paste. A game of what is the right dose of which medication.

"Back in Michigan," I said in answer to his question. "I haven't heard from them in several years. His father is a well-known sociology professor and his mother worked for a national kidney dialysis company as regional manager. She traveled a lot. Really knowledgeable people. Smart, engaged... they tried everything they could think of for Jeffrey. I think his drug use finally wore them out. Cocaine specifically. Who knows for sure. That is how I put it together. In fact, I saw an article his father wrote in a medical journal on his personal journey as a parent with his son's mental illness. The article took me by surprise since they appeared to want to keep things under wraps for so long. Maybe they wanted to protect Jeffrey and just finally realized how serious his illness was. Maybe they decided the best protection was going public?" This was a complicated business, and there were both public and private narratives for family affairs that spilled into our front doors. The narratives morphed out from the cocoon of family secrets into semi-public, awkward, embarrassing, financially devastating, humiliating, destructive, demanding, and lifelong family sagas. Rarely were the two narratives the same—nor should they be.

Mahendra sat quietly in his chair and turned his full attention to me. From where we sat in a glass-enclosed room, we could see 360 degrees from the waiting room into the interstices of the psychiatric emergency space. He had a gift of making you feel you were the only thing of importance in the room and on the planet when his gaze switched onto yours. I knew he had a big private practice and worked late into the evening every night. I was surprised he hadn't left Bellevue some years earlier for the siren call of a lucrative private Manhattan psychiatric practice. This was concierge or boutique medicine, the opposite of what we were doing every day. When I asked him why he'd stayed, he said it was because of his father.

"My father was a successful businessman in Pakistan, in retail clothing, and came to the United States and washed dishes. When he was in Pakistan he had unlimited offers to participate in widespread corruption and make a small fortune. He never once participated." He continued, "He told me, 'Son, if you go down that path even once you are doomed. What do you care about and what do you want to be? Just answer those questions and you will always make the right decisions.'

"I bought my parents a house a few years ago, and he lives a few blocks from my apartment. My kids hang out with him all the time. It is the best I can give to him and to them. That is why I've worked here now for over twenty years. The line between health and illness is a thin line, very thin. You never know which side of the line you will be on and when or who will be there to look after you. Everything else is myth."

"You know, I met Jeffrey over twelve years ago when he first got admitted to Bellevue," I said. "At that time he was a Princeton gradu-ate student. He had just completed his doctoral exams and was on track for his thesis, in religious studies in fact." Mahendra fell silent. It was now my turn to fill him in on the patient under his watch.

"I got a call from the mayor's office, the Giuliani era. 'Call Jeffrey Torkelson's father. His son is in CPEP and call ASAP.' The deputy mayor and Torkelson had been in college together. He was gracious on the phone and asked, 'One, can you assure me he will get the best care you can provide? Two, can you keep an eye on him?' I think some of it was the public hospital thing. Private must be better. The more you spent, the better it was. Like single-malt Scotch. You know, *Law & Order* crap. *Take them to Bellevue.* Like who do they think is sit-ting in the Hartford Retreat or McLean, the Bobbsey Twins? And if it is the Bobbsey Twins, then they're fratricidal meth-snorting pederast twins!" My riff was over.

"I came here and sat talking to your predecessor, Harold, now long gone into an academic psychoanalytic practice in Upper Manhattan. Jeffrey had taken a bus to New York City from Princeton. He went to a local Midtown hotel to check in. The clerk asked to see a credit card. He said he didn't need one. They pressed him a bit and called the manager. Jeffrey lowered his voice and confessed that he was 'God and God doesn't need a credit card.' He was on a journey to find Scarlett Johansson, who was Mary, the mother of Jesus. It was his mission to protect her from evil forces that were going to kidnap her into a

parallel *Matrix* world until the end-of-time apocalypse when everything would be exterminated in a Singularity, the Big Bang in reverse.
There was no Rapture for the holy in Jeffrey's delusion. A white powder would be all that remained of the universe."

"Sounds like 9/11 to me...," muttered Mahendra.

I finished, "He was clear that the world would end as it had begun
in a Big Bang, a Singularity, that created all matter and over billions of
years the earth condensed out of elements forged from primal hydro-
gen atoms. Scarlett Johansson, aka Mary, alone had the power to prevent the Apocalypse, and the rain of white powder that would be all
that was left of an eon of creation. The hotel manager said he would
get him a room and picked up a phone in the next room and called
hotel security and the police.

"It had been Jeffrey Torkelson's first psychiatric hospitalization. His
parents were on the next flight from the Midwest to LaGuardia Airport and showed up on the inpatient psych unit shortly after I did.
They were your ideal couple. Everyone was thanked numerous times
for our caring and considerate work. They were here during every visiting hour. They rented an apartment a few blocks from the hospital
and embedded themselves in their son's new ten-thousand-square-foot
locked universe. It was around this time that Jeffrey started calling
himself 'Jain' after the Indian religion that extolled all life, insect to
human. The Jains placed their dead on wooden platforms reaching to
the sky. The cadavers were eaten by vultures feasting on human flesh.
They circled the Towers of Silence, riding the warm air currents, while
waiting for their next meal.

"'Jeffrey switched from physics to religion in college,'" his father
told me when we were sitting in a small conference room off the 18
North psychiatric unit where his son was hospitalized for sixty-two
days. 'We didn't think that much about it at the time. You know,
they're related in many ways. Thinking about ultimate causes, trying
to unite everything into one grand unifying theory. That is the stuff of
physics. The idea of a unifying theory drove Einstein to distraction,
and he didn't accomplish much after his *annus mirabilis* except to try
to disprove quantum mechanics.'

"At the time, I remember appreciating the father's intellectual approach to his son's case. But I also wondered where the emotional side to this tale lay, the rawness, the sadness, guilt, pain, anything. His son was an inpatient on our psychiatric unit for an acute schizophrenic break and I was sitting in a room high in the air, in my Tower of Silence, overlooking Gotham in all directions, discussing particle physics, Brownian motion, string theory, and how many dimensions are required to satisfy a totalizing explanation of all of reality. Jeffrey's father and I were pretty much in a 'real' reality now, weren't we? Or maybe not? That was the question.

"Mr. Torkelson and I sat in that small room filled with pegboards, schedules, phone numbers for different community agencies, and Manhattan's best take-out restaurants, given gold stars by the staff. He took me through his son's medical history. 'Jeffrey was always sort of a math prodigy since grade school and he got interested in optics in middle school. The speed of light fascinated him. Why it was a constant and how it fit into Einstein's equation about mass. The relation between mass and the speed of light squared inspired his imagination and he got stuck on it. Our other son was always fascinated by sports. He collected things, memorized things, and obsessed about sports teams, ice hockey in particular. It was totally normal stuff. Not Jeffrey. By the time he was in middle school, he was reading Richard Feynman, the quirky Nobel laureate whose taped CalTech lectures about QED or quantum electrodynamics are cult classics. We talked to the school counselors, and they said he had a special talent and not to stress over it. *Like a kid who has great musical skills. Support it and let it go where it goes.* The school itself didn't have enough to offer him so I took him to my university where colleagues let him sit in on classes as a personal favor. I had no idea what this stuff was about and still don't. The math is beyond my capacity. He was a high-maintenance kid. We wrote it off as pre-adolescence, then as puberty, then post-adolescence. I guess we were fooling ourselves.' He was very matter-of-fact and presented a police dossier about his son. Like Inspector Maigret. I was not clinically involved and decided to leave those conversations to his doctors, social workers, psychologists, and nurses.

"Mrs. Torkelson had entered the room cat-like and sat down without making a sound a few minutes earlier. She went for long jogs along the East River, up past Roosevelt Island and the huge Soviet-style buildings of the Manhattan Psychiatric Center. She ran early in the mornings no matter the weather, 'to clear my head and get in the right zone for the day.' She would stay until late evening reading fiction and autobiographies and writing in black ink using artist's pens in unlined notebooks. She said, 'I have to be close to him and didn't want to be a bother. Just please let me hang out here. I won't get in anyone's way.' We were more than accommodating since so many of our patients didn't have anything resembling the all-American family. The families of our patients were more typically fraught, complex, dysfunctional, and compromised. So the idea of having a Midwestern couple in matching J.Crew outfits, with sharp creases in their jeans, hanging around the unit for a few weeks was a minor variation on novel.

"It took more getting used to from our side but after a week she was part of the social milieu on the unit, bringing coffee, thousand-calorie half-pound all-chocolate cupcakes with red sparkler candles for a social worker's engagement. The couple was very discreet. They studiously avoided other patients' business and affairs. I ended up talking to her when I had a moment. Even when we weren't discussing Jeffrey, he remained a heavy black storm cloud over everything said and not said. She was writing about her son's illness, tracing it back to her pregnancy. She was racking her brain for clues missed, opportunities squandered. A mother's guilt on hyperdrive.

"'He was always a complicated kid,' she told me. When and where? Her versions of events came out at first tentatively, then more assertively. 'He was very artistic and creative even before first grade. But he needed me with him and got frightened easily. So I took him everywhere after school and on weekends until he went off to college. Over the years he did very well in school and participated in many activities and we traveled together a lot. Maybe too much,' she said hesitantly, weighing her words carefully. She spooned them out in small doses.

"I asked about his emotional control: Was he easily upset, irritable? Could he relax, calm himself down? I had touched a button. Both parents started to talk at once. At that point it was clear that Jeffrey had been a handful, a kid who burst into uncontrollable rages for no apparent reason. His distress escalated until he wore himself out. They had experienced him as both tightly wound and at a high-normal range of intelligence. He displayed a sensitivity both artistic and scientific. They provided a very tight web of family interactions and participated in all aspects of his life. It wasn't clear much separated his life from theirs even when he went through puberty into full-blown adolescence.

"Now Professor Torkelson took up the narrative: 'He was a very irritable preteen. Sometimes that lasted months. Then it would suddenly wear off and he would be fine. During those bad periods he didn't want to see any friends. Stayed in his room, drawing and reading. We would hear him puttering in the middle of the night in the kitchen. He had trouble sleeping for months on end. Then we would have a holiday and he would melt down in front of family and friends and completely lose control, thrashing and banging his head against a wall, crying uncontrollably, just losing it. We would rub his back, read to him, and gradually, if we were lucky, he would get back to his baseline. It was like it never happened. We lived on edge, always expecting something to happen.' This was a common story I had heard from so many parents. The emotional regulatory system had short-circuited. The ultimate diagnosis was unclear. Too soon to tell.

"'We took him to the best specialists in Ann Arbor, to Chicago, even to San Francisco and the Mayo Clinic,' continued Professor Torkelson. 'We heard a lot of different diagnoses. There weren't two that were the same. He was a very sensitive kid and seemed normal in many ways, whatever that was. *Just let him grow out of it* was the advice from the head of child development at Stanford. And from a Chicago specialist, *Your son has serious developmental issues that are indistinct—undifferentiated* was the precise term she used—and could develop into anything and everything from depression, to ADHD, to borderline personality disorder, to drug addiction. No one mentioned schizophrenia.'

"'Everyone wanted to know if he was sexually abused,' Mrs. Torkelson interrupted. 'One doctor spent an enormous time trying to recover his memories of childhood sexual abuse. And finally one day they did...with a babysitter who looked after him for a year when he was about four years old, really a nanny-type person, a totally lovely human being. It was inconceivable to us that this had happened. But the moment was difficult. It undermined us completely. We doubted everything from our parenting, to our love for our kids, to our marriage.' She was at the edge of her seat and agitated, wringing her hands at this point. The professor waited to make sure his wife had finished and then continued, 'It was very difficult. Just at this time in California, there was an epidemic of child abuse cases coming out in nursery schools and day care centers. Prosecutors were out for blood.' A national contagion, it spread and caused a lot of damage. Of course it was disproven, but not before it took down a lot of careers and lives in a modern version of the Salem witch trial exorcisms.

"Mrs. Torkelson picked up the thread: 'We were confused and didn't know what to do. Maybe the doctor was right? But something held us back, and we just let it sit there never quite sure. It made Jeffrey more anxious.'

"'And of course there were all the questions about whether there was domestic violence. *What did he see, witness?* The questioning implicated us deeply in his mood swings. We started to go to therapy ourselves. Our marriage had never been a problem. We never thought so at any rate. We had doubts and even considered splitting up at one point.' The less professorial professor emerged, like a tortoise poking its head out for a peek around. He glanced at his wife, checking to see if it was okay to have emoted. She gave off no signals I could detect, and I figured they were past some private marital pain. Maybe it was a relief to have a diagnosis. Any diagnosis. A real road untraveled lay ahead. I had jumped ahead and stopped myself. Better to listen and to try to hear."

I was sitting talking to Mahendra in the glassed-in intake room surrounded by thirty-three patients in various states of decompensation, mania, drug-induced delusions, suicidal depressions, personality disorders littered with ruined relationships, Wernicke's encephalopathy from alcoholism, and a woman who had jumped off the Brooklyn

Bridge and lived to tell the tale (with some broken bones). And that was just the north side of CPEP. They all had complex stories. Deep histories, archival material we would never recover.

Mahendra was engrossed in the story of Jeffrey. He had known him as a street person, one who needed to be deloused when he came into the emergency room. Jeffrey's delusions made him King of the Jains. He swept with a small fine broom in front of his steps to avoid trampling invisible insects, and Jeffrey covered his mouth so he wouldn't inhale organisms thoughtlessly, ending their tiny lives. Whenever he entered the CPEP, he bellowed furiously when the guards took the broom away. As compensation, they offered him a surgical mask for his face, but Jeffrey threw it on the floor in disgust. Mahendra had the imagination and experience to know that behind every single patient we saw was a much larger story of a human being, of humanity. It was the thin line his father had told him about. He asked me to continue. "Eric, so the family suffered because no professional told them that no one can predict where these early symptoms might lead? You just cannot know. There are no predictive tools or models." I wondered how many more Jeffreys were in the room. He had all of the advantages of a supportive family, more-than-adequate financial resources, and access to the best specialists. His family had sacrificed time and effort to keep him functional and flow with his emotional roller coaster, providing the guide rails to keep him on track, hoping that time was on their side, that he would indeed "grow out of it."

"Mahendra, the conversations with his family that I'm telling you about were almost fourteen years ago, and the guy you are seeing through the Plexiglas talking to himself was twenty-four years old. He had finished two years of graduate school. He looked like a rower on an Olympic team. In fact he was a compulsive marathoner on a special diet and fastidious about himself to a fault.

"What made it exceptionally difficult were the unpredictable aspects of Jeffrey's emotional irritability, then moodiness, then exuberance, and then his impulsivity. There were scarcely two days in a row when he was what anyone might call stable. They felt drained totally. They were transfusing him from their own emotional reservoirs. If he was down, they pumped him up. If he was up, they calmed him down, and everything in between. They were exhausted emotionally but committed—even as they pursued their careers and tried to keep their marriage intact and maintain friendships. Emotional vampirism. When they added up the psychiatric consultations and visits over the years to a couple of dozen specialists, they concluded what you just admitted: No one knew.

"A neighbor offered them the best advice. She was a high school guidance counselor married to a professor at the same university. She had witnessed their distress and been silent. One day they went home and found an envelope from her under their door with a two-page typed letter. The first paragraphs apologized for her forwardness and the letter itself.

"Mrs. Bernier lost a thirty-year-old son to a congenital heart disease, hypertrophy of the ventricle, some abnormal heart muscle that triggered a spasm of electrical short-circuitry. A sudden death lying at his pregnant wife's side in bed on a winter night. 'I never thought she would recover,' said Mrs. Torkelson, recounting the moral of the letter, 'but she did. That letter was the best thing we got from anyone.'"

"What did the letter say?" Mahendra asked.

I paused to channel myself back to the time on the inpatient unit, talking to the Torkelsons when they had flown in from the Midwest, sitting in front of some take-out menus stuck to a bulletin board years earlier.

"In the letter, Mrs. Bernier talked about the kids she had counseled over the years. She mentioned the emotional growth and development the kids were going through. There were two things in the letter that hit home. Something like *Your son has an inability to regulate his emotions, so you are providing him with an environment to regulate them. That is all you can do. And you have to wait and be patient. What will evolve will evolve, or he will outgrow most of the behaviors. You cannot ask more of yourselves. Most of the kids I have worked with over the years would be blessed to have parents who could provide them with the love and nurturing that you have provided. The psychiatrists have no idea, and no way of knowing what will turn out. Worse for you, they cannot say this to you. They simply don't know and their way of saying they don't know is what you have heard. More consultations will be more confusing.*

"Professor Torkelson continued, 'At that point we stopped looking and searching and started to relax a little even though we knew we might be looking over a cliff. I mean, here we were at the edge of the cliff. We could lose our son and not be able to do anything about it. We finally accepted it from a woman we hardly knew.'"

"The hardest lesson for most parents, if they ever get to this point at all," said Mahendra.

"I asked them how Jeffrey made it through college since they weren't there anymore. He had gone away to an Ivy League university that was very demanding academically. 'In a way,' Mrs. Torkelson continued, 'we had nothing more to offer. I was exhausted and perhaps had kept him too confined, too much under surveillance. We were relieved he went away to university. You know the punch line, Doctor. We feel stupid, like idiots. He couldn't cope, it was too much to hope for. His doctors are telling us now he is schizophrenic. We have spent close to twenty years with Jeffrey monitoring all of his activities, thoughts, and relationships. Trying everything to keep him okay. Adjusting things constantly the best we could, spending a small fortune to get the best advice in the country about what he might have and what could be done. We knew schizophrenia was on the list of possibilities. But it's like on a bottle of aspirin that lists all the possible side effects. You don't think you're going to get them all or probably any of them, really.'"

Mahendra interrupted me. "You know, Eric, all parents feel so guilty when they find out their child has schizophrenia. How much of it is genetic? How much environmental? Why this kid and not another? It's hard to know. We have those 'weak link' associations. Some have to do with the age of the father at conception. Some hint at the use of marijuana. In 1943, the Nazis controlled half of Holland and cut the calories per person from eighteen hundred to six hundred in retribution for partisan activity. The Allied half of the country had ample food rations. The rate of schizophrenia in the starved half of the country went up by orders of magnitude. Pregnant women in Jerusalem during the 1967 War had a higher rate of schizophrenic kids. History gives us these 'natural experiments.' But how does that explain Jeffrey?" Mahendra always wore a white doctor's jacket and carried a stethoscope, unlike the rest of his psychiatric peers. He insisted he was a doctor first and a psychiatrist second. As he would often remind me, *"What do my patients with severe and persistent mental illness die from?* Diabetes, heart disease, strokes, kidney disease, all the common things that go untreated, under-recognized, and basically neglected by both my psychiatric colleagues and internists." Like me, I realized.

I continued, "The problem that the family had to deal with pretty soon was that Jeffrey refused to believe he had an illness. In fact, while he appeared to be fine on his medications to the rest of the world, he felt the subtle side effects were daily reminders of an illness he did not have. He gained twenty-five pounds, he was always hungry, and he had a subtle restlessness that increasingly made him uncomfortable. The conventional response of his doctors was that this was a 'small price to pay' for control of delusions, to finish his doctorate and have a life to share with other people. He took the medications for a year and then stopped them."

"Well," Mahendra concluded, "the smarter you are, the harder to accept treatment. I prefer the Bellevue patients to my Lexington Avenue patients in terms of drug adherence. They understand that mental illness is like diabetes. It is for life!" He knew as well as I did there was a relapse rate of better than 80 percent a year for patients who stopped their medications. They were now entering into the world of a chronic disease where accepting the illness and adhering to the drug regimens were the major challenges. As one of my psychiatrist colleagues at Fountain House on the west side of Manhattan said to me, "Eric, it is all about the medications."

"Did he have any relationships?" Mahendra asked.

"No. A few guys he occasionally went out with. Pizzas and Chinese takeout most nights. Pretty normal for geeky mathematicians, physicists, computer scientists, and engineers. But by this time he had switched to studying religion with a mathematical twist. Ancient

languages and hidden messages in texts were his thing. He was studying Aramaic, deciphering Kabbalah and Midrash, when he came to
New York City by bus to find Scarlett Johansson or the mother of Jesus.
Meanings within meanings, hidden symbols in abstruse texts in dead
languages completely absorbed him. Physics and religion were one and
the same."

I realized that I had seen Jeffrey over a long period of time now and
watched his schizophrenia or what we call the natural history of an
illness in real time, up close. After his initial psychotic "break" he had
been treated with a combination of medications and psychotherapy,
with excellent results. As one of his therapists told me, "You couldn't
tell he was schizophrenic—he had that good a response." From his first
psychiatric admission as a graduate student to the unkempt Prophet
before me unfolded a tragic series of downhill steps.

French researchers developed the first anti-psychotic medication in
the 1950s while looking for a way to assist anesthesiologists in preparing their patients for induction, to make them drowsy just before
giving them a general anesthetic. The Thorazine class of medications
was serendipitously noted to change the mood of patients and reduce
psychotic delusions and hallucinations. Executives at the French pharmaceutical company Rhône-Poulenc recognized the possibilities and
an entire class of medications was developed over the next ten years
and licensed to Smith, Kline & French. The remarkable had happened.
There was a pill for psychotic patients. The barbarities of a generation
of frontal lobotomies and insulin-induced hypoglycemia were finished.
Over half a million patients with serious and persistent mental illness
were warehoused in state hospitals across the country in conditions
that were more reminiscent of the Gulag archipelago in the old Soviet
Union than asylums conceived by nineteenth-century sanitarians.

A nationwide movement followed to "deinstitutionalize" these
patients and move them into community settings over a decade. The
lack of adequate resources, and appropriate oversight, however, along
with the exponential growth of a prison industry enabled by the war
on drugs, shifted the newly deinstitutionalized patients onto the street,
into the prisons, and into poorly regulated facilities in a booming new

"industry" of community therapeutic living. The comprehensive community mental health resources promised by President Kennedy never materialized as the Vietnam War spun out of control and siphoned off both the will and the dollars. While there were many success stories, and Bellevue worked closely with many of these community patient-based organizations, the full dark story has yet to be written aside from the occasional scandal of sexual abuse and another state politician being prosecuted for funneling funds to family members.

Mahendra and I went into the common room together. I went up to Jeffrey and said hello. "Do you remember me, Jeff? This is Dr. Mahendra, he's the head psychiatrist on the emergency unit and will be in charge of your care here." I spoke to him softly and slowly.

He looked at me and said, taking his time, "I know you." His eyes skittered around the room, rimmed in red. With his tangled graying beard and pungent smell, it took imagination to make out the young man I had met twelve years ago behind the wizened weathered face that bore the marks of street-years like intergalactic light-years.

His urine tox screen was positive for cocaine, speed, alcohol, and benzos. This was the cocktail in different combinations that each time led to his "relapse" and progressive deterioration over the years. The CPEP team had put him on sedatives to mitigate drug withdrawal symptoms, along with a rapid-acting anti-psychotic medication that dissolved under his tongue to quickly bring the frenzy of psychotic thinking under some kind of control, along with its more general sedating effects.

This was an all-too-common scenario for so many of the mentally ill patients in the large room. Unable to get a handle on their meds, they became recidivists, frequent fliers, high utilizers of health care dollars, cycling in and out of the medical system. The staff knew them well, down to a fine-grained level of detail about their lives—the lost families, careers, wives, and children, and their delusional systems. Their medical histories were filled with the most common diagnoses of hypertension, diabetes, obesity, high cholesterol, and, for three-quarters, heavy tobacco use. The statistics were revealing. Average age at death was twenty-plus years younger than among patients without serious mental illness. These common undiagnosed and untreated medical conditions were the bread and butter of an internist's practice. All were treatable with access to quality medical care, and the consequences were all preventable. I decided to see Jeffrey on the inpatient unit when a bed was available.

Our visit was abruptly interrupted by Isabel Humala, the middle-aged veteran head nurse who poked her head in from the nursing station door: "Captain Stanley needs to talk to you guys right away. Mr. Snickers is on his way. And to make your lives sweeter, he has finished his sentence and needs to be placed on a civilian unit! I knew you guys were blessed. *Suerte, amigos míos.*" She let the door shut behind her with a heavy bang and was gone before we could say anything.

Mr. Snickers. I was not thrilled to have this patient transferred to Bellevue at any point, regardless of our expertise and position in the public health system of New York City.

My first inkling of his existence was a phone call from my counterpart at another city hospital over a year ago. One of the psych nurses had nearly been killed by a prisoner who refused his anti-psychotic medication. He used her head as a battering ram on the floor until six health tech aides could grapple and manipulate him off her limp body. It took a prolonged hospital course and a long period of rehab for her to recover physically. The emotional toll would last a lifetime, and the contagion effect through the system was profound and instantaneous. The newspapers picked up on the story briefly and then let it drop. It was much more salient and clearly financially more rewarding to report on our imperfections and mistakes than when one of our own was caught in the line of fire doing her daily job.

At the time of the assault, Mr. Snickers was in prison for a parole violation and possession of marijuana. The additional assault charge was made a misdemeanor. The result was that he finished his year at Rikers Island with some intermittent hospitalizations for psychotic symptoms when he stopped taking his medication. His delusions were a mix of Old Testament imagery, garden-variety paranoia, and his response to watching Hassids annexing large swaths of his Crown Heights Brooklyn neighborhood.

And now he was back, unmedicated no doubt. Six foot four and weighing three hundred pounds. Maybe the Prophet could talk him out of thrashing living beings. The legal rules of engagement allowed prisoners to take their medications or not, even if they were severely psychotic. Their legal right of refusal was sacrosanct in the system of public health law that used the "least restrictive" test to decide whether they should have the medication or not. For many prisoner-patients at Rikers Island, it was rational to refuse medications—counterintuitive as that sounds. The medications are sedating, and the challenge of survival meant you needed your wits about you at all times. Better to have racing thoughts and command delusions ("that guard is teleprompting messages to my temporal lobe") than a jailhouse rape or loss of your hard-earned cigarettes.

Mr. Snickers had been at Bellevue a couple of times in the last year, both on the prison forensic unit, where we were used to violence-prone patients in the throes of a hallucinatory storm. Despite having Department of Corrections officers present and a staff trained for this type of work, the triggers for violence were often subtle, and our people were not immune to attack, beatings, attempted rapes, inappropriate touching, and every type of verbal harassment. An amicus brief, the Reynolds Agreement, brought by local and national patient rights groups supporting prisoners' rights, had "pulled" the Corrections Department from its traditional role of first responder. We were in a sea change of managing undertreated and undermedicated patients with a cornucopia of mental illnesses and drug addictions, criminal records from insignificant parole violations to homicide, and a textbook of medical issues. All of the patients had histories filled with shame and humiliation, the substrate for a volcanic rage that seeped to the surface with seismic results.

Physicians could (and did) get a judge to sign a court order mandating that a patient take medication despite "refusal" when harm to self or others was imminent. The court at Bellevue met every Tuesday. Our lawyers helped with the Treatment Over Objection paperwork, and the prisoners were assigned lawyers provided by the Department of Health of New York. We invariably received the okay to treat the patients, usually after a ten-day delay to get to court while the patient's brain was in a psychotic short circuit, burning through neurons. Being psychotic was not a free lunch for the hippocampus and the billions of neurons and their packets of neurotransmitters. Untreated or partially treated psychosis led to profound and permanent cognitive decline and a loss of intellect.

Captain Stanley, a compact and meticulous officer of corrections, found Mahendra and me in the warren of small glassed-in offices off CPEP proper. He was impeccable in his deeply creased trousers, polished black shoes, and custom-tailored white shirt.

"Gentlemen, Prisoner Duprey will be here in an hour and I understand you have chosen 18 North for him. Excellent choice since the team there is first-rate." The captain had a Jamaican accent that softened his stern exterior.

I let Mahendra break the bad news: "Captain Stanley, we are packed, in fact we are over census. The only place we can provide adequate space and supervision for Snickers is 18 South."

Before Mahendra could explain further and justify the choice, Stanley was off and running. "That is not a good decision and I cannot support this decision. We planned for 18 North and worked with the staff to ensure everyone's safety."

"Captain," I said softly, learning over some years that when things heated up we needed to lower the temperature, "I have worked closely with the South team and they are completely prepared to provide excellent psychiatric care and a safe environment for Duprey. Besides, they have had a lot of experience with violent patients. I know it is an Asian unit, but at any one time a third of the patients don't speak a word of Mandarin, Cantonese, or Fukienese, so this is not an exceptional circumstance." I then said the one thing that he couldn't and wouldn't argue with given his paramilitary training, even though my pants never saw a crease. After all, I was the "captain" on this ship. "I accept full responsibility for this decision, Captain Stanley. It is a done deal." After a few minor pleasantries—he was a gentleman after all—he turned and left us alone in a crowd of thirty-five patients both voluntary and involuntary, ten staff members, five police officers, a hospital security guard, and a Mexican guy with a wispy beard and mustache who just showed up with four pizzas in a red insulated bag, with white stuffing showing at the corners.

I put off going to see Jeffrey for a few days. The brief visit to CPEP had been unsettling. He was admitted to the eighteenth floor two days later. Mr. Snickers was there as well, so far without incident. The chief of the unit called and invited me to their community meeting. An email followed with a full-page color invitation for Chinese New Year with food and karaoke. What made me cancel some meetings to spend some time on the unit was a call to the trauma slot. Another Chinese woman had jumped in front of the Q train.

Dr. Rosalinda Estrada, a Filipina psychiatrist with mainland Chinese ancestry, greeted me at the door to the unit. A number of years ago, a bad incident at a state psychiatric hospital involving a monolingual Chinese-speaking patient had forced some facilities to reserve a small number of beds for chronically ill patients with staff that could speak Mandarin. Bellevue had responded by creating an "Asian" unit on 18 South with a polyglot staff fluent in many of the dialects that echoed the waves of immigration. The last twenty years saw a movement of Tibetan patients from political persecution and poor rural Fukienese-speaking immigrants who were not participating in the Chinese capitalist "miracle." Many borrowed the eighty-five thousand dollars from extended family and Snakeheads—as the human traffickers are called—to make the long and hazardous journey.

Rosalinda smiled broadly, put on her white coat, took me by the arm, and opened the door to the day room just as the meeting was getting under way.

Patients trickled in over ten minutes and sat in the semicircle of hard-backed chairs. Half were in pajamas with bathrobes and slippers, half in street clothes. The day room was a functional recreation room for movies, television, group therapy sessions, parties, and celebrations. There were signs in Mandarin and English reminding patients about the Chinese New Year celebration with red cutouts hanging from the ceiling and "Year of the Ox" spelled out for English speakers like myself. The room had been impeccably cleaned, and rectangular tables were being readied with paper tablecloths for the take-out Chinese food feast in the afternoon.

Jeffrey walked into the room in Bellevue garb, cleaner and with his hair combed. He took a seat next to a tiny Chinese woman in her sixties, fully clothed including a black parka with a red scarf wrapped around her neck. He had shed a few years in the transformation from CPEP homeless street person to a middle-aged, out-of-shape, down-on-his luck everyman. Mr. Snickers, or Mr. Duprey to use his real name, was sitting to my left quietly talking to himself between a behavioral health technician and a young white man, good-looking, with a full black beard Taliban-style. The Osama look-alike wore a plaid bathrobe, and his legs jiggled constantly as he carefully appraised everyone in the room.

The translator tried to keep up with the small woman. "My husband was mistressing...with the U.S. military...he stole my children and all of my possessions...I have to leave here and torture him...I have a new husband"—pointing to a black homeless man sitting quietly by himself in a chair, all six feet plus and skinny. He ignored the woman, who went on for a good ten minutes before Rosalinda asked her quietly but firmly to cede the floor to the next person with a hand up. This was a schizophrenic Chinese man who had been a model patient taking medications delivered to the Chinatown kitchen by the Bellevue community outreach team three days a week. A trivial illness forced him to miss two days of work, prompting an automatic layoff. He was sent to Maryland by a Chinese "distributor" to work in another fast-food establishment. He had missed his medications and rapidly become delusional. His wife worked in a laundry in Ohio. She came to Maryland, picked him up, and dropped him in our CPEP before she took the Fung Wa bus from Chinatown back to the Midwest to avoid being laid off from her job.

Half of the Chinese patients were delusional and refused to take their medications. Some had been on the 18 South Asian Unit for over a year waiting for beds at psychiatric state hospitals where turnover is measured in geological time. We hadn't placed a Chinese patient in a state facility in five years. Discharging patients caused enormous ethical problems. The staff knew that the risk of suicide was very high—given the number of relapses, the lack of adequate services, the stressed-out and humiliated families where mental illness meant shame and certain social death, and the relentless financial pressure to pay off the Snakeheads. The Chinese embassy was not helpful. The officials required elaborate documentation, though the papers were unobtainable.

Mr. Snickers had his arm in the air halfway through the monologue of the tiny Chinese patient dressed in her overcoat and ready to leave at a moment's notice. The unit chief called on him. "Mr. Duprey, welcome to 18 South. Would you like to share anything with us?"

Duprey stood up. At six foot four, in civilian clothes he looked like a linebacker for a pro football team. His voice was soft and nonthreatening. "I want to learn the secret languages here," he said, looking around the room.

The psychiatrist said, "These are Chinese dialects, Mr. Duprey, not secret languages."

"Whatever you call them, I want to learn the languages. I learned a secret language in Crown Heights. Jewish people, dressed in black, spoke in tongues. It took me some time, but I learned to decode what they were saying. I broke the code. I learned their inner secrets." He looked at the Chinese woman who had finished her comments.

Jeffrey at this point had his hand up and was waving it to be noticed. "Yes, Jeffrey, you can speak if it is okay with Mr. Duprey since he still has the floor." It was Robert's Rules of Order on the units to keep a semblance of organization. Duprey nodded that it was okay with him, and Jeffrey stood up.

"I think, Mr. Duprey, you are on to something by decoding these languages." Jeffrey addressed Duprey respectfully. "I have been studying codes and have worked out the unity of all the forces in the universe back to the Singularity. Life speaks. You have to listen carefully," he finished and looked at Duprey.

Duprey's eyes were wide open. "You can break codes?" he asked Jeffrey.

"I have been working on codes for two decades and have made

major breakthroughs. The essence of life is what is being revealed."
He paused for a couple of seconds, collecting his thoughts for Duprey.

"The rabbis have had deep insights into the workings of the world,
and Kabbalistic and Midrashic knowledge is part of the entire base of
the understanding. Like Planck's constant—"

Before he finished, Duprey asked him, "Do you know the Kabbalah? I have studied it for some time myself, and the riddles have given
up their meaning to me."

I was briefly teleported to an anthropological book, *The Three
Christs of Ypsilanti*, whose author had observed three self-declared
Jesus Christ figures sharing their delusions. Fast-forwarding to the
present, I was sitting in the common room of a psychiatric unit in the
clouds facing south exactly where I had once watched the Twin Towers
smoke and collapse in an inverted mushroom cloud of fine white dust
on a crystal-clear Tuesday morning.

Jeffrey quickly jumped back in. "The Kabbalah has some of the
codes. It is foundational to the knowledge of the origin of all life and
the Apocalypse."

Duprey was enraptured and had his mouth open to continue when
Rosalinda interrupted, "We have to let everyone speak, this is a community meeting," a statement she repeated in Fukienese and then
Mandarin. Duprey listened intently, his mouth still a gaping hole.
Rosalinda fascinated him as she switched Chinese dialects, chatted with a Filipina nurse in Tagalog, and switched into Spanish with
the housekeeper, who was sliding his bucket of water and mop into
the room. "I am so glad we have two new patients, Duprey and Jeffrey, who can share a lot together and maybe with the group again
tomorrow?"

The staff got up and made noises about moving to group meetings
and activities. Duprey took some tentative steps toward Jeffrey, who
was looking at him. They slowly closed the ten yards separating them.
When I left a few minutes later, they were gesticulating and talking
while an aide discretely sat on the piano bench.

During the long community meeting on 18 South, I sat quietly in my
metal chair listening with one ear to what was being said and the other

to what was unsaid. I felt overwhelmed by the enormity of the distress I sensed and how complicated the journeys had been to this particular "singularity" on this particular morning. On the path forward, these patients would come into contact with overextended caseworkers, long waiting times, imperfect decisions larded with a big dose of hope. In a society based on instant gratification, instant treatment with a pill, or instant redemption through rebirth, there would need to be another way to measure an inch forward. The relief of suffering was the only pertinent principle in this broth of human misery and fractured lives. One's frame of reference needed recalibration. Mine did.

After the community meeting I went with Dr. Estrada to talk to Mr. Duprey. She introduced me and apologized profusely as she ran off to a family meeting.

Duprey, or Mr. Snickers, wore an extra-large OR gown since he didn't fit into hospital-issue pajamas. He looked a lot younger than he was, almost like a teenager. He needed a haircut and a shave. He didn't look at me and he offered nothing spontaneously. I had asked a tech to sit outside the interview room; I wasn't Braveheart. A few days had passed since his admission.

We had persuaded Duprey to take his medications in exchange for a steady flow of Snickers and Mars bars. The nickname coined by the tech who discovered the sweet tooth stuck, and the candy modified the raging hair-trigger temper. While the drug companies were developing look-alike drugs, the Mars company seemed to have hit on the magic ingredient for some of our patients: Abilify or Geodon plus a Baby Ruth. Or lithium and Depakote plus Hershey's Kisses. I was going to try to remember to email the scientist who detailed the emotional maps in brain neuronal circuitry to try dribbling the active ingredients in Mars bars on rat amygdalas to see if it blocked GABA release and allowed a little forebrain electrochemical activity to make a choice to not strike first.

"Duprey, how are things going here?"

He looked up and said, "Okay, but the food sucks." I asked him what he liked to eat, besides Snickers. "Pizza, Doc, with pepperoni and a Coke and garlic knots." He was a little more engaged.

"What has it been like for you on the streets?" He had been robbed at men's shelters numerous times, so even when it got too cold to stay outside he had decided it wasn't worth the hassle. The rooms were large with bunk beds but no place to secure your possessions. "You get your dinner and breakfast and there is heat, but they kick you out all day, and your stuff is gone. I am not a walkin' Macy's, you know. They call me a fucking SPMI." Pronounced *spemy*, the term was an acronym for "serious and persistent mental illness." "I told them to go fuck themselves. You fucking satanists, beasts, and I spit at them."

So he lived off the streets and had hot spots where he could keep his stuff and sleep. He got his meds when he was in the shelter, but he didn't take them anyway for some time. He mouthed the pills and spit them out or sold them on the street. The pills made him disconnected. Like he had a fog in his head, full of smoke. One of the meds he was given a couple of years ago had given him the creeps. He was jumping out of his skin. Like it was full of ants, worms, and crawling things. He scratched himself so raw that his legs got infected, and he had to go to the hospital. That wasn't too bad. A friend came in and brought him drugs and cigarettes. He stole some from other patients in the rooms. He got some food, and he was warm. The meds he was taking now were switched and he didn't feel the restlessness but he didn't care since he wouldn't take the meds anyway when he left.

He looked at me, sensed he'd said too much, and pulled back completely into himself. The temperature in the room changed. I got up slowly and moved quietly out of the interview room. The next day I brought him a slice, Coke, and garlic knots and left them with the head nurse.

I went back to the day room and saw Jeffrey sitting near the window. I asked if we could talk for a while, if I could catch up on his life since we had last seen each other. He was insisting everyone use his delusional sobriquet, Jain. I think he agreed to talk with me more to break the hospital rhythm than from any desire to establish a relationship or satisfy my curiosity. He was back on his medication, after the judge had signed the order.

He had been in the courtroom at Bellevue on the nineteenth floor about ten years earlier. Back then he was just several years into his illness. He refused to let us talk to his family about his care and did not want them to come and visit him in the hospital, though they continued to pay the bills. Jeffrey at this point had been in the hospital three times in a year and qualified for the AOT program—Assisted Outpatient Treatment. His hospital-assigned psychiatrist came in and took the stand surrounded by the volumes of Jeffrey's medical records. Jeffrey came in with his lawyer, provided by the state department of mental health. The room had wood paneling on one side and plastic maroon chairs with paper signs taped to the backs to "Keep Your Feet Off The Chairs" with speckled brown linoleum flooring. Two armed court security officers dozed against one wall in full battle dress. The judge sipped a large latte from an orange paper cup. There had been three cases earlier, each one lasting fifteen minutes. The hearings involved outlining the "evidence" against the patient—his or her inability to take medication without supervision and stay out of the hospital or avoid behavior that might lead to an arrest.

The murder of Kendra Webdale by a schizophrenic young man, Andrew Goldstein, who pushed her in front of an oncoming subway train, had led to a law in New York State (Kendra's Law) that created a legal space for outpatient commitment. A novel approach to treating patients whose histories indicated that they could not self-manage their disease, it provided an alternative to hospitalization.

Jeffrey had refused to take his medication following each hospitalization. The psychiatrist was a young Chinese doctor, articulate and precise, who did not need to refer to all of the documents piled in front of him. He knew the case by heart.

The judge asked Jeffrey Torkelson if he had anything to say. His lawyer, a young woman dressed in fashionable Soho black chic, said he did.

"Judge, I have been taking my medications faithfully during the thirty-eight days I have been in the hospital. I have had no problems and fully cooperated with my treatments, community activities, groups, and my therapy. I have a stable apartment, good social supports outside the hospital, and graduate school to return to when I am released. The intrusiveness and supervision is gratuitous and unnecessary. It provokes anxiety and is infantilizing. I certainly understand why some of your clients require more onerous treatment regimens with teams of providers overseeing their care and well-being. However, I do not qualify in any respect for this type of program." He took a pause and looked around the room for a few seconds.

Back then, he still could pass for a graduate student. He had curly hair worn a little long, wire-rimmed glasses, a well-trimmed beard, a buttondown shirt in sky blue, and pants that hung well on his six-foot frame. It looked like Kenneth Cole, just like my suit. He wore brown tasseled loafers and no socks. Judge Garland shifted in her chair and started to open her mouth. Jeffrey jumped in, "I am in the middle of a very important project in my doctoral work. The AOT program demands are unacceptable and will interfere with the progress of my breakthrough." Jeffrey spoke carefully and clearly to the room.

"What breakthrough, Mr. Torkelson?" The judge was straying from her script, but her schedule was repetitive, and she had someone she recognized from her background in front of her now.

"Judge, Einstein failed to create a theory uniting gravity and quantum mechanics. He spent over thirty years trying unsuccessfully to unite the known forces of nature into one unified field theory." Even the guards were awake at this point. I didn't know if it was Einstein that got their attention or quantum mechanics. Jeffrey continued, "It is all in the Singularity. The truth of the cosmos and human existence are united in the primordial matter, energy, and massless state that existed before everything else billions of years ago. I am approaching that synthesis in my work."

I realized when his delusional system escaped into the open air that the judge would sign the order. Whether or not he was a danger to anyone, whether or not he would take his medications and follow the directions of his team, was irrelevant. Hidden behind this yuppie facade was a ramifying delusional system that made up his private world. And the branches of it protruded like an extra eye or arm when he was on his medications and fully flowed unedited and unadulterated when he went off them.

"Mr. Torkelson, you are a wonderful, brilliant young man. Your whole life is in front of you with such promise and hopefulness, and I applaud the great progress you have made here. However, you have been hospitalized three times within the last year and each time you stopped your medication."

Jeffrey stood up and started, "Judge—"

She raised her voice and said curtly, "I am the judge and you are not to interrupt me. Sit down and be quiet please. I am signing the order for AOT for six months. You will have another opportunity to meet here to review the order. Think about your decisions and the implications. It is not safe for you to be unsupervised at this point. Dismissed." She picked up her latte, turned toward the clerk, and started chatting. Jeffrey got up slowly, his lawyer patted his back, and they turned and walked down the aisle and out the back door.

I remember breathing a sigh of deep relief, though looking at the Prophet now I knew how momentary that relief would prove. But one of the core aspects of schizophrenia is the lack of insight the patients have about their illness and their lack of volition or forward movement to do anything about it or to take charge of their life. Some experts have even defined the illness as a volitional absence. Was it as elemental as a lack of desire?

"How are you doing here, Mr. Jain?" I wanted to know where he was coming from, thinking back on that crystallizing moment years earlier.

"Doing? You know how I'm doing. I am locked up and under observation. Look, I am an adult and know my rights. I can make my own decisions and do not want to be supervised and checked on like a prisoner or a child." He was emphatic.

"What about the 'relapses' your doctors went through in some considerable detail?" I didn't mean to play verbal chess with him. Just get his take on the ups and now more downs of his emotional life.

"A relapse for you is not a relapse for me. What you find problematic is not a problem for me. It is a matter of definition and power. At the end of the day, I am here because the state has the power to keep me here. Let's get real. You have the power to lock me up. I get it." The psychiatric diagnostic bible was pathologizing everyday life from shyness to menstruation. He had a point, and I could feel his tension and anger.

Despite existing as long as humanity, mental illness has not escaped strong public and private censure, stigma, and shame. Psychiatry as a profession was and is seen as something less than a hard science built on biopsies, CAT scans, and blood tests. Its bible of diagnostic categories, the *DSM* (now going into its fifth iteration in committee), is a phenomenology of signs and symptoms bundled into disease states. It is used by insurance companies for billing purposes and as a justification for disability claims, insanity defenses, access to Social Security, longer time for SAT exams, early retirement, and World Trade Center compensation. If you don't fit a category, then you don't exist as an entity. Thus the "fight" to be legitimized as an illness continues in the back rooms of lobbying groups and in the psychiatrists' committees themselves: Legitimization follows funding, and powerful players in the field control funding. It is a work in progress very much embedded in politics and payment systems. Thus a solipsistic system with complex eddies and histories that reflect the times as much as scientific discovery.

Mr. Jain and I talked for an hour on 18 South. As we spoke, the steps of his decompensation over the fourteen years I had known him flickered through my consciousness like an old black-and-white movie on celluloid. Despite the wear and tear, glimpses of his younger self would punch through and stir up an old memory.

"Mr. Jain, have you spoken with your parents?"

"They have interfered with my life from before I was born. You are not allowed to talk to them under any circumstances whatsoever. I have written commands not to allow them access to any of my health information. My lawyers have all of the information." He looked at me in the eyes for the first time.

"I understand and respect your wishes. Do you have anyone you want us to contact?" I knew the social worker had been down this road with little success.

"I have fired all of my so-called friends," he said with ferocity and a little spittle forming on his lower lip.

"I remember Dr. Fountain and you had a long relationship for almost fifteen years." I brought up the name of his longtime psychiatrist. I wanted to know why Jeffrey destroyed this long-term connection with the man who had hung in with him through more detoxes and bailed him out of jail half a dozen times. Dr. Fountain had gone well beyond the limits of the doctor-patient relationship for his generation of traditional Freudian analysts.

"He fooled me for a long time. I mean he didn't really fool me. He deceived me into believing that he could be trusted. I made a big mistake in pretending to myself that you can trust someone else. The bastard was going to take my ideas and steal them for himself. The son-of-a-bitch had been taking notes, filling notebooks with things I had told him in confidence over a decade. He put them in code and was going to use the information to decipher the last ultimate steps of the Singularity. There was no fucking way I was going to let that happen once I found out his dirty little secret." The spittle flew in my face and onto my black suit.

So that was why he'd ripped Fountain's office apart. He had been high, flying in fact on crystal meth. His brain had been rewired again, paranoid on top of the unmedicated paranoid delusional baseline. I had seen enough of these patients in our emergency room to know the power of these drugs. I had told families enough times that their kid was in orbit and might not land safely.

"I want to get out of here and be left alone. No shelter, no apartment, no home. Just leave me alone and let me get out of here. You pretend to be well intentioned, but you're jailers. Really that's what you are. I have my work to do and this is bullshit. All of it."

After an hour and a half of chatting with Mr. Jain on 18 South, I said good-bye, I knew for the last time. He would be released in a few days or weeks and disappear under an overpass or into the tunnels that riddled the palimpsest that lay under the skyscrapers, subways, water mains, and sewage gutters. He would join the sandhogs scraping and blasting the rock. Maybe he would find his Singularity once and for all.

CHAPTER 9

Trauma Detroit

The call to the emergency room had come in from the fire department dispatch just after midnight. The ambulance was four minutes
out with a young woman hemorrhaging badly from a gunshot to the
left groin. A passerby had called 911. He was coming out of a liquor
store in the Lower East Side, just south of Houston Street, and saw a
woman screaming, going down clutching her left side. Blood spurted
like a fountain into the air. Her male companion was frantically pressing his hand to her side and pleading with her, too stunned to call for
help. A couple of hoodies were running south down the street and cut
left at the corner toward the Baruch housing projects.

The EMT driver and his partner had been getting a coffee and
falafel when their radios went off. They ditched their food in a trash
can, sprinted to the ambulance, engine idling in front of a fire hydrant,
made a U-turn with their lights and siren on full throttle, and headed
to Houston Street. They could see the woman on the sidewalk with
a man clutching her as they pulled down the street. A cop car was
pulling in from another direction and blocked the street just as they
pulled up with their sirens screaming. A crowd had already gathered
around the pair lying on the sidewalk. The techs ran up with their bags
as the cops came out and cleared away the crowd and two other cop
cars and a fire truck pulled into the area. The streets are narrow in
this part of Manhattan, and even after midnight the traffic congeals,
barely moving.

The Lower East Side is a funky area in transition. It had the reputation of being a beat-up no-man's-land when I was growing up. Everyone
avoided it except junkies and the Puertorriqueños and Dominicanos

who lived there. *Loisaida*, they called it. That had been changing rapidly as New York City morphed over the last dozen years. Very little was left in Manhattan that had not been colonized by wealthy young couples and their children in Ben-Hur strollers. The rents had skyrocketed, pushing out the mixed generations of locals. Hipster restaurants, pubs, bars, and single-outlet specialty clothes shops lined the streets. After dark, and particularly after midnight, it was nearly impossible to walk down a sidewalk. Legions of twenty-somethings took over the streets and stood smoking unfiltered Camels in tight new pants outside the clubs. Squads of out-of-town young men and women cruised by in late-model black BMWs and Mercedes with New Jersey license plates looking for the right place to score and chill. To see and be seen.

The edges were still a little rough. Avenues C and D in Alphabet City had some dark areas that could be tricky late at night. Toward the projects near the FDR Drive below Houston there were plenty of drugs going down, plenty of dealers. The suburban middle class came to buy cocaine, heroin, and crystal meth. There was a squadron of undercover cops who looked scarier than the pimps and real drug dealers. The only things differentiating them were the gold detective badges dangling from their necks and the Glocks strapped under their baggy jackets. They would bring in their busts, wilted yuppies in withdrawal looking a lot less glamorous than when they'd left Short Hills or Great Neck.

It only took a few seconds for the EMT crew to realize they were dealing with a traumatic injury to a major artery with a massive hemorrhage in progress. The woman was covered in her blood. She was no longer screaming. She was very quiet and lying still, though conscious and responsive. Her companion moved to the side and allowed the EMT guys access. They asked him to keep pressure on her left groin as they put an intravenous into her right arm with a bag of saline, or saltwater solution, running flat out. They checked her pulse and blood pressure, listened to her lungs, and—with the help of her companion and one of the cops—quickly raised her onto the narrow stretcher they had retrieved from the ambulance. They had her in the ambulance within a couple of minutes, and one tech looked at the man covered in blood. "I'm her husband," he said in answer to the nonverbal question. The tech pulled him inside and slammed the doors shut. A cop car started to clear a pathway as they circled the block with their sirens on full tilt to get the stopped cars to move across a red light. It all seemed to take too much time. The teams were frustrated at their inability to make it to First Avenue and ride the long wave of yellow cabs up the twenty-seven blocks to Bellevue. There were a couple of other hospitals in the vicinity, some too small, some limping along on support from the Catholic Church or Albany handouts, but none with the capacity to handle this kind of trauma. Finally, after what seemed like much too long, they made it to First Avenue, a cop car still leading the way. The driver called into the FDNY call system and got patched through to the Bellevue emergency room.

"Woman down, around thirty, massive bleeding left groin, gunshot, tachycardic pulse 150, blood pressure now sixty over palp, thready and a respiratory rate twenty-five and shallow. We will lose her soon." His last words hung in the ear of the emergency room attending.

She was becoming less conscious and less responsive as they sped up the wide avenue with Alphabet City on the right and Greenwich Village on the left, into Kips Bay/Murray Hill and Stuyvesant Town. There were a dozen cabs lining the east side of First Avenue both north and south of 10th Street outside the Islamic Council of America Madina Masjid Mosque. The drivers congregated outside on the street in multicolored salwar kameezes and white skullcaps. They all looked up in unison, as if in a Broadway play minus the Lion, as the FDNY ambulance headed north. The traffic was finally moving, and they blasted through the red lights on 23rd Street. Just at the corner of the old medical examiner's office on 30th Street they turned right and drove down a long block.

The ambulance turned right at the East River and swung into the bay outside the Bellevue emergency room. Doctors were waiting outside the automatic sliding doors for the patient. The back doors popped open and a dozen hands reached in to help the stretcher out. The EMTs popped down the wheels and ran holding the IV bags over their heads, making a sharp left down two doors and into the slot in the second bay. The entire trauma team had been activated through their pager system and was waiting for "Trauma Detroit," as she had been named. A pre-numbered medical chart had been activated, one of the hundreds we have for emergency admits when there is no time to ID the patient. Standard operating procedure for trauma centers, using alphabetical code names for unknown arrivals when time to treatment often equaled survival.

There is a small intensive care unit of twelve beds, the emergency ward or EW, adjacent to the slot. The nurses in this area are critical and trauma care experts and enter the slot through a side door to titrate as much nursing care as needed for each situation. They have a window into their other work area so other staff can be activated directly.

The husband followed his wife as she was being rushed into the slot. The night nursing supervisor coaxed him toward the visitors' waiting room a few doors down. "You'll only slow things down in there," she convinced him. "I'll keep you informed. I promise," she had to add to ensure he would stay put in the small room. He looked for a chair, but it was standing room only. There were thirteen traumas that weekend, mostly broken bones, bicyclists hit by cars or pedestrians hit by bicyclists, and two jumpers in very serious condition. The administrator rounded up a few more chairs and brought some coffee for Trauma Detroit's partner.

The call to me came a little after four in the morning. It was Larry, the night supervisor for twenty-plus years. He had called me more times in the middle of the night than anyone else. My wife knew him well; they would sometimes chat for a few minutes with a diagnosis and treatment plan of her own as she waited for me to get the phone. Tonight he wasn't chatty. "Eric, we have a problem. You'd better get down here *prontissimo*."

At four thirty in the morning the Bellevue buildings were lit up and empty, like a circus tent from *The Twilight Zone*. I gave the middle-aged Sikh driver, his graying beard tucked into his red turban, ten dollars, told him to keep the change, and walked quickly to the swiveling doors then down the long ramp into the central atrium toward the bright-colored New York subway-style signs that welcomed you into the labyrinth of the F-Link, C and D Buildings, administration, and the main hospital building.

There were a few overweight hospital guards in dark blue uniforms chatting, a family leaving the building, and a middle-aged couple sitting on the stone benches desolate and tearful staring into the emptiness. I had no time to find out what loss they had suffered and kept half jogging into the labyrinth. I cut through the walk-in clinic outside the emergency room, swiped my card at the double metal doors, and headed past the ambulance bay to the slot. Larry was waiting for me in his pressed yet well-worn chinos, de rigueur L.L. Bean shirt with pocket flaps and perpetual *been there, done that* smile. He was a hardcore Vermonter at heart.

Cops and detectives were milling around outside the slot. An investigation into the shooting was already under way. The husband had been taken upstairs to the doctors' lounge, a very quiet area with computers, lockers, a shower, and fifty white doctors' coats hanging on pegs at the entrance. His mother-in-law had arrived to keep him company. His wife was in the PACU, the post-anesthesia care unit.

"What's going on?"

Larry quickly summed up Trauma Detroit's situation, her bleeding out, the emergency surgery. So far, standard. Why was I up in the middle of the night? Then came the kicker. "She received eight units of the wrong blood type."

I was stunned.

"She was dying," Larry continued. "We had to give her blood or she would fibrillate, a cardiac arrest."

The nurse jumped in: "We gave her two units of packed red cells from the refrigerator in the slot that were O negative. We tubed her samples to the blood lab for type and cross." Bullet-shaped hollow plastic canisters the size of seventy-five-millimeter howitzer shells hurtled through a vacuum system filled with specimens connecting the patient areas with the laboratories and pharmacy.

"That blood wouldn't have hurt her. That's the universal blood type for transfusions." I still couldn't understand what had gone wrong.

Larry added: "It wasn't enough blood. She was bleeding out. Trauma Detroit had cleared the slot and was on her way to the operating room. Just then, another trauma came into the slot, Trauma Houston, a Brazilian lawyer hit by a cab, his leg held in place by a leather belt. The guy was still gripping his belt with both hands. We had to cut the belt off, he was so traumatized he couldn't let go, like a rigor. The trauma B team attended to his needs and immediately sent off blood to be type-and-crossed for ten units of packed red blood cells. He had no identifiers so another premade chart was assigned, Trauma Houston."

Jon, one of our top anesthesiologists on Trauma Detroit's case, joined us. Tall, lanky, and self-confident almost to a fault, he was clearly rattled. He cut in. "The surgical team proceeded immediately with a cutdown at the left groin site, first controlling the blood loss with a clamp around the femoral artery and vein above the injury. The site was a mess and several nerves had been severed. As they worked away, the plastics team showed up. So did the vascular surgeon. This was going to involve several team members each providing their special expertise sequentially.

"At this point," he continued, "I was totally focused on Trauma Detroit's vital signs and resuscitation. Everyone in the room was concerned about losing her from overwhelming hemorrhagic blood loss from the gunshot wound. The room was tense and there was a profound sense of urgency in the atmosphere. We rushed an order for blood and sent one of the residents down the hall to go get it. When the resident returned with the first four units of blood I took them immediately and hung them to run in rapidly 'wide open.' Fifteen minutes later another four units of packed cells arrived and I ran them in sequentially. I know. I know. I didn't check the labels." Jon was distraught and so was I. Trying to avoid a death by cardiac arrest from life-threatening bleeding, he had skipped a key step in the *thou shalt* protocol for transfusions.

"Once the bleeding was controlled by the surgeons," Jon continued, "we settled into our usual routine to assess and repair the damage to the blood vessels and nerves using magnifying lenses. The patient was being transfused, there was plenty of staff in the ORs, and the patient was young. She would make it and they would do the repair, taking their time. After two hours the patient had received all of the units of blood and the group had settled down into a calmer routine. The nurses shuffled around the room tidying up from the controlled chaos of the first hour. A circulating nurse, in charge of supplies, cleanup, and getting items from other ORs and storage, asked to talk to the head RN in the room and one of the attending surgeons not involved directly in operating. She said it with some urgency. She showed them several empty bags of blood. They reviewed them and compared the blood type on the bags with the blood type on the patient's chart, name, and medical records number. They got all the empty blood bags and asked to talk to me. The surgeons who were still operating asked what was going on.

"Trauma Detroit got the wrong blood, all of it. It is the blood from Trauma Houston." Jon said it slowly and deliberately, allowing the full effect to sink in to the team.

Larry picked up the thread and explained that a second-year surgical resident had been sent from the operating room to pick up the blood. He ran to the window at the blood bank, agitated. The trauma patient in the OR was dying. He needed the blood. He had shouted through the old teller-style opening in the Plexiglas window. The two women who staffed the lab overnight asked to see the Blood Request Form. He didn't have it. He became increasingly agitated. "She's going to die," he insisted. He started yelling at them to "fuck your forms! If she dies, it's on your head."

Even with their combined experience of thirty-five years, the idea of a young patient exsanguinating on their watch was too much. They had blood from a designated trauma patient they were working on at that moment. They got the blood for that case and pushed it through the opening in the glass window to the resident. They were agitated, angry, and felt demeaned at being treated so disrespectfully by a trainee the age of their children. They wanted this guy to get away from them as fast as possible. They took his name down from his ID and decided to report him to their chief in the morning when shifts changed. This was not rare bad behavior. But there was a zero tolerance for abusive behavior of any kind. The tides had changed in medicine. Just how much verbal abuse were they supposed to take at their pay grade, at any pay grade?

"So"—I finally understood—"the lab gave the resident the blood. The wrong blood. Houston's blood." So many errors. The resident's. The lab's. The anesthesiologist's. I felt very tired, and not only because it was four forty-five in the morning.

"How is Trauma Detroit doing?" I asked. The critical question now was whether she would have a major reaction from receiving the wrong blood—lung injury or renal failure and bleeding.

"We're not sure," said Jon. "Too soon to tell."

"And please tell me Houston didn't get Detroit's blood."

"No," said Jon. "The mistake was caught while the surgeon was talking to Houston about the odds of saving the leg."

"Thank God," I said, too frustrated, even angry, to say anything else. "Let's talk later today. I have to give a talk in a couple of hours. After that. Call Patty to find a time."

Back in my office, I threw my coat on the table, flipped on the espresso maker, and collapsed into my chair in the dark. I was beside myself. I thought of calling Diana and then remembered it was only a little after five a.m. I flipped through my phone and then threw it back down. I stared out the window at the first streaks of morning light. If a mistake could happen, it would happen. The possibilities were endless, no matter how many systems and forms and cross-checks we had in place. I knew being angry would not be the professional way to proceed. And it wasn't good for me, either. At moments like this, I wondered if my cancer hadn't been produced by all the stress I confront every day. For many reasons, I had to calm down.

A long career is littered with cases of things gone wrong—"bad outcomes" or, in the most sanitized, medical-speak version, "adverse events." Sitting in the control center of a hospital can be a very depressing experience. Sometimes it is like being a psychiatrist when all your patients have complaints, bad behaviors, and emotional angst. I could easily slip into the diagnosis that humanity itself is little more than an auto-induced or socially induced mess of unmitigated suffering. I could forget the thousand and one acts of generosity and selflessness that go unnoticed every day. Enough bad things happen to reinforce a vision of a Hobbesian world both unforgiving and untrustworthy. It happens to police officers, corrections officers, social workers, judges, doctors. Why not medical directors?

Yet as I sat brooding, it also occurred to me that constantly being aware how many bad things could happen was the best preventive medicine, a mental strategy that prompted a kind of hypervigilance. It wasn't the only thing that was needed, but we did need it. I decided that would be the subject for my talk today to the hospital staff. One aspect of my job was patient safety, maybe the most important part of the job. I decided to talk about what I had learned from mistakes I had seen firsthand over my career. It would not be hard to find the cases. I ripped up my prepared comments, consigned them to the trash can. I quickly jotted down one through four with a couple of words after each number in block red letters on the back of an announcement for a fund-raiser with the Greater New York Hospital Association. I had given up on the ubiquitous omnivorous PowerPoint presentation years earlier. Stories told the tale better than multicolored Disney-style animation—all distraction and faux entertainment.

A couple of hours later, heavily fortified with caffeine, I got up in front of a conference room packed with four hundred people in uniforms from various areas of the hospital. Maroon scrubs, blue scrubs, gray scrubs, white lab coats, surgical booties, and gray double-breasted suits lined the walls around the edges. "I want to talk about things I have learned in my career from a few cases that I think about nearly every day, and some that have been uninvited guests in my sleep. I am sure you all have similar cases that you have known in your broad and varied professional experience.

"My first case involved a prominent surgeon. Let's call him Dr. P. Dr. P had decided to do a case in an operating room that he and his team were not familiar with. They were an outstanding group who had worked together for many years and had a reputation for clinical excellence. A different hospital's surgical program had expanded and P had volunteered to operate on the first case in the new environment, to guarantee its success. The first patient was carefully selected, and the preparation was exquisite enough to make this a non-event. What had not been considered, however, was that Dr. P's experienced team was not familiar with this particular operating room. Operating rooms are not like 747 cockpits. They are not all identical. A pilot does not need to know what kind of plane he or she is flying. Planes don't have local nicknames or lists of peculiarities. But, unbelievable as it sounds, we know that each operating room is different. All the equipment is different, from different companies, different vendors, different arrangements, setups, electricity outlets, computer systems, supplies, and doors. So everyone's rhythm and circulation in the room differs in each OR. The lighting and spatial arrangements all vary—and some variations are so subtle, they are beneath the radar, really invisible.

"So Dr. P and his hand-chosen, experienced team were working in a new OR. A tube got hooked up incorrectly. A tube that had been hooked up a thousand times before by a senior technician who could do it during REM sleep. A seemingly routine operation turned south in a nanosecond, and the patient began tanking. The banality of the error was so apparent and so inevitable given the circumstances. I was in the back of the OR that day in crisp blue scrubs and a sweatshirt—they like the temperature at sixty degrees—excited about expanding the new program. I was a fly on the wall. There to celebrate lots of hard work and hard-earned success. I learned more in five minutes about how and why things can and do go wrong than I had learned in decades of practice." The room was quiet. I stood behind the lectern looking around the huge room at my colleagues individually and talking slowly.

"The second case is about magical thinking in medicine—the magic of technology. The prevailing national myth is that technology equals progress; that it can and will fix everything. Another dose of technology will eliminate all risk and eliminate the effects from global warming, food scarcity, water shortages, peak oil. Everything. The fact is, however, that every technological solution introduces another set of problems, and some are worse than the problems they are supposed to solve. It bypasses the need to work better together. The technology often outpaces our ability to manage it, socially, politically, even prac-tically. But I am jumping ahead.

"All of you have walked through an intensive care unit. If you're like me, you're struck by the complex and exasperating monitoring equip-ment sending real-time signals to the staff caring for a patient. Elec-tronic signals via beep, blip, flashing lights, and monitors transmitting huge amounts of data inputs that continuously add information. If the computers detect findings outside normal limits, they set off an alarm. The constant noise, lights, and beeps are nerve-racking. Like the car alarm that rattles your sleep in the middle of the night and that the entire neighborhood ignores, safely assuming it's a mistake.

"Alarm fatigue follows the same logic. Too many alarms and they are discounted, downgraded, and sometimes out of sheer frustration just turned off. A top nurse was trying to get his work done at his desk. The steady beeps and flashes for trivial occurrences, like a line falling off when a patient moved, were overwhelming. He turned off the beep status on the monitor. Guess what? The patient died. We plug and play and don't understand what we have just spent millions of dollars on. There is no quick fix. There is no plug and play. There is no such thing. These are myths and legends I read to my grandchildren." They all got it and hands went up. I said please hold on, I had two more examples, and then we would talk.

"A number of years ago, data on our infection rates was on the agenda for a routine meeting in my office over coffee and bagels, New York–style. Lots of data and flow charts full of information. I kept turning the sheets upside down. The curves made no sense. I was told by my expert that we were doing fine. Our infection rates were where they were supposed to be. Well, they might have been where they should have been if I held the paper upside down. So I said, 'You mean to tell me the graphs are not upside down?'

"He explained to me, 'The worsening performance is normal when you have our kind of patients. They are sicker and more com-plicated. We are actually doing better because it should actually be worse.' Sounded like the phalanx of bankers and government econo-mists talking about the recession aka depression. Infections and errors were inevitable. Part of life. The way the planets circled the sun." I paused and let the words penetrate. "This was flat-earth thinking. Pre-Galileo. Maybe we needed an Aztec calendar specialist, 2012 is here. Why do anything at all?

"I flipped the charts upside down and said that this is where we had to be without exception. No errors. No avoidable infections. Not one. Never. Period. I told him our patients were exceptional but not in the way he was describing them.

"Probably the biggest improvement in intensive care in this country has been the introduction of pencils and paper into ICUs. The now famous checklist. These are the five things you have to do twice a day to prevent infections. These are the five to prevent pneumonias on ventilators. Paper and pencils. The Luddites may win yet!" People rustled, smiled, and nodded. "Who was Dr. Luddite?" I heard from my right side. "And the real point of the checklists is to get people to talk together! It may not matter what is on the lists!"

The final case I presented had happened some years ago early in my career, but it still haunted me. "A patient was transferred from a hospital on Staten Island for specialty treatment. The woman had a benign brain tumor that was giving her migraines. Benign or not, anything in the brain can be deadly, trapped in this bony vise we call a skull. The only way to relieve the pressure was to press down into the narrow canal where the nerve fibers exit at the base of the brain, where the spinal cord begins. We examined her and repeated the CT scan and observed her in an intensive care area under close and careful observation by an experienced team.

"The nurses became alarmed when she started speaking in Mandarin, like speaking in tongues. She had always spoken in English before, although she was multilingual. They regarded this switch as an ominous sign. They paged the physicians in charge to move on the patient right away. Her exam was otherwise unchanged. After much discussion and review by the physician team, it was decided to continue to observe the patient. The nurses were not happy and continued to lobby for more aggressive intervention. To them, the language shift meant that the benign tumor mass was pressing on her brain stem. Too much pressure would cause herniation—that is, it would force this most sensitive part of the brain against the canal's hard bony walls. Two hours later, the patient was in the operating room, having lost consciousness. She died. The organ donor team was activated the next day. Many lives were saved, the woman's legacy.

"These are just a few examples from hundreds. They are icons of what the core challenges are for all of us. So number one: A great team cannot make up for the lack of a standard set of procedures in a standard operating room. The only thing that had remained the same was the music in an old CD player they brought from their old OR to this new one. There is a lot to be learned from your next flight to Miami. Variation within the medical industry is inherently unsafe and potentially lethal.

"Second: Hardware and software are amazing. But they have serious limitations, and they introduce their own set of problems. We all turn childish in front of the promise of solutions from blinking lights in a shiny metal container. Our own electronic medical record has been rechristened at least eight times as the industry consolidates and it is purchased again and again. Once you think you own it, you are owned by the vendor, unless you know as much as or more than they do.

"My third example shows how vital it is to set our own bar high. When we start to rationalize mediocrity, then we are condemned to it. Mediocrity. Multimillion-dollar investments were not necessary to turn around that upside-down graph. The questions on the pads of paper or tree bark force us to talk to one another, to answer the same questions, every day without exception, face-to-face.

"And finally, I couldn't tell a patient's story in front of two hundred nurses in one room without including a doctor's number one lesson: We all have to listen to our nurses. Listen to the people who spend all of their time at the bedside. You really don't need gray hair to figure that one out. But you will get it prematurely if you don't!"

I ended the conference in the twelfth-floor Rose Room conference center with a Circle Line boat making its way north up the East River, the deck packed with tourists as it cruised past the Waterworks Restaurant on a barge jutting into the river. The sun was glinting gold off the UN directly to our north. A helicopter was landing. My colleagues were chatting in clumps, some waiting to catch up with me as we strolled to the elevators and back to work. Normally, I would have invited someone to have coffee with me back in my office. But not today.

First, I stopped to see how Diego Matta was recuperating from the amputation. The international phone calls had started as soon as he arrived at Bellevue. Matta's mother had flown in overnight from São Paulo, a formidable matriarch. She informed me the rest of the family would be arriving today, and I promised to stop by later.

Then I checked in on Trauma Detroit. Her husband was in the doctors' lounge just off the OR main entrance. The nurses had found a spot for him to sit quietly and where they could find him. He was sitting with his winter coat over his shoulders. He looked exhausted. His mother-in-law slept in a well-used armchair in the corner. He was on his cell phone when I walked in. He wound up when he saw me come in with my white coat and scrubs. "I will call you back. One of the doctors is here." I introduced myself and gave him my card. "I'm Charles. Chuck Reed," he said, standing up.

We shook hands. I gave him an update, leaving out the most glaringly important detail. That would have to come later.

I went through her injuries and what the surgeons had done. The major vessels had been repaired; the bleeding had been controlled for some time. They were making sure all the damage was controlled and a plastic surgeon with skills in microsurgery was looking at the nerves and doing a repair through a microscope. She was stable and we were hopeful. Youth had put her in the likely-to-make-it column. Hemorrhagic deaths were not common, but they did happen and we did not want one on our watch. Ironic, I thought, given what had happened.

I asked if I could spend some time talking about what happened in the Lower East Side. He gave me a *You too?* look. "The cops," he told me, "have been at me for hours. Did I know the shooter? Do I buy or use drugs? Does she? On and on. Like I'm going to have someone shoot my wife? Fuck." He looked over his shoulder at an older woman wrapped in a blanket, but she was still asleep. I let Chuck talk about his interactions with the police, but then he said he didn't mind going over the events one more time.

The crux of the story was that two men had tried to snatch the woman's bag and she had resisted. They shot her, grabbed it, and ran off. The rest I knew.

"How long have you guys been together? Tell me a little about her," I asked, quietly keeping Detroit's mother in view and avoiding the detectives' line of questioning.

Reed came around. "Susanne is a dancer. She came to New York City ten years ago from the suburbs. She worked part-time in different gigs. They went nowhere really. She used up her savings after a few months. Luckily she found an office day job at a private school to pay the rent and tutored high school preppies in French. Pretty much like everyone else we know in New York City. We live in a world of waiters, bartenders, special-event caterers, grave-shift doormen who are artists, singers, musicians, and dancers trying to hack it here." Sounded pretty similar to my kids and a lot of our friends. The great immigration to the city to find yourself and pursue a dream, a fantasy until reality imposed itself—financial reality that is.

"So what's she like?" I murmured.

He smiled, then remembered where she was. "Susanne is the quiet and introverted type. Super intelligent and sensitive. She shouldn't have messed with those guys who were robbing us. Who cares about the money, a cell phone and stuff? It doesn't matter. She responds, reacts first. That is how she is wired. She goes from hypervigilance keyed up to low, moody, pulling away. She cycles like that." *Like what*, I thought.

"So she can be pretty reactive, huh? Got to be careful in the city— like any city, I guess. Life can get pretty cheap depending on the situation. Two dollars and change during the crack scene in New York." One of my doctor colleagues had been killed in the parking lot at Kings County at high noon for the change in his pocket.

He agreed and said, "Yeah, I do know all about that."

"What do you mean?" I asked him.

"I am retired military, army, on disability now. Iraq and Afghanistan multiple tours. Fucked me up pretty much. I'd been living with my parents in New Jersey when I met Susanne." He seemed like he wanted to talk. I just listened.

"I spent four years overseas. I had been married before I was sent overseas, the stress of the two tours killed off the relationship. Can't blame my ex. You sit and wait and you form other relationships. It was painful for sure but like the common cold everyone suffers from it over there or when they come home."

"Were you injured?" I knew it was a meaningless question even as it came out of my mouth. So many vets came back with the invisible injuries. They were rewired by the experience.

"The command were running us really close to the Pakistan border. There were some advanced bases to support some ops going into the Northwest Frontier Province, the 'stans' as we called them. I was on a small base running patrols for the groups going deep on reconnaissance trips. We would even get stuff from Peshawar, the capital of the wild west." I could start to imagine the isolation, cold, and fear from being way out there with a long helicopter ride back even to what passed for civilization in an armed camp.

"We got shot up pretty bad and had to evacuate the camp. Burned everything and blew it up. We lost some guys. I was burned on my legs." He pulled up a pant leg where he had the telltale marks of third-degree burns and surgery. "Bad shit going down."

"Did they ship you back to the States?"

"Yeah. I've been through rehab after the surgeries and grafts. They did a pretty good job. By this time I'd been out of the military for a year, had disability, and was back with my parents to continue rehab and psych treatments and try to figure out where my life is going. There were lots of times, sitting in my childhood bedroom, I had no idea if it was going anyplace."

"Susanne?"

"I lucked out. Some friends dragged me into the city one weekend to just get me out of the house and from in front of the television set. There was a party for a friend's friend who catered big expensive parties for wealthy people. Music, drinks, a barbecue out back. Susanne was there alone and we just picked up a random conversation standing in line for smoked ribs dripping in chipotle sauce—which I promptly spilled on her."

"So chipotle brought you two together?" I smiled at Reed. He was looser and slightly more relaxed.

"I was terrified of what she would think of me when she saw my legs and thighs. I ain't pretty."

"But everything is working okay, right?" I asked him.

"Most of the time," he shot back. "She didn't care. I looked like an armadillo. That's what she said. But not making fun of me. I was like a wounded bird that she looked after. I did need looking after." He added that matter-of-factly. And then continued without prompting.

"It hasn't been easy at all. Not just my burns. Sometimes the complete meaninglessness of life in these dead-end communities sucks my soul right out. People getting blown to bits so suburbanites could sit in their SUVs waiting to go through the Holland Tunnel for under four dollars a gallon? Shop to support the troops? Nobody here has a clue what is going on and really doesn't care. So much for the volunteer army."

"Do you have trouble sleeping?"

He started with a list of complaints—anxiety, flashbacks, the fitful sleeping, hypervigilance. Clearly PTSD. He started talking about the treatment programs, the cost, the medical opinions and prognoses. The program that had worked the best was a virtual-reality one in which he had gradually been able to reenact the explosion. He explained about wearing the goggles as the therapist walked him through the scenario, again and again, slowly adding more and more realistic details. Increasing the dose of trauma a drop at a time while monitoring his pulse, his reactivity.

"Are you on meds?"

He stopped talking for a moment. Maybe the cops had asked him the same question.

He looked over his shoulder at his mother-in-law. She had opened her eyes briefly then dropped back into semi-consciousness.

"Yes," he said, "I've done all the meds. But believe it or not, I'm feeling better. With Susanne. She has been the best treatment. I mean I was in emotional hibernation. She woke me up."

I smiled and promised to come back with an update in a few hours. The cops were returning as I was leaving.

I went to see how Trauma Houston was doing. The decision to amputate Matta's leg was not difficult. Everything below his knee was mangled, the vessels and nerves shredded by the steel bumper. I met him in the intensive care unit, heavily sedated, his mother by his side. Everyone understood he was a high-profile patient. She demanded every assurance that he would receive the finest treatment. Her children were just beginning to arrive from Brazil. She employed all of them and the in-laws in the family's enterprises and kept a careful watch on everything and everybody. They were all exhausted. After I assured them that Diego would be well looked after, I promised to come back and left the room.

I called Marion from crime victims on my way down to my office. "Look, Marion, we got this trauma case overnight. Patient is in the OR and husband is a vet from the Middle East with a long history. Can you swing by soon and let me know your thoughts later. This is a really fragile situation."

"Of course, I heard about the gunshot on 1010 WINS when I was checking for delays on the Long Island Expressway so I could plan my assault on Manhattan and how much coffee I would need, one gallon or two. I'll check in and call you later." Reed would need someone to talk to and sit with through this time when his wife's life hung by a thread. Our therapists had seen just about everything that one human can do to another and helped to reconnect the pieces. They could help moderate the police interrogations and bring in additional help if and when it was needed. I couldn't assess how vulnerable he might be, but there were people at Bellevue who could.

Patty knocked on the door of my office later that afternoon and ushered in Jon and the trauma surgeon, Elias. I shut the door. "Have a seat. Let's go over Trauma Detroit from a couple of different points of view."

Elias led off, "We think she's doing pretty well at this point but things will be clearer by tonight and certainly by tomorrow. Transfusion reactions are usually pretty quick."

"The surgical repairs? How are they going?" I asked.

"She's back in the OR. Jamie is repairing the nerves now. It will also take time cleaning her out and looking for re-bleeding." Our top surgeons were in on the case—that was a relief. Their experience came from the limb reimplantation program we had. Arms, fingers, limbs cut off by band saws, subway trains, machetes, knives, firecrackers, you name it. The limbs would arrive, packed on ice, in a cup, a bucket, wrapped in a towel, a lunch box; the team would spend the next twelve hours fitting the pieces together, vessels and nerves, bones and muscles, tendons and skin.

"Elias, for the record, what's up with the other trauma case, Houston? I just saw him but I don't have all the details. He was hit by a cab in Midtown, something like that. I have lost track."

"Yeah, he stepped off the curb in front of the Parker Meridien just as a yellow cab screeched in to grab the spot. Bastard driver didn't even get out of the front seat. He would have driven off except he was boxed in by a limo. One of the guys from the Meridien, the guys in the suits and top hats, pulled him out through the window and nearly took his head off. Ex-marine. Houston had his right leg de-gloved to the knee, all of the skin was flayed off, and crushed the vessels and bones below. We couldn't repair it. It would have required twenty operations and even then it would probably still have to come off. Not worth it at the end of the day in my humble opinion. Houston opted for a guillotine, straightforward amputation." His opinions were never humble, but they were dead-on accurate if you could discount the presentation style.

Jon jumped in before Elias finished. "Houston's a young guy and will be playing tennis on a titanium prosthesis in a year or running in a marathon down in Rio. I heard he is a hotshot lawyer." I'd figured from my glimpse of the family that he was a somebody. Besides, the Parker Meridien is not the local YMCA.

"Look, we need to talk about what you are going to say to the

Trauma Detroit family," I said to Jon and Elias. "This is complicated and the husband needs an explanation. Not only is he dealing with the near death by exsanguination of his wife, but he's also getting inter-rogated by the police like he's some perp or part of a drug cabal." I stopped at that point, and let them pick it up from here.

Jon jumped in. "Look, I fucked this up and will talk to him and explain what happened. I have been doing this for nearly twenty years and never, ever bypassed the sequence of checks before." He was anx-ious, but I thought a little relieved to see that the goal of the meeting was not to hang him from the nearest lamppost. The old days of shame and blame in front of your peers had died a quiet death. There was nothing like public humiliation to burn a hole in your brain for a life-time. It didn't accomplish anything except make it even harder to find out what had *really* happened. It was the *Rashomon* effect, one event and ten different stories about what passed for reality.

"Guys, we saved Detroit's life with rapid treatment, controlled the bleeding, brought in the best crew of über-specialists, and she will go home and have a normal life. I don't know exactly why we have to beat ourselves up over this mistake." Elias was out there on this one.

"Elias, we don't mention anything about the transfusions and wheel her out of the door in a week and bask in the glow of another job well done? You have to be kidding." I was getting tachycardic myself.

He jumped back at me. "Mistakes happen all the time, Eric. Do we apologize for giving a Tylenol instead of an aspirin? Do we flagellate ourselves over a chest X-ray done twice on the same patient because the order was picked up two times? Do we need psychotherapy for delays in getting patients to the operating room for their needed pro-cedures because cases like this pop in and Jamie has been up for over thirty hours and can't stand up anymore? Just tell me where you draw the line?" He was on a roll.

"I draw it at wrong blood for Detroit, for Christ's sake, Elias. I know very well there is no black and white in the work that we do. Shades of gray, counterintuitive rules, lots of uncertainty, an over-reactive regulatory framework, complex systems of care, diffusion of responsibility, lack of clarity, a punishing legal system. I see the same

1-800 Sue Your Doctor signs on the subways that you do. I can also smell the trolling ambulance-chasing lawyers in their cheap baggy suits and shitty haircuts in the coffee shops hustling families for a piece of the action. Come on, I get all of that. But you cannot lump together mistakes of no consequence with this one. And by the way, every one of those mistakes of no consequence is an indicator. It sends a message. The next time it could be something a lot worse, a Detroit. Remember, we call them 'near misses.' Even the stupidest-appearing incident can send a message if you can hear it." I was angry at Elias now. Jon got it, and was mortified.

"Her life was saved by outstanding medical care is my point." Elias was retreating.

Jon joined us. "Look guys, Elias, we have to tell the patient what happened. In fact I have to tell her myself and not just for her but for myself as well. I've always considered myself a perfectionist. A lot of my colleagues call me a perfectionist asshole. Well, the asshole just got tighter. Let's go."

There was something to the personalities in the room that I deeply respected. Despite the bluster, it takes determination to get out of bed every day to do what they do with all the risks and at times terrible outcomes...then get up and do it again the next day. Decisions have to be made. Drugs have to be given. An electric cautery slices deep into a nearly blind space. When things go down it is in a split second. My job is easy.

Elias finished, "Jon and I will go and talk to the husband. We will go over the facts of the case from the surgery to the blood product errors. No apologies, just the facts and how she is doing. And we will keep him posted regularly and kept up to date." I knew he got it all along. He had been furious—how to reconcile almost killing her when he'd been doing everything possible to save her life?

"Irony of ironies," Elias continued sotto voce, "if she doesn't have a substantial reaction it may very well be because she hardly had any of her own blood left in her vascular system." I let it sink in as they left. She survived because she nearly died? That was the world we worked in.

I sat back in my chair and closed my eyes. It happened to be Tisha B'Av, the day of mourning, the Day of Lamentations for the loss of the Second Temple in Jerusalem over two millennia ago. I only knew that because my daughter, Marina, had been a religion major at college and had a project to educate me about my tribe's history, rituals, and beliefs that began thousands of years ago. My mind traced a series of seemingly discordant dots. They left a contrail in my brain that I tried to stay with, to make some sense from the apparent randomness. Detroit's veteran husband was being treated by being exposed to the trauma that had turned his legs into "armadillo" skin. The treatment was reimagining the event again and again, a little more each time, like turning up the sound, the brightness, until it lost its edge, its power, its force, its ability to dominate. This led me to the duty to "never forget." The day, the loss of the Temple, the scattering of a people who lived cataclysms over and over again. But wasn't this commemoration a form of transmitting trauma itself? A group psychopathy, passed from generation to generation. A vicarious type of PTSD visited upon the youth by the parents? How could re-exposure make you get better if continuous re-exposure could create the disease? It was confusing, and I was confused. Forgetting was a source of healthiness, or could be. Some treatments required remembering for trauma. Others required denial and forgetting for trauma. What about Detroit herself after this? Infusions of traumatic memories titrated to her heart rate? Or a pill that would obliterate her consciousness?

A few days after Diego's admission, I went to the unit in the midafternoon. While still in the hall, I paused when I saw a willowy blonde sitting upright like a ballerina in front of a hospital adjustable bedside table covered with white linen, a bottle of red wine, bone china, and silver laid out like a four-star restaurant. She was eating slowly and methodically, as if this were the most natural thing in the world. A gourmet midafternoon lunch with views of the Empire State Building, Chrysler Building, and beyond all backlit with cumulus clouds lazily drifting to the east. Diego was prone in bed hooked to a morphine pump and intravenous fluids. His bed was covered with stacks of newspapers in Portuguese, financial magazines and legal documents. His family was in absentia.

I hesitatingly slid the door open and entered.

The Mattas were from São Paulo; we communicated in Spanish since English was their third language. Diego looked up and said, "Hola, Eric, this is my girlfriend, Gabriela."

I went over and shook the dyed blonde's soft manicured hand. Her English was perfect, with a slight British accent. "Good afternoon, Doctor. I was expecting you. How is Diego doing? When will his wound be closed? When can we get on with therapy and a prosthesis?" She smiled. Too many questions, she acknowledged. We went through the basics and she continued to eat slowly and poured a glass of claret into a cut-crystal wineglass. On closer inspection, she was closer to the age of Diego's mother. The visible effects of a fine plastic surgeon's scalpel had removed age lines and the crow's-feet around her made-up eyes. Without blinking, her vaguely expressionless face looked me over. The family's absence was clear over the next couple of days. This was a family crisis, and the matriarch was not approving despite the blonde's wealth from previous marriages and the bona fide beauty, certified by national pageants (thirty-plus years earlier). Half of the Brazilian government cabinet flew to New York to pay respects in the next few days. I figured if "wine and spirits" had been on the pharmacy list at St. Vincent's hospital to prevent alcoholic church officials from going into withdrawal, then who was I to cork the bottle of deep purple Argentine Malbec Reserva and spoil the party for a family friend?

The next morning when I got to work, I met Susanne's mother sitting in a chair just inside my office and shook her hand. She had arrived the night before. She was in her late fifties, wearing a designer knockoff, one of those non-wrinkle generic outfits adaptable enough to wear to shop, work, travel, or visit your daughter in a critical care unit in the oldest hospital in the country. The fatigue was leached from her face, which was carefully made up, everything in place. "My name is Margarita Ben-Habib Laurent. I want to talk to you about my daughter." Her accent was French. I nodded *of course* and arranged the chairs so we could talk comfortably. I offered her a coffee but she didn't want anything, just my attention. I asked Patty to block all calls and visits. Patty didn't say a word; she got it and quietly shut the door, leaving us in silence.

I decided to not say anything. This was her time, and I would go with her lead. "I saw Susanne this morning. She was awake. I only stayed two minutes. The nurses were in the middle of changing her sheets after the doctors had looked at the dressings. Just really poked my head in and we looked at each other. She needed to know that I am here." I looked at her and listened closely.

"We've had a difficult time as a mother-daughter...team." She got it out.

"I mean we have had a tough time. We communicate. We talk. We see each other. It has been so difficult. I got the call from Charles and all I could feel was guilt. A huge wall of guilt washed over me. Doctor, there were many times in the last few years when I didn't care if I saw her again. Really, I know I must sound like a monster mother, not a human being really." She looked up at me. Her muscles were tight, as if she were sitting in a vise. She was sitting at attention.

"Margarita—is it okay if I call you Margarita? If you don't mind my asking, where are you from?"

"Yes of course, I would prefer that you call me Marga. I am French, from Algeria originally. We moved to the States when Susanne was a teenager. My husband, or ex-husband, is Algerian and teaches at the university on Long Island. I tried to reach him. He is on sabbatical in the Middle East now. I don't know where exactly."

"What was going on with Susanne? What made being her mother so hard?"

"I don't know where to start. The beginning or backward maybe is better."

"Don't worry, we can put the pieces together. It doesn't have to be all right now."

"Things started to get crazy when we were divorcing. I don't blame the divorce, but I do think the house was poisoned in ways it took me a long time to 'own up to,' as you would say in the States."

"It can be a pretty painful time for everyone in a family. There can be a lot of wounding as marriages unwind."

"Her father had wide-open affairs with his students and made nothing of it. I was supposed to watch, suffer in silence, and continue with our suburban pretend family life as if nothing was happening. I refused one day. He went crazy. He ranted, he broke things, he hit me and told me to get out, that I could figure out how to live on my own and could crawl back to clean up his 'shit.'" More left unsaid than you could put in an encyclopedia. The details of domestic dissolution were too painful. Humiliations recycled and introduced with surgical precision. Self-abasement, drop by drop. Extreme stress pried open doors into people's lives you would never otherwise get an opportunity to enter. It was perhaps the greatest privilege of being a physician. Confession, but face-to-face, not hidden in a wooden box.

"Susanne was a teenager. She got caught up with other kids, her friends, and stopped coming home regularly. I didn't know because she was split between two homes. A mother who had a studio apartment and spent her days, MetroCard in hand, climbing cement staircases in four boroughs as an itinerant French teacher. I was a backup, a stand-in adjunct for subsistence pay seven days a week. A father who flaunted his new sexual freedom like a teenager, with a twenty-year-old college senior sleeping in my old bed.

"Over the next few years—it is all blurry now, and it doesn't matter really all of the details, I know that—she tried drugs of all kinds and overdosed a couple of times. One time she was saved by chance. Another addict had a syringe filled with a medicine that brought her around. She had stopped breathing. That close. She got pregnant twice, more crises and abortions with pills and mini surgery." The tip of dozens of other issues. What could be said hid a lot more that couldn't. The social workers and the team would have time to tease out what was current and what was history.

"I did what I could. School meetings, therapists, hospital visits, emergency room middle of the night, taxi rides, advice from friends, group sessions for parents who had similar lives. We careened. We didn't live a life. We were like random planets bouncing from an exploding star. That was my daughter. That was me." A phase change. From the outside, it was invisible. Normal family. A trivial incident brought it from liquid to gas like water to steam. A fraction of a degree of difference.

"She stayed away from me. From her father, too. She wouldn't talk to us. She hated us. I couldn't understand. I have to say, I stopped looking for her. But more than that I hid myself away in a protective cocoon. I had to do something to hide myself so I did not get damaged beyond repair as she fell apart. Her father never stopped. The good parent, I guess. Or maybe not." She looked at me, enigmatically.

"Until I got Charles's call. It all started to flood back again. I had to talk to someone," she said, looking at me. "I did a terrible thing. I didn't do anything. I abandoned my daughter."

"Your husband? Is he involved? Will he care or want to know?" I wasn't sure which layer of Detroit's story I was encountering now. It was getting more and more complicated—and I hadn't even met the patient! The only thing I did know for sure was that I hardly knew anything at all. Medicine is a forensic science. It hardly prepares one for this. This, life that is learned the hard way.

"I really don't know, to tell you the truth. He is and isn't involved with Susanne. He can be cold-blooded one minute and generous and warm and outgoing the next moment. He is two people in one. You never know which one will be there with you. It is a sort of terror. Will he be doting father number one or father number two who likes young girls?" Marga was leaning toward me with her elbows on the table. The cords of her neck muscles stood out like cables of the Brooklyn Bridge.

"Marga, are you saying what I think you're saying?" I didn't know what to believe. I had seen so many stories turn into their opposite.

"I don't know what I'm saying." She looked away.

"You emailed him?"

"Yes, I sent him a message. I called his department. He is in Europe and then to the Middle East. North Africa, his life's work."

"Marga, what about your daughter and Reed? You talked about a teenager in trouble."

She paused a moment to take a couple of breaths. "She has gone through a few partners including a marriage to a guy who wanted a green card from a *gringa*. That lasted until the paperwork came through and then he was packed and gone. He was too young, too tattooed, too much into marijuana, beer, and uppers and downers. Stoned all the time and played the guitar all night long. Not a bad person, not vicious or violent. Zero motivation. Zero reason to get out of bed. But one day he was gone."

"It sounds like Susanne doesn't know who she is."

"Doctor, I really don't know myself. I was hoping you could help me while she is here, I mean help her. She is like a wounded bird and I think she found another wounded bird to look after. He is a nice person—don't get me wrong. I mean he has been through terrible injuries."

"So maybe that is not so bad, if they can help each other? There aren't a lot of opportunities for caring and loving out there in the cold."

We had patients, deeply wounded souls, who had stories of betrayal of the most intimate kind. Fathers preying on their daughters, selling them to strangers and watching television while they were being violated with broomsticks. We sewed them up, re-operated half a dozen times, and tried to figure out the puzzle of why and how. How could someone stay with anyone so evil without repeating the cycles of violence? Many of the stories, we couldn't understand at all. We were at a loss.

"Did something happen to your daughter when she was a kid? Is there something you are trying to tell me?" I had no idea if I was way out there, even becoming inappropriate, thirty minutes into a family meeting. I rationalized that Marga had opened the door, kicked it open in fact.

"That's what I don't know. Precisely. I mean precisely what I don't know. I have been terrified that I was there and it was happening in front of me but I didn't see it or want to see it. He had me in some kind of a grip. A fog or something. I was afraid of him. Totally afraid. I anticipated everything so as not to trigger something that might set him off into that other person that lurked inside the one I had married. I must be confusing. You would think I had married two men."

I had never jumped out of a plane. At that moment I felt I had been pushed out of one.

It took a few days to get our review team together. Susanne was out of the PACU and into the surgical unit and doing very well. For a woman who had been bled nearly to empty, she was in good spirits and liked the nearly full-time attention of the care team that fluttered around her bed. She was in a chair when I went to see her again for a few minutes by herself.

"Hey, Susanne, not bad now. Up and moving around. Impressive."

"Doctor, I am doing okay. I just spent another hour with Marion. She walked me through the events. It was like talking about someone else. I was out on the street corner, there was yelling, and then nothing." She had a slight hint of a French accent and spoke Arabic with one of her doctors from Baghdad.

"The good news is that your body goes into a complete survival mode and in the process wipes most of the memory banks clean. Pieces may come back, but overall it will be about recovery and getting back to your life." Here I was on less firm ground, but I held my voice firm.

"The doctors have come by several times to go over the transfusion mistakes. I don't really know what to say. I am okay. Evidently nothing bad happened to me. So in the scheme of things I guess I got great care and a big dose of luck."

"We are going through what happened to make sure it cannot happen again. I will let you know what we put in place," I added.

"I know they feel terrible about what happened. But they did save my life. My husband was hit and burned and he was evaced to a military hospital. Did he tell you about the medication combination that gave him a very high temperature, something-malignant syndrome? His legs get burned and he survives and then nearly dies from medication side effects that burn him up to a temperature of nearly 107!"

"No, I had no idea, but I'm not surprised unfortunately. The combinations of medications can be pretty nasty." Just then Reed walked in and I said good-bye, promising, as always, to come back. He bent over her and gave her a warm smile, and a warmer kiss.

My office wasn't big enough for the meeting, but it was serviceable.

The people involved in Trauma Detroit were squeezed around the table, ready to discuss what had happened. The mortality from mistakes in the five thousand hospitals around the country is equivalent to a 747 going down every other day. What industry had this as a business model? Or a permissive attitude: "That's the way it is," a variation on "shit happens." The feds were finally coming out with *Never Events*. They finally refused to pay for avoidable complications ranging from pressure ulcers acquired during a hospitalization to infections from contaminated poorly maintained intravenous lines. Unless quality and safety standards were hardwired into the regulatory and payment rules of engagement for medicine, it would take decades more for the profession to adopt them. The awkward truth was that medicine was slow to come around to embracing safe practices, from hand washing to standardizing equipment.

"Thanks for being here," I started. "I want us to go over the case and get down to the underlying issues right away, before the trail gets cold and events become blurry. We have the written details of the case, and you have talked to everyone involved. Ozal first, please."

"The error occurred in my department," she said. "Senior attending who knows what to do and made the mistake. We have been over the procedures and processes again and again. They are crystal clear, there is no ambiguity here about hanging blood." We were a long way from the days of heat-seeking missiles looking for the single person to blame and shame. In my day, I recalled, similar discussions had felt like group initiation rites, obligatory rituals of cutting and bloodletting.

Our senior surgeon chief, Greg, jumped in. White hair and beard, permanent blue scrubs, forty years of experience, and he still had a sense of humor. "Things get really complicated in the operating room, and many of us are pure adrenaline junkies. I am not joking, really." He looked at all of us and made sure we were paying attention. "Life-threatening trauma activates everyone around here at a gut level. Even good doctors lose their common sense. It's contagious." I think he got it just right. Technically everyone was a black belt. In a moment of extreme stress I wasn't so sure. These were known, competent people, and they still made a major mistake.

"So," I said, "we have these policies and procedures in nice shiny red vinyl binders and online. What do we do?"

"The irony," Saul the head of trauma put in, "is that the traumas are way down. The big stuff, I mean. Yeah, the orthopedic guys get motor vehicle traumas but real trauma, the stuff we grew up on, is down. People just don't see enough of it. You take that plus the residents having to leave in the middle of a procedure, who will see enough trauma cases? It doesn't come in on a schedule like your dentist's office." He was rabidly opposed to the new work hour rules for interns and residents that prohibited them from working more than a specified number of hours a week. Yes, exhaustion would cause certain mistakes, but the many handoffs during procedures caused other mistakes. The young medical staff did not get to see a case through from beginning to end, and so wouldn't get a sense of ownership and responsibility. "It will take ten years to train a surgeon," he continued, "just so they see enough cases."

"We need to practice and video everyone in mock traumas," Greg said. "We play it back and debrief. It is part of training and competency. Period, done. That's the only viable alternative, short of sending all surgeons-in-training for a tour in Kandahar. We are a long way from see one, do one, teach one. The way I learned medicine."

We'd covered a lot of territory by the end of the long meeting. The airline industry had cleaned up its safety record by standardizing its procedures, putting all of its pilots through extensive simulations, and developing a system for pilots to report in problems and errors that created a database mined regularly for improvements. We all knew the practice of medicine was a complex ballet, and every patient had his or her own vagaries and responses. But we also knew that the profession had hid behind "My patient is different" for too long. It had delayed our ability to respond to the overwhelming similarity of patients. The journey was long, complex, and only partially under way.

My office was a mess strewn with coffee cups and half-eaten cheese Danish. My cell phone went off with an unknown number.

"It's me, Marion."

"Hi, what's up?"

"Eric, you have to come upstairs right away. We have a real problem." She was not prone to exaggeration. Zero alarm fatigue.

"What is happening and who are you talking about, Marion?" We were following several patients together throughout the house.

"Susanne's father called her. He will be here tonight to see her. She just passed out in the hall. They called a code, for God's sake. Fortunately Pam from cardiology was there before they put the paddles to her chest. She is almost catatonic." I headed upstairs to meet with her on the unit.

So he was flying back to see his daughter. What did that mean? This case was operating on multiple levels, and all were increasingly complex. On the one hand we were coming out of a near-lethal trauma and a near-lethal complication. The medical part was starting to look easy, though, as the focus telescoped rapidly onto a family dynamic that was at first blurry and suggestive, confusing and yet increasingly worrisome for another kind of violence.

I wasn't prepared for the possibility of uncovering a bottomless well of emotional trauma inside a fairly routine Saturday-night-special gunshot case. The fragments and loose ends flying around started to line up like iron filings around a magnetic field. "Can't she block his visit?" I asked, starting to glimpse the outline. We found a niche to talk privately.

"She won't block his visit." Marion was back to her professional demeanor.

"Better to black out? Become catatonic?"

She gave me that look, the one that meant *We see this. It happens. Sometimes there is nothing we can do about it.*

Marion had an intimate knowledge of the gravitational pulls of intimate violence and abuse. Years of working with the police department, social work, advocacy in professional organizations, and training the next generation plus thousands of emergency room visits had given her a critical third eye and an extra sense. The attachments could be so deep they completely defied sense, except if you spent your days and months in this world. It was children's services, inpatient psychiatry, day hospitals, crisis intervention teams, addiction centers, adoption agencies, family court, juvenile prison, and Rikers Island rolled into one. This was not just the Stockholm syndrome, but a Greek tragedy linked in a death-rattling spiral that contaminated everything around. "I don't get it, Marion, what is real and what isn't?" I asked her like an innocent.

"We ask ourselves as well. We go over it again and again. It looks like abuse and acts like abuse. Was there abuse a long time ago that ended? Once you start dissociating or splitting your personhood to survive, how exactly do you stop? It becomes second and third nature. Incest..." She stopped for a few seconds. We looked at each other.

"The ties that bind," I said to her. "Can last for decades?"

She nodded. "The bonds that tie can last a lifetime if the person is undermined so badly. Real threats or even suggestions of violence and the cycle continues. The most we can hope for is that her husband can help her get out of it. The mother certainly hasn't helped. Probably made matters a lot worse, in fact."

Like broken shards from an archaeological dig, the outlines started to emerge over a series of interviews and visits over months after discharge and during Susanne's physical recovery. The black hole at the heart of the family leaked a little light through its overpowering gravitational field, but never enough to let us know with complete certainty. Only the 99 percent kind of certainty you got from watching the shadow dance of people caught in a slow-motion drama.

The fog of memory sets in almost immediately. Stories change, events once clear become more confusing, time erodes details, time lines, and specificity. The outside world and its codes of conduct and rules of engagement implacably intrude like an unwritten law of physics. Every day squared becomes the distance to travel. It is not linear. Whether it is exploring the details of a bad event in a hospital with a dozen participants or carefully weighing the hints of a family in a four-alarm fire of distress, the window is open for a short time only.

The trail gets cold.

CHAPTER 10

Index of Suspicion

The name was familiar, Hugo Beltrán. Where had I heard it before?

We were in the middle of making patient rounds on 7 West, reviewing all the cases on the unit with the entire team, when his story came up.

"Hugo Beltrán is a forty-seven-year-old Hispanic male with TB and HIV, a D-5 who was transferred from 15 North Surgery one week ago today." The resident, Don Liu, wearing a rumpled buttondown shirt, had been on service for a few weeks and was well versed in both his patients and the routines of this special locked unit. He had been up all night with a new admission hemoptysizing, coughing up blood, and had a casual way of presenting his cases without any sleep that belied a complete command of all of the facts. He made it look easy.

"Beltrán's biopsy came back from pathology positive for tuberculosis from a partial lobectomy or lung resection specimen from his trauma surgery. His fever is down to ninety-nine degrees. He has no more night sweats, and his appetite is coming around. Asked me where he could get decent Chinese food when I made rounds this morning."

"So what are we waiting for?" the chief said to the group. "Let's get this guy home soon."

"His home is on an island...," the social worker Linda looked up from her clipboard and said matter-of-factly. "Rikers Island."

"Everyone has a home. An apartment, a shelter, a cardboard box, the street, and even Rikers." The chief did his half-smile thing, undeterred.

"Besides, they won't take him back until he is not infectious, and for some reason he is a D-5 now, the highest level of detention for tuberculosis. So he is ours until we say he can go home, whenever that may be." Liu jumped back into the conversation. He continued.

"We are waiting for the AIDS team to come by and discuss when to begin treatment. His CD4 lymphocyte count is fifty-four, less than one-tenth of normal. Risk factors include unprotected sex with prostitutes, drug use but no needles, cocaine, marijuana, crystal meth, poppers, and alcohol. He was under DOC, Department of Corrections, but has been transferred to D-5 courtesy of the Department of Health and Hospital Police." He said it again for emphasis. More complicated than the usual HIV-positive, TB-positive, homeless prisoner hallucinating about Jesus and the end of times.

Fragments of the case fell into place when Dr. Liu mentioned the DOC or Department of Corrections. Beltrán had been admitted a couple of weeks earlier, delivered by a screaming fire department ambulance to the Bellevue emergency room. He had been stabbed in the chest at Rikers Island in an "altercation" with another prisoner. From the trauma slot he had gone directly to the operating room. The collapsed right lung was compressed by blood accumulating rapidly in the pleural space that surrounds the lung like a slippery second skin. An emergency thoracotomy or lung operation had cost him a piece of a lobe and left a long clear drain coming from his chest into a bubbling water-filled plastic container hanging from his bed rail. The microscopic review of the specimen revealed rice-size nodules embedded like a hailstorm everywhere the pathologist looked. There wasn't any untouched normal lung tissue. Mycobacterium tuberculosis or TB was the diagnosis.

I had barely seen him while walking through the surgical intensive care unit and recollected several corrections officers outside his room along with two New York City detectives in dark suits. The nurse mentioned to me that he was under a John Doe alias since the attempted murder had been gang-related. FBI officials came by for a private chat with a couple of us. Beltrán was in that netherworld between prison and a Witness Protection Program. Apparently he was an informant related to national-level gang activity. I hadn't seen so much police activity since Son of Sam was in G Building, the Gothic psychiatry monolith at Kings County. The Maras, the deadliest gang in the Americas, attacked him at Rikers. They would find out he wasn't dead.

So his real name wasn't Beltrán. He was recovering from the stabbing and the "incidental" biopsy showed widely disseminated tuberculosis, the miliary variety from the millet-size lesions. You could make it out on his chest X-ray as a gray haze where it should have been jet black. The CT scan showed golf ball–size lymph nodes surrounding his trachea and main bronchi along with the rice-size lesions peppering what lung remained after surgery. His drug screen had come back positive, and some astute history taking in the recovery room two days later made it clear he had plenty of risk factors for HIV infection. Consent was obtained, and his blood test came back HIV-positive. TB usually lived a quiet dormant existence for many years or a lifetime after an initial infection. HIV's targeted destruction of immunologically active T cells brought it to life.

D-5 was reserved for patients who demonstrated that they were not compliant with their treatment through multiple treatment failures. TB treatments last from six months to two years, depending on the relative resistance of the strain. New York City had passed public health laws in the early 1990s when a TB epidemic surged from the confluence of immigration from vulnerable areas of the world with significant TB and the HIV epidemic that was celebrating its tenth anniversary. The public health detention laws were a last resort, implemented to protect John Q. Public from infectious patients who could or would not participate in treatment regimens. The reasons for screwing up on treatment regimens were many: isolation, mental health issues, fears of being deported, hostility to authority, drug or alcohol abuse, and the long-term medication compliance that a TB cure demanded. The bugs were killed by the TB antibiotics during their reproductive cycle, which was very slow compared with those of other germs. The laws were controversial; civil rights advocates butted heads with the power of the state. Even Typhoid Mary had not been incarcerated the first time she infected her customers. Only after she killed again did the authorities finally get wise and quarantine her on an island in the East River.

There were a lot of pieces missing from the unknown patient's story, but they would have to wait until after rounds. The team continued to go over the rest of the cases before we started walking and talking.

Chin continued the tour: "Mr. Thierry has paraspinal TB with two large abscesses that are drying up on treatment. He is receiving medications for toxoplasmosis—a germ often complicating AIDS infection, with a propensity for attacking the brain. His CT scan shows persistent lesions. He will be here for another few weeks. Still requesting narcotics for the pain. He's a fringe guy, a vagabond who bounces around from Jersey to Connecticut to New York City. Has a long history of going from hospital to hospital." Gratuitous comment for a D-5 patient, I thought. And they weren't all vagabonds.

"Okay, let's get the pain people by to see him. At least that will make him happy and get us out of the bad-cop-of-the-day role." The head nurse usually didn't say too much during rounds, but when she did the suggestions were on target. Patients on this unit stayed from weeks to years, and she and her staff lived with the patients 24/7. Angry, manipulative, antagonistic patients made the unit impossible to work on or provide decent care. She believed in negotiating and giving the patients what they needed if possible. Her philosophy was simple: If you were reasonable, the patients would be reasonable no matter their social challenges and backgrounds. She was proud that none of the staff on her unit had developed TB in almost twenty years—thanks to meticulous attention to protocols. She wanted to keep it that way.

There were several other patients on D-5 hold. Mr. Castro had an obliterated left lung, a whiteout on a chest X-ray from tuberculosis. It looked like a black-and-white photograph from your grandmother's collection of a heavy snowstorm in Vermont. You couldn't see any normal tissue at all. He also had heart disease and the merest suggestion of a lung tumor sitting in a bronchial tube. He was too weak to take care of himself. The main issue with this patient would be making arrangements with a nursing home after he was non-infectious. Patients were non-infectious after several weeks of treatment with three to four antibiotics. Itinerant Department of Health TB caseworkers would bring their medications to them several days a week. Long-term residential facilities were not enthusiastic about having even a treated TB patient

in their midst. We were held hostage to both staff's and society's pho-
bias around AIDS, famine, and starvation, Russian prisons, and old
novels.

I drifted down the salmon-pink hall with scraped orange bumper
wall guards toward the cluster of guards outside Room 36, home to
Beltrán. It was change of shift and there were two cops from the local
precinct talking to two gentlemen with buzz cuts and off-the-rack
suits. I came over and introduced myself.

"Heard about you, Doc," said the senior police officer in a dark
chocolate-brown suit half a size too small. I fished my business cards
out of my pocket and handed them around. They scrutinized the rectangular card with minute attention. "Detective Swann, glad to meet
you, Doc. Detective Keller." He pointed to the other detective to his
right. We shook hands. "Officer Jones and Officer Peralta here are just
switching shifts right now." We nodded.

"Are you guys all 13th Precinct?" I asked matter-of-factly.

"The two officers are, yes," Swann said quickly. "We are from
Police Plaza, downtown," he added, to make sure I understood the
command order.

Most of the time, we had an amiable relationship with New York's
Finest. We needed each other and never knew when something might
happen. In essence, we were doing a lot of the same work for a lot of
the same people. Being a first responder for humanity's less-than-finest
moments was challenging. Plus a hurt cop's place of choice was our
emergency room.

"Hey, Doc," Officer Keller asked, "how long does this guy have to
be treated? I mean so he is not infecting anyone around him? I mean so
you can't catch what he has?"

"You mean so you can't get infected?" I got to his point. "Six
months at the minimum if his TB germs are the usual suspects. We
test for resistant bugs and will know pretty soon from the lab what
antibiotics we are going with for the full treatment. We have seen some
recent strange new TB strains in the Garifuna population from Hon-
duras and Nicaragua who now live in the Bronx. With DNA extracted
from the bugs, we can type where the strains came from. Just like what

your forensics techs do with DNA at the lab next door," I answered quickly.

A soulless rectangular reflecting glass DNA lab had gone up on our property post-9/11, a gift from an ex-mayor to the chief medical examiner. "And by the way, he has been treated now for over two weeks so you guys don't have to worry about catching any red snappers from him." I was alluding to the appearance of TB under a microscope.

I saw they were still jumpy when the door opened. A doll-like Chinese nurse came out wearing blue latex gloves, with the tight-fitting mask sealing her nose and mouth. She peeled off the mask and threw a big smile in our direction. "Good morning, Officers and Dr. Eric. Anything I can do for you?" Her diminutive size, youth, and creamy complexion made the cops' fear more than a little ludicrous. They mumbled and relaxed a few notches. The square air filtration box hanging off the wall near the door with its buttons and dials and lights didn't reassure them, but this was the key to controlling contagion. All the rooms had negative air pressure that recirculated the air and sucked, vented, and diluted it into the atmosphere. Plus people wore special fitted masks to keep them from inhaling the germs. The city invested in rebuilding public health TB infrastructure in the early 1990s.

"You're okay," I repeated to them. "We will look after you. You look after this guy." I jerked my head in the direction of the room. Beltrán—the details were coming back to me—was a very bad actor. I left it at that. I wasn't sure what they all knew.

While the cops' fears of catching TB were irrational, they were understandable. The germs were aerosolized with a cough, dispersed and inhaled by whoever was in the room. Infection wasn't limited to junkies shooting up in dank abandoned Bronx tenements littered with stained mattresses and broken glass. Worldwide, TB remained and has remained an enormous challenge, with millions of new cases a year. The development of several "miracle" anti-TB drugs in the 1940s and early 1950s gave hope that it could be eradicated with medications. Tuberculosis hospitals, sanatoriums, and the public health infrastructure built around the comprehensive management and isolation of the disease were gradually downsized and shuttered. By the 1970s there were only a few centers specializing in TB diagnosis, treatment, and control nationally. My personal training at Kings County Hospital between Bedford Stuyvesant and Crown Heights had included regular rotations in a six-hundred-bed TB hospital that closed a few years after I finished my residency.

Since its triumphant return, my colleagues and I had seen every kind of TB. From TB of the skin to TB meningitis, TB of the ureters with renal failure, and Pott's disease or spinal bone TB. Cavitary TB or TB of the lungs was highly infectious since millions of the organisms sat in the liquefied destroyed lung tissue or cavities and with each cough were aerosolized in a fine mist. But as TB "died out," so did the specialists who knew it so well. The protean nature of the disease created a subtle, confusing masquerade of other ailments. Patients' presenting symptoms mimicked cancers, blood clots, common infections, and masses in ingenious ways. Fevers of unknown origin. Night sweats without any focal symptoms. A solitary lesion in the brain. A swollen abdomen filled with fluid in an alcoholic with too many lymphocytes. The pericardial sack around the heart swollen with infected fluid and no bacterial growth.

I marveled at the disease's variety, its trickiness. It would hide encapsulated by an auto-fortified rind for many years. Decades of normal healthy life would pass by as the bacilli created a shell and liquefied the tissues within so they could not be engulfed or attacked by the host's immune system. Throw in aging, an innocuous viral infection, treatment with steroids or immuno-suppressants, however, and the long-dormant bacilli would become active. The TB bugs began to multiply and spread beyond their redoubt, usually in the lungs. HIV's explosive entry on the international scene in the early 1980s brought many infectious diseases that were medical textbook curiosities, like a two-headed circus snake, into front-row seats. The HIV virus crippled a class of immune cells of its host. TB erupted on main street in a society that had temporarily banished it to the margins in areas of destitution, drug addiction and alcoholism, clandestine immigration, malnutrition, and economic vulnerability. The democratic HIV virus knew no such restrictions.

"Hey, Doc, TB, but also HIV?" added Officer Jones to make sure I understood the risks they had undertaken sitting ten feet from the hermetically sealed door of his room behind a small desk covered with the *Daily News* and the *New York Post*, thumbed beyond recognition. A fat green-lined notebook in which they recorded the comings and goings of life on the unit lay open. The medical issues were complicated but parsed out by our specialists into options A, B, and C as the gang member's responses to the treatments and their interactions evolved.

"They travel together a lot. Wherever you have TB, you find HIV," I said. "South Africa and prisons around the world—like Russia, for example. If you have the HIV virus, your immune system isn't working fully, making you more susceptible to the TB germ. Most people who have TB don't know it. They got it as a kid and it hides inside them until something damages their immune system and then it takes off." Short course on TB for the guys in blue.

Swann interrupted one of the officers about to continue the commentary on TB and HIV infection. "Doc, he needs to be treated here for the entire time until he is cured, right? I mean the TB. You can't cure HIV yet, right?"

"We hold the D-5s here until their TB is totally cured. Remember, D-5 was created for that tiny group of patients who don't or can't take their medications for the full course. Taking the medications intermittently also makes it likely the bugs will become resistant to the usual treatments, which by the way are not easy to tolerate. It's a lot of pills to take. How many times do you guys finish a course of penicillin from your local family doc?"

No one answered.

"Like I said, if it's the usual kind—sensitive to the tried-and-true pills—that would be a six-month to nine-month course. The HIV infection makes it a little more problematic since Beltrán's own defense system is partially down. We will have our AIDS group come around and help with that decision." They were doing some mental arithmetic trying to figure out his remaining days at Bellevue.

By this time everyone was more relaxed. The infections were scary to the cops whatever their grade. Their Glocks and the weapons strapped to their calves wouldn't help, and they knew it, so everyone's fears were operational here. Wearing black rubber gloves was one thing, part of their modern culture post-HIV. With an invisible respiratory pathogen and a virus like HIV, all bets were off from their point of view. They were counting on us to keep them safe. The air filtration, the tight masks, the antibiotics in combination, the tests and X-rays were what was going to protect them and their families.

The officers did their shift switch as I put on a mask to enter Room 36 on 7 West. I looked like a cartoon version of a *Star Wars* Imperial stormtrooper.

The mask fit snugly over my lower face as I pushed open the door to the negative-pressure room. I wasn't worried about the TB. The little I knew about the patient I was going to meet made me queasy. Gangs, narco-trafficking, hit for hire, Central American military to the United States? Like a puzzle turned over on a table, the pieces scattered everywhere. The air circulated multiple times a minute then was vented out of the building and diluted in the New York City air. There were ultraviolet lights in each room delivering lethal frequencies to the DNA of any errant airborne bacilli.

Beltrán looked up from *El Diario* as I came in with a whish of the door. He was midforties, fleshy, full-faced with a mustache and thinning black hair slicked back with pomade on his large head. He wore pale blue pajama bottoms and hospital-issue slippers. His upper body was swaddled in white bandages. He had an empty can of Pepsi and some take-out Chinese food containers on his bedside sliding table. Chopsticks stuck out of a white take-out carton of partially eaten brown rice that was already turning black at the edges. It attracted a fly that had miraculously made it into the air-filtered room.

"Beltrán," I said, and then introduced myself. "How are you feeling? Any pain, fever better, breathing, cough, sputum color, moving around okay?"

"Señor Doctor, I could use some more pain medicine. It is hard to cough with the stab wound in my side and my ribs cracked by the surgery. I can barely move." His accent was not Mexican, that was clear.

"I will talk to the nurses and see when you are due for your next medication dose. You got a narco tablet just an hour ago. It should be fine now. You are two weeks post surgery, *verdad*?" He smiled and realized I had gone over his records in some detail, so we could skip the games like conning me for extra pain pills.

"Where are you from? Your accent is not Mexican," I stated matter-of-factly. "Guatemala?"

"You have a good ear, *jefe*," he answered, looking at me carefully, as if I hadn't had a blue mask covering half my face. "I was born in Alta Verapaz near Copán."

I knew a little about his hometown—a place where many Germans had settled in Guatemala in the nineteenth century looking for business opportunities in the flourishing international coffee business. A couple of hours north from where my patient Soraya had grown up and ultimately fled in horror. A friend of mine, Father Ricardo Alemán, had spent nearly twenty-five years in that area until the day he was notified by the Vatican that he was on a death list. He was in Guatemala City on some personal business when an albino man in dark glasses came to his hotel, handed him an airline ticket to Newark, and drove him directly to the airport. There were two Uzi-armed bodyguards in the backseat. His infraction was being a liberation theology Catholic priest suspected of "supportive attitudes" toward the "communist insurgency."

The military was after him. Copán had been and continued to be a very dangerous area. Alta Verapaz bordered Chiapas, Mexico. It was *Ganglandia*, infiltrated by narco-trafficking and immigrant kidnappings, and in a permanent state of low-grade civil war against its own population of Mayan and Ladino or mixed-race Highlanders.

The room was spare and reminded me of the bare prison cell of a hotel I had stayed in near Rabinal in Guatemala south of Copán. Diana and I had gone to the festival of Rabinal Achi that occurs every January, and there were no hotel rooms to be had. In the pre-Columbian drama, a warrior from an invading Mayan tribe is captured by the Achi Mayans and offered his life in return for marrying one of their princesses and becoming an Achi. He is given a year to travel on his honor and think over their conditions. He returns a year later and refuses the offer of life with forced/voluntary conversion. He is sacrificed according to the terms of the agreement. He was respected as an honorable warrior. And he knew he would die when he was captured. A little different from the post-modern narco-violence that percolated into the U.S. newspapers, offering scenes of tortured policemen and heads stitched up as soccer balls.

"So, Beltrán, tell me how you ended up in Manhattan getting Chinese takeout? A guy from the boonies of Guatemala?" I teased him from underneath my mask. My wife and I had been obsessed with this part of the world for decades. Diana spent months every rainy summer in San Cristobal, Chiapas, working with Tzetzal-speaking Mayan women. We had a deep history here.

"It's a long story," he said, debating whether to put down the newspaper.

I didn't have to tell him he would be our guest for a long time.

Over the next few weeks we talked many times, and I pieced together a story that may or may not have been the total truth—in fact, I was sure it wasn't, but the truth for this guy may never be known. He had lived a life of disguises, of hidden lives inside of hidden lives. He had molted identities so many times, he might not actually know which one was which at any one time. The identities were adaptable and served as survival tools depending on the circumstances.

My familiarity with his childhood haunts and even some of the characters in his community, including Father Alemán, whom he regarded as a wonderful human being however misguided he must have been—"Perhaps naive, Doctor?" was the way he put it—gradually made it easier for him to talk to me. The hours on the unit went by slowly for him. He was not a difficult or complaining patient. In fact, because he was a "special" guest of the city or federal government, he had cable television, a cell phone that received incoming calls only, and access to unlimited take-out food that he bartered to other patients for favors, cigarettes, candy, music, and other things, as I would later find out. He had a loose-leaf binder next to his bed, filled with menus coded by country and cuisine. We were in Manhattan, after all, the take-out capital of the free world.

One night Beltrán developed a raging fever of 106 with drenching sweats. He had been a model patient clinically, improving on schedule. Adhering to the textbook version of what was supposed to happen. His TB was being treated with a standard four-drug regimen. You always began treatment with multiple drugs to avoid the emergence of resistance, and then modified the combination under the careful eye of our HIV specialists so the medications would not interfere with one another's pharmaco-metabolism. His T cells, HIV virus–infected, or CD4 count was coming up to normal. He looked so good that I had thought his lead doctors were overly cautious when they talked of a shoe about to drop. When I came in that morning, I had an email from our diagnostic prestidigitator warning that *B has a rash, looks like Pox to me!!! IRIS syndrome!!* The subtext was obviously *I told you so.* Chickenpox.

Chickenpox in an adult is no small thing. He was covered with a papular itchy red bumpy rash on his back and chest and was clearly miserable from muscle aches, nausea, a headache, and a temperature close to 107. The team had started him right away on intravenous acyclovir, an anti-viral medicine that was safe and effective in preventing complications not uncommon in adult men (with HIV and TB), and towels soaked in cool water. He was convinced he was going to die from chickenpox. Not the tuberculosis saturating every millimeter of his body. Not the HIV virus hog-tying his immune system. Chickenpox!

The cops guarding his door didn't know what to make of it. Would he die? Would that be a good thing? Or a bad thing? Would they catch chickenpox, on top of everything else he was offering them?

"WTF?" they asked me as I came out of Beltrán's room later that morning.

"Excuse me?" I couldn't make out what they said.

"What The Fuck? Doc, WTF?"

"He should be okay," I said. I wasn't sure if they were relieved.

"Though this can be really serious. The timing of his HIV treatment is tricky. I know it sounds bizarre, but when you treat TB and AIDS, the patient's crippled immune system starts to work again." I felt like I was teaching in school. They all looked at me intently. "I mean when we put Beltrán on HIV medications, his immune system started to recover, the T cells rebounded and started to attack his infection—and his body did an overshoot. It looks like his TB is active again, but it's not."

The looks on their faces made me realize why we needed physicians who really knew these diseases in all their granularity. Every case had a unique twist. Textbook cases were cartoons, averages, generalities. They were not substitutes for real-life experience. The disease had escaped my internist capabilities some time ago. It was like an oncologist's job now, teasing out regimens, side effects, testing and rebalancing and keeping up with an avalanche of new drugs and treatment regimens. Studies were ongoing for a morning-after sex pill and for a daily preventive pill. Plan B for HIV disease from your local pharmacist, like oral contraceptives. If you had HIV and access to HAART (highly active anti-retroviral therapy) or the comprehensive treatment regimens, your life expectancy was normal. In twenty years it had become a manageable, chronic disease. The *if you had access* piece was the big variable.

"Doc, you mean you treat the guy, he gets better and then gets worse?" The chief of detectives looked at me and then his entourage.

"Yes, Detective. Precisely. We call it IRIS, immune reconstitution inflammatory syndrome, a mouthful, I know. It is strange. But it means he is getting better. His immune system is healed and exploding. We will watch him carefully and treat the syndrome." The detectives and officers were listening and trying to figure this out. It was counterintuitive, like a lot of what we did in medicine. Less is more. More is less, and on and on. Revisited in every generation.

After a week, it was clear Beltrán had survived that setback. I came by regularly while he sweated and moaned away. Now he wanted company. Chickenpox got him to talk about what his life had been like and how he had ended up in a seventh-floor room on a locked tuberculosis unit in a city hospital in custody of the U.S. justice system. A pause for some reflection on the meaning of it all?

"Have you heard of the Kaibiles?" he asked me a few days later, after his temperature came down.

"*If I advance, follow me. If I stop, push me. If I retreat, kill me.* Those Kaibiles?" I responded, my ears now wide open at the mention of Guatemalan military, special ops. Ruthless.

Beltrán repeated in Spanish, "*Si avanzo, sigueme, si me detengo… Apremiame…, si retrocedo…Mátame.*"

"My wife and I took a trip up the Usumacinta River from Yaxchilan in Mexico near Palenque in the Yucatán. We were traveling to Tikal in the late 1980s. Not the regular tourist flights from Guatemala City or overland from Belize. We were stopped at a checkpoint at a military camp that might have been *El Infierno*, Hades. Los Kaibiles had their 'motto' prominently displayed on a wooden sign: *Bienvenidos. Si Avanzo…Sigueme. Si me detengo…Apremiame…Si retrocedo… Mátame.* After that introduction, how could I not have heard more about them?" I asked him back. Diana and I had actually stumbled on a black-ops training camp deep in the jungles of the Petén, the large Guatemalan province that juts northward into the Yucatán Peninsula. The recruits were young men trained to be killing machines through psychological and physical deprivation and brutality. A fourteen- or fifteen-year-old with a machine gun pointed at our faces had stopped our dugout canoe.

As Diana and I sat for hours on a wooden bench waiting for our passports to be returned (and our guide to resurface), we could see young boys, fifteen or so years old, beat one another to a pulp while older men surrounded them in a circle, cheering and taunting them. Young Kaibiles in training. We drank a Coke under ads and calendars graced by beautiful blond women and children and wondered if we'd ever see our kids again. During the thirty-plus-year civil war in Guatemala that "ended" in 1996 with the "Peace Accords," many Kaibiles left as mercenaries seeking other "opportunities" or were decommissioned into civilian life. Over 250,000 civilians were dead in a war that left the country in a collective state of post-traumatic stress. The perps were granted immunity. I wondered where he was going with Los Kaibiles. I was feeling uneasy at this point.

"I was twenty years old and had no skills and no future. The civil war had decimated the Highlands. Family was turned against family, friends against friends. I decided to enlist. Just like the guys your age who enlisted to go to Vietnam from the poor barrios of New York." He threw that in gratuitously. By this time we were not wearing masks anymore, literally and figuratively. He was non-infectious, having completed several weeks of TB therapy. He would need a full six to nine months to finish the complex four-drug regimen ensuring that all of the slow-growing bacilli were moribund.

"So you joined the elite of the elites? The Navy SEALs of Guatemala?" I asked him if they really bit off the heads of live chickens, and drank pulque, the local fermented alcohol, out of recently fired mortar shells. And I asked if he had CIA advisers in his years of training.

"*Jefe*"—he must still have had his military reflexes since he called me "chief"—"we did a lot of weird and stupid things. Part of the harassment and way they break you down. You ever see the movies about Jason Bourne?" He loved the movies, evidently a Kaibil fascination. I smiled, some of my favorite action movies of all time. The protagonist is so destroyed in becoming a killing machine that he doesn't know who he is or what he has become except through short flashbacks. "I would have thought you were a *Terminator* fan." The pirated CDs littered the markets of every Latin American town.

"I left when the Guatemalan Peace Accords went down in '96. A lot of us left at that point. It was a poisonous time for the military and particularly the 'elites' as you call us. The Truth Commission was putting a report out and it wasn't clear who would be sacrificed, except that it wasn't going to be the top commanders for sure. The United States was pulling dollars out of its intelligence operations. You couldn't trust anyone." I reflected on the concept of trust for an ex-black-ops guy suddenly cut loose from the decades-long fratricidal killing rampage.

"So what did you do then?" I felt like the psychiatrist from *The Sopranos*. Short questions, non-judgmental. Psychopathic killer sitting opposite with charm and a sense of humor.

"There was another game that had been developing in Guatemala and spilling over from Mexico and El Salvador. Narcotics. If you were ex-military and weren't freelancing, there was only one thing you were capable of doing and that was the security service industry that was growing around everything like a *matapalos*." The *matapalos* were killer vines in the jungle. They started innocently climbing a tree and ended up strangling it—killer vines, like the Guatemalan military.

I remembered a long conversation with our driver from Guatemala City to Rabinal through the back gravel roads winding our way over mountains and through small pueblos. His previous career had been in private security as a driver and guard. After a few cycles of layoffs, Rafael ended up chauffeuring an ever-diminishing tourist trade. For unemployed security employees, there was only one other option to have a steady income. The narco trade was the growth industry and the networks were all ex-military and ex-security, almost one and the same. "The government tolerates a high rate of crime so there are not more unemployed security personnel on the street," he told me. You could drive through the Zonas or neighborhoods in Guatemala City and not see a soul. Barred windows and doors gave the impression of prison cells without roofs. Rabinal was a cluster of white buildings between two rivers in the distance as we zigzagged down the clear-cut mountainsides, the few remaining trees hugging the steepest banks and arroyos like their life depended on it.

"What is freelancing for ex-Kaibiles?" I asked straight back.

"Like the Zetas," he said, referring to the elite units of the Mexican military that had defected around that time and taken up positions as the paramilitary enforcers of the Gulf Cartel before freelancing in the narco business. They were notorious for their cruelty and their creation of new forms of barbarity. Narco-messaging was an art form. They communicated using corpses and body parts they left hanging from lampposts or overhead bridges. They mutilated the decapitated bodies beyond recognition. *Posole*, corn soup, was a concoction of vats of acid where they melted bodies to the consistency of stew. Heads stitched to look like soccer balls were left on playgrounds.

"Like Zetas, like Kaibiles and the Colombian paramilitaries. Some common buddy system across international lines?" I pushed a little further.

"We all worked together all the time. Remember, our commanders trained in Panama and then Fort Benning at the School of the Americas run by your government, *amigo*. They all knew one another and developed close ties between countries, like classmates from college. What do you call it, a fraternity, *una cofradía*. The borders were porous." *Esponjoso*, spongy, was the word he used. "We helped one another all the time. Collaboration. I think the Fortune 500 call it teamwork." He was having a good time with me.

"And Las Maras, just how did they fit in?" The puzzle was starting to fit together.

"Las Maras came into Guatemala across the border from El Salvador. They networked right up to the frontier with Mexico and extended a spiderweb north into the heartland of the United States. Remember, Los Angeles is their ancestral land. During a civil war, their parents fled Central America to California. The kids were born north of the border before they were sent back to El Salvador. But now as pretty hardened gang members to survive the tough turf battles and life without jobs. Many sent back did not even *hablar* the Spanish. They were distributors, independents, human traffickers, *sicarios* (guns for hire), and Mafia, all in one, not specialists. They couldn't become an independent cartel in Mexico. The Mexican cartels were too powerful and well established, so they worked in the spaces between the major cartels and worked with the cartels. There is always room for some independent contracting. This is a very advanced form of capitalism."

He smiled broadly at his political message to me. We were talking in codes, but there was truth in his throwaway line. There was plenty of money being made on the War on Drugs north and south of the border. The United States had recently signed a multibillion-dollar "Plan Merida" of "assistance" to the Mexican government. This would go to U.S. contractors to service the border, providing armaments, motion detectors, and drones. What U.S. congressman could object to that list of familiar requests? These weren't earmarks, after all.

Two converging lines brought the drug cartels into open and

brutal competition—violence that has left a body count approaching fifty thousand in the few years since President Calderón of Mexico announced a military operation against the major cartels. The first was the loss of elections by the long-term single governing party in Mexico, the PRI, to Vicente Fox, the former Coca-Cola executive, in 2000. The loss of the near-dictatorial rule of the PRI, which had managed the country with a form of distributive payments for votes and compliance, combined with the closure of Florida as a transshipment zone for South American cocaine, left the traditional areas of the Mexican drug trade now awash in unlimited sums of money and zero government "cacique" or strongman controls over the "plazas," the local drug distribution centers.

The second converging phenomenon was the North American Free Trade Agreement or NAFTA concluded in 1994. The net effect of the treaty was a time bomb for Mexico. It devastated the agricultural sector, pushing millions of peasants into the cities and sending them in a northward migration as agricultural subsidies for corn were withdrawn in Mexico and the distributive land or *ejidos* (unsalable) from the revolution was revoked. Millions of people lost their means of livelihood. The maquiladora phenomenon on the border—zones of businesses that assembled refrigerators and televisions for U.S. consumption—was eroded by lower Chinese labor costs and created the phenomenon of "nini": "*Ni empleo, ni estudios.*" Neither work nor studies (education). Generations of unemployed, uneducated young Mexicans with nothing to do and increasingly nowhere to go. The U.S. post-9/11 militarized the border and increased the border patrol from four thousand to over twenty thousand members, with drones and temperature-sensitive detectors. The most insidious was the criminalization of immigration. Crimigration. The creation of a vast new industry of privatized detention centers run by Immigration and Customs Enforcement, part of Homeland Security, has placed over four hundred thousand immigrants in its centers.

Undocumented immigrants are summarily convicted of a misdemeanor and deported or spend a few months in detention. The next offense is a felony with up to twenty years in prison. As the United

States is facing a prison crisis domestically while state budgets reel from the loss of tax receipts from an enduring recession and it can no longer afford to keep 2.5 million under lock and key, a parallel private detention system is growing in hundreds of sites in rural America, competing for jobs and political favors, off the radar screen for most Americans. Tough justice for complex socioeconomic problems that are not amenable to tough-justice solutions. Just as the War on Drugs has not solved the "drug problem" and has ignited a reign of violence in our neighbors to the south. Here I was talking to one of the warriors.

Beltrán knew about it all. Not just the common-knowledge stuff—Las Maras shaking down the billion-dollar business in human trafficking from Central America to the United States. Not just that they specialized in extorting the immigrants and killing them if their relatives in the north did not pay promptly, or that they sold them to other gangs, drug cartels, or the police. The way he told it, both the U.S. and the Mexican governments were involved in making sure that these immigrants did not make it north to the border. They supplied the gangs with weapons. "Mexico," he said, "is an enormous cemetery for immigrants trying to reach the United States. This is a free-fire zone. You have shifting rules and allegiances among gangs and local and state governments and international police and intelligence forces. A perfect business for the cartels and the narcotic transshipment business. Like Vietnam, Doc. The same playbook. Did you ever see *Apocalypse Now?*"

I was thinking an ex-Kaibil could offer a lot. After all, hadn't Blackwater Inc., rebirthed as Xe based out of the Emirates, been a haven for highly trained former U.S. commandos providing guns for hire in the Middle East and around the world? Wasn't the Sunni Awakening purchased with dollars? A nurse's aide, Sharma, came into the room. "Mr. Beltrán, time for your medications soon. Let me get the room cleaned up first." She was carrying clean white sheets and a fresh towel, threadbare and the size of a large washcloth. Sharma was in her midfifties with a soft beguiling smile, a lightly freckled face, braided hair, and a voice just above a whisper. She had been at Bellevue for many years and felt comfortable on the TB unit. She had obviously developed a good relationship with Beltrán. They talked about the weather, where to get the best Chinese food, the art class that afternoon. Sharma had been in exile for years in a Nepalese transit camp for displaced Tibetans. The 1959 Chinese invasion of her Himalayan country left her an orphan.

She trained as a midwife in the sprawling camp filled with international NGOs and through "fate" was befriended by an evangelical couple visiting from Michigan. They sponsored her application for asylum and helped her settle into a community. The growing Tibetan enclave in Queens—covering more square blocks and surrounded by Indians, Pakistanis, Colombians, Peruvians—became her home. The final maneuvers of perilous journeys to the United States through a hundred different back channels, each with a unique story. The trickles of people from distressed areas around the globe were messages in a bottle—wars over land, oil, diamonds, rare minerals, timber, grazing rights, religion, population explosion, water, environmental degradation, drugs, and shattering local economies. And then the petty thugs like Beltrán. He was no Pablo Escobar negotiating to pay off the sovereign debt of Colombia for immunity. I wondered if Beltrán knew anything about her story, and what he would say if he did. A deadly contagious disease had brought us all together. That had to be one of the messages.

I saw Beltrán again a few days later in the activity room at the end of the long corridor on the west side looking toward the Hudson River. I swiped my ID card, which deactivated the electronic lock and let me onto the unit. That was after I went past the hospital security guard behind his wooden desk. The idea of forcible controls on patients had a checkered history in public health circles—from forced sterilizations to withholding treatments for syphilis in the Tuskegee "affair." Recent headlines broke the story of U.S. public health service physicians infecting Guatemalans with syphilis and gonorrhea to test penicillin's efficacy during World War II. The poorest and most deprived members of society had borne the brunt of "control" efforts. In many ways, New York City had been a pioneer over the last hundred years in a more enlightened approach to public health that resulted in improved health for its citizens. The issue of civil rights violations was appropriately on the forefront of legal activists' agendas.

I had come to respect the amicus brief, the legal actions taken by interested third parties on behalf of clients who could not mount their own defense. *Brad H. v. New York City* was in response to a lack of outpatient services for mentally ill prisoners upon their release from Rikers Island. The prison system had become the de facto "mental hospital" for SPMIs (the seriously and persistently mentally ill) following de-institutionalization fifty years ago. The practice of releasing prisoners at three o'clock in the morning, underneath the 59th Street Bridge in Queens, the flickering white lights from a fast-food outlet spreading a halo over the scabrous concrete sidewalks of Gotham's netherworld, with a couple of dollars and a MetroCard warranted an intervention. A tiny ecological niche of pushcarts, prostitutes, and drug dealers stuck like lichen to the grit.

Beltrán was seated at a beat-up rectangular brown plastic table with three other patients in their hospital pajamas. Julie the "therapist" aka artist who had worked on the unit for many years guided the group, who responded to her calming presence. Months being cooped together in a potentially charged atmosphere of forced conviviality could be combustible. After serving everyone instant coffee or tea, she handed out paper and brushes. "Let's paint today, guys. What would you like to make the theme of your drawings?"

Everyone was working with watercolors that day. Mr. Alonzo, a Puerto Rican gentleman and former city transit authority employee, had severe sarcoidosis, an inflammatory disease with no known cause; he required high-dose steroids to control the worsening pulmonary fibrosis that had activated his otherwise silent tubercular infection. Clear plastic nasal prongs delivered oxygen from a small green tank hanging off his wheelchair. Nguyen was a young Vietnamese man, thin to the point of vanishing in his pale pajamas held up with an extra piece of red shoelace and a striking shaved head. His arms were heavily tattooed with snake motifs in blues and red scales. He was the son of well-to-do Saigon merchants who became Vietnamese "boat people" fleeing the North Vietnamese takeover of Saigon in 1975. He was born in a Thai refugee camp, where his family had re-created their business buying large burlap bags of rice and sugar, dividing it into small plastic portions, and pocketing the price differentials. They were granted asylum in the United States after four years. They now lived in Texas, the proud owners of an expanding chain of fast-food stores.

Nguyen had fled "bourgeois" capitalist life to street life and drugs in the Big Apple. He started as a musician, a bass player in a band, and got hooked on free-flowing cocaine, then graduated to heroin. We were getting him invested in multiple treatment options to see if he could break the descent. His TB was almost certainly a reflection of the crowded chaotic living conditions of his early childhood and the reactivation of an otherwise silent pulmonary infection from repeated drug use and malnutrition. He didn't want his parents to know where he was and went to great pains to obscure his location and treatments.

The final patient sitting at the table hunched over a piece of paper and drawing the apartment buildings and skyscrapers outside the window was Ngugi Yusuf. He had emigrated from Francophone Africa. As far as we could tell he was a businessman, but the details of his life were unclear and changed constantly over the time he was in the hospital. He had fled from Mauritania to France and then to the United States for asylum. He was a D-5 detention case who had failed multiple attempts to treat his cavitary TB (highly infectious lung variety) by evading and avoiding treatments with Department of Health caseworkers. After the fifth attempt and six months of trying, the team had the case reviewed by the TB bureau chief, who promptly signed an order of detention. We had decided he had much to hide and possibly to lose by letting anything out about himself. His biggest fear was ICE, the post-9/11 immigration service now a subdivision of Homeland Security. He was convinced all the authorities were interconnected and there was one giant computer that notified officialdom everywhere of his movements, including tracking his cell phone. We did not regard this as a paranoid delusion with Google Earth on our desktops, a GPS chip in our phones, drones flying over Helmand province piloted from

Nevada, and a secret court in Washington that determined access to any information from all sources.

We made it clear we were not interested in his legal status, only in treating his tuberculosis. Resistant tuberculosis was not uncommon when treatments were partial or incomplete. He had now earned extra months of treatment, additional second-line medications including daily injections, and the enhanced scrutiny of the Department of Health epidemiologists who found his case "interesting." The last thing you wanted to be in medicine was "interesting." Yusuf had of course made himself more widely known than would be conceivable if he had just swallowed his pills twice a week at the DOT (directly observed therapy) clinic and quietly gone about his business, whatever it was.

I sat down with the group at the table and said hello. They had seen me around the unit enough to know I was "*jefe*" and let it go at that. Julie asked if I wanted some paper, which I declined. Beltrán looked up and said, "I never joined Las Zetas. You couldn't anyway if you wanted to." Nobody at the table spoke Spanish except Alonzo, and he was deep into his painting and chatting with Julie.

"So how did you get into the Mexican end of things?" I asked him.

"I left Alta Verapaz through Tapachula like every other immigrant on their way out of whatever hellhole they had found themselves in. I went to meet some army buddies who had left and gone to Guerrero."

"Pretty dangerous place, even for an ex-Kaibil," I said.

"I knew guys from Las Maras in Guatemala whom I had helped out, and they put in a word for me. You needed someone to make you trustworthy." He looked up again from his drawing out to the distance.

"So...?"

"I ended up working with them, doing some jobs, protection, collections, stuff like that. You Americans call it muscle."

"So when did it fall apart? You weren't Maras and you weren't part of the cartels. Trust is all relative and is a finite resource." I kept at him, interested in his journey from hunter to hunted.

"That's for sure. My colleagues decided they needed to make some money. We got paid nothing in the military, really nothing at all. A few quetzales a month, ridiculous when you saw what people were making including my *comandante*."

"Independent contracting?" I asked him.

"Exactly. The Kaibiles are good at killing but it is not a business school, and we were out of our league and over our heads. Dealing on the side was punishable by death."

"They found out?"

"I never knew. I left one afternoon when I sensed something wasn't right and headed up north by bus and car. I never looked back. I knew they knew somehow. I dumped my cell phone and kept going. You get a feeling and go with it. You hesitate and end up as *posole*."

"Where did you cross?"

"Jesus, they have everything covered at the borders. You have to be really careful. The *halcones* are everywhere"—falcons, or lookouts for the cartels. "Once you are in it, there is no way out of it. Alive that is. I had to go to the States for my own safety."

"Pretty ironic, hey, Beltrán. You can't go back to Guatemala since Las Maras are everywhere, and you can't stay in Mexico since between them and the cartels you are a dead man. So you came here to be safe?"

"Yeah, but funny no. They are here as well." He lifted up his pajama top and showed off the bandages over his right rib cage.

He was right, of course. Rikers Island prison system was a filter for many things in American society. For one, it was the largest prison complex in the United States, with eleven prisons; each had a capacity for two thousand prisoners. It was filled with black and Hispanic prisoners waiting for trial, serving sentences of less than one year (or they went upstate), and had a full complement of mental illnesses, HIV, and addictions. Las Maras hit the East Coast some years ago. The new generation was less obvious, avoiding the heavy tattoos and having them removed with laser treatments.

A few weeks later, I slid into the booth at the coffee shop with Detectives Swann and Jones. They were in the middle of the Towers specials and being looked after by Danny in the farthest corner of the coffee shop.

"You guys look pretty good. How are things going?" They always wore the same clothes and looked the same no matter when.

"You heard about our prize patient here?" Swann mumbled with his mouth full of the *shawarma* special. The white yogurt sauce gave him a mustache like the television commercials for milk.

"Yes. For sure I heard. In fact the head nurse on the unit stopped by my office to fill me in on the news."

"Look, we will take care of the officer who was asleep at the switch. He has been reassigned already. No excuses, but the patient has been off isolation and can wander around the unit. Right?"

"Yes, Detective, of course. But I thought you were protecting him?" I added and then, "Hey, I know. It happens. We cannot guarantee we can stop someone from killing themselves if we are more than three feet away round the clock. We get it completely. Surprised you guys think it could be otherwise." I mentioned a truism no one seemed capable of digesting who didn't work in hospitals.

"Really. So much for one-on-ones. Not bulletproof, that's for sure," he said, swallowing hard and taking a sip from his Dr Pepper. He let the protection comment go by.

"Nothing is bulletproof in medicine, Detective. Maybe in your world but not in mine. We aren't running a prison except on the nineteenth floor, and that's under DOC control. You enter their universe. Families, friends, girlfriends bring in drugs regularly. Should we do vaginal inspections on female visitors? It is not an uncommon place for cocaine in a plastic lunch bag. I had a guy overdose on 17 North recently in the bathroom when a patient from the next unit sold him some narcotics in front of the nursing station. Another patient found him slumped over on the toilet with his pants down around his ankles."

"Not in mine, either." He looked up from his fries. "No guarantee, that is."

"Explains his HIV, though, doesn't it, though it probably doesn't need explaining." Detective Swann kept going, and it was time for me to go.

I wished them a pleasant afternoon and walked to the cash register, paid the check, and headed back to the office. Swann was referring to

Beltrán's sexual adventure with a new patient on the unit. So much for high security. Next time I saw Beltrán he was being escorted back from a mandated "fresh air" break on the metal cage on the hospital roof. He marched down the hall with his personal police officer in tow.

"*Hola, jefe.* How are you today? What brings you to such a special floor on such a beautiful day? You have so many things to do in such a busy place. You know, I could see New Jersey and the planes landing at LaGuardia, Kennedy, and Newark. Like I was the chief air control *comandante* for all of New York City." The thought gave me pause. Reagan redux on steroids.

"Hi, Beltrán. Have a few moments to catch up?"

"Sure. Come on in. Let's have lunch and sit for a while." A white plastic bag with an orange smiley face filled with Chinese food had just miraculously shown up, brought in by the hospital security guard for the police officer and our patient.

"Aren't you sick of take-out Chinese by now? There are a few other eating establishments on this narrow island, you know?"

"In Los Kaibiles we had a Indian worker bee who cooked Chinese all the time in a real wok. A change from *Moros y Cristianos*, rice and beans. Your bread-and-water prisoner rations. I got used to it. I like the taste soaked in soy and hot sauce in my *boca*. I guess the salty soy taste brings me back to my youth in *El Infierno*, the hellhole in the Petén, *my cuña*, my cradle." He grinned at me.

"So I hear you have a new friend here on the unit, Beltrán. He is a kid."

"Hey, *jefe*, none of your business. And he is not a kid and I am not a fucking *maricón* faggot, either." He was more than a little exercised. The muscles on his neck stood out.

"Look, I don't care about your personal sexual habits or interests. None of us gives a flying fuck, to use an expression I know you are familiar with. Except this is a hospital and I am responsible for what goes on here. And number two, we see a lot of patients here who are really damaged goods by the time they make it through the front doors. Many have been trafficked and severely abused physically, emotionally, and sexually as they make their way from Haiti, China,

Africa, Guatemala, to wherever they are dumped. You know damn well what I am talking about. Probably too well. And these are the ones who are not dumped in *narcofosas*, pits filled with the dead bodies of immigrants taken off buses, kidnapped, and killed for no reason whatsoever."

He stared at me blankly. I had no clue what ideas were brewing behind the flat look, but nothing good, I imagined. Yet he betrayed nothing.

"Look, you eat your pizza and your Chinese takeout while you are here. You don't pay for sex here with cash or slices of pizza. You don't prey on the other patients. You don't get off, jerked off, or anything else by some kid who is totally fucked up. I guarantee you the rest of your time will be under control of the DOC on 19, and then we will see who is fucking whom. You will have hoisin sauce in parts of your body you never thought possible. Do I make myself clear, Beltrán?"

He still looked blank.

Then he smiled. "Okay, okay, chill down, *jefe*. I won't do it again. Promise." The smile and promise chilled me more than his stare. He was an unsentimental killer. Smile, listen to merengue, put a bullet in a skull, then finish dinner with a beer.

"Look," he said, "I'm the victim here. I was a bit player for a few years between the drug cartels and Las Maras. Remember, I got squeezed between the two of them and ended up an immigrant myself. It is something, huh? I came here fleeing violence and certain death, not too different from the woman you told me about from near my hometown who fled the gun-toting *motocicleta* narco-violence and out-of-control machismo in her family eh. So I was part of the military elite who got blamed for everything, every bad fucking thing that happened in Guatemala was put on our head. You live without rules. Except the rules dictated by your commander. Unconditionally. You deviate and you are punished within an inch of your life." He held out his fingers and indicated a millimeter between thumb and forefinger.

"You learn to kill and put it behind you pretty quickly," he continued. "You kill one minute and have lunch the next, next to the dead body. On the dead body. After all, who trained the elite killing squads in Latin America, *jefe*? You invented them in Vietnam and practiced them on us. If you want an advanced degree in black ops or whatever, where do you get it? So let's not get too crazy about who is doing what to whom without some looking in the mirror." Again that smile. He pushed both hands through his hair and arched his back. He had a script and had it memorized. He would give up what he had to and not a millimeter more.

"So you come to the United States seeking safety like the rest of the patients at this hospital. Many here have been driven by the violence and kidnapping and mayhem of the cartels and Las Maras and the corruption that has all but taken over their societies." I almost felt stupid saying the obvious. How could I be playing the *your fault, my fault* game with this killer?

"*Jefe*, you are a smart guy. I am a smart guy. We both know the system is much bigger than we are. It extends over all the borders. The U.S. buys the drugs, sells the weapons, and launders the fucking money, after all. We all know that. It is the foundation, the basic shit 101. I participated in some bad stuff. I never hurt women or children, *jefe*, never. I was raised too good for that. I am a Christian. Like Father Alemán. He was my hero. I had partners that were really bad and did those horrible things. I have seen it firsthand." At least he didn't say he was just taking orders. I gave him credit for that. But I wasn't sure if I could believe him, either.

I stayed a few more minutes and then left. Beltrán completed his TB therapy after several months and was on his HIV-suppressive medication when he was escorted from the hospital by federal officials to an unknown destination. He disappeared one night. Detective Swann was uncommunicative when I saw him a final time a few days before Beltrán's discharge at the elevator bank on the main floor. I felt uneasy months after he left the hospital.

I swore I would never eat Chinese food again.

CHAPTER 11

The Unloved Woman

It was business as usual as I went on rounds with the trauma team. I did not put a name to the half-visible face lying in the intensive care unit for several days what with the tubes, color monitors, layers of hospital gowns, and black hair plastered to her head.

A clear plastic tube arched from her mouth to a high-tech ventilator, a computer attached to an electric bellows. The machine shushed her chest up and down like a metronome in slow motion. While semiconscious, she "bucked" the ventilator and her oxygen levels dropped. Insistent alarm beeps and flashing red luminescent warnings up and down the unit brought the trauma team to the bedside. Pancuronium, a curare-like drug, was "pushed" into her IV, and the drug paralyzed every muscle completely. The patient's oxygen levels normalized. Lunch-box-size computerized pumps clumped on IV poles lined up like the masts on a model sailboat collection controlled blood transfusions, intravenous solutions, and half a dozen medications all titrated to her lab results and instruments that monitored her in real time. An empty plastic bag hung from her left side rail. The shock of her injury damaged her kidneys. A dialysis technician, wearing a navy-blue Bellevue sweatshirt to ward off the proverbial chill of the ICU, hovered over the dials of a white console on wheels. Blood-filled catheters snaked from the patient's right upper chest and fed the insatiable kidney machine. The insistent hum of the electric pump circulated blood through a filter canister like a liter of blood-red milk.

Erika, the social worker on the intensive care unit floor, came by my office the next day. She had gone through the electronic medical records and seen my outpatient office notes. The patient's name had not registered with me during rounds with the surgical team. "Eric, you know Trauma Miami. Her real name is Alicia Rittner. She is an old patient of yours."

I had gotten the call a few nights earlier to accept a transfer. It had been about three a.m. A small community hospital in Brooklyn called our trauma surgeons about a case they couldn't manage; they needed an emergency transfer "right now." Our chief of surgery apologized for waking me up and got to the point. "Eric, look, I know this is unusual. This is a private hospital. But they have a young woman just out of the operating room who is still bleeding from a lacerated liver from an assault by her common-law husband. They are over their heads. She will die if we don't take her, and she may very well die if we do."

"Send her over. Do we have staff in the house and a bed in the recovery room after surgery?"

"Yes, we are fine there, no problem. By the way," he added almost as an afterthought, "she was twenty-nine weeks pregnant. They did a quick C-section and the baby is in their neonatal intensive care unit. I don't know the status yet; we will find out tomorrow."

"Jesus, Saul, got it. Let's get her over. ASAP." I would call about the baby in the morning. I knew their medical director.

I couldn't get back to sleep and didn't even try. I slipped out of the covers trying not to wake Diana and went into the kitchen to look at the lights over Manhattan, Queens, and Brooklyn. There were plates, glasses, and empty wine bottles piled up from a dinner with friends who were Chilean émigrés that ended only a few hours earlier. They had come to New York to escape from the terror unleashed as Pinochet commandeered the government on September 11, 1973. There were other 9/11s; we were not the first. It was strange to think that as I stared at the remnants from a dinner where we had covered the state of the world, life, love, all of our kids and their lives and loves, somewhere an ambulance was threading its way down Ocean Parkway to Flatbush Avenue and over the Manhattan Bridge. There wouldn't be any traffic. I made myself a quadruple macchiato. As the red light on the machine stopped blinking, I wondered if she would make it or not. Assault or homicide? That was the question.

The next thirty days were rocky for Alicia Rittner. The trauma from direct blows to her internal organs bought her a few trips to the operating room to find and tie off more bleeders. The patient had been discovered after neighbors had heard the screaming in her apartment and called 911. The restraining order was hanging from the refrigerator by a seashell-shaped magnet when the cops and EMT crew arrived and found her semi-conscious. Her husband was picked up by the police at a corner bodega buying cigarettes. Her pregnancy escalated *ordinary* domestic violence into another category. Jealous male rage followed typical patterns, and a pregnancy was a potent trigger. We had seen an uptick in home abuse as unemployment rates went up and the stock market went down.

Meticulous nursing and hypervigilance brought Ms. Rittner around. The turnaround was quick. The bleeding, oozing, and coagulopathy— the inability of her own blood to stanch the wound—stopped. The final signal appeared one day as rust-colored liquid appeared in the catheter bag at her side. Her kidneys, hit hard by the shock of low blood pressure and protein breakdown products from the assault, were coming back. "I told you guys to be patient." Omar, our trauma surgeon, looked satisfied on rounds as he lifted the bag and showed everyone the good news. Like the ancients looking for signs in the entrails of a slaughtered goat, this was a sign, a save. By putting her body into a kind of stopped time, we had allowed it to revive, rally, and begin to mend.

She now sat up in bed and was moved gingerly to a large lounge-type chair where she could be repositioned to look out the windows toward the blood-orange sunsets courtesy of the oil refineries in northern New Jersey, or toward the glass sliding doors where her doctors and nurses huddled several times a day poring over her medical record and the waveforms on her monitors.

Her baby, a preemie girl, was in stable condition and had been transferred to our NICU. There would be time for them to meet later. I went up early in the mornings just after the team made rounds or late in the afternoons when things were a little less hectic on the unit. I pulled up a plastic chair. "Alicia, I thought you left the city completely.

I have thought about you many times. You sure gave us a run for our money on this one."

"Sorry about that, Eric. Missed my last appointment, so I decided to take an ambulance to see you." I hugged her gently.

Alicia and I had met in the Bellevue general medical clinic years earlier when I still treated patients. The electronic printout for the day listed "Rittner, A." buried in the middle of twelve other patients, with hand-written "add-ons" taking me through lunch hour and early evening. I ran behind before I got started.

Alicia was in her midtwenties, pretty, with long dark hair, an inno-cently seductive smile, and a self-deprecatory sense of humor. I had a cartoon-like outline of her background despite prompting her for more details. Her middle-class, South American family were originally Jewish émigrés from Europe who had fled during the Nazi *anschluss* or annexation of Austria. They had settled in whatever country would take them, a rapidly shrinking planet lottery. Scarce Argentine visas were purchased, and her grandparents settled in Buenos Aires. At some point in her teens, she became pregnant. She decamped for the United States with the child's father and ended up in a poor Bronx neighborhood. A couple of one-liners was all I had.

Over the next few years, I saw her frequently. Alicia became an "overbook"—a patient squeezed in between scheduled patients. Dur-ing her first visit she had complained of migraine-type headaches, with nausea and vomiting and no obvious trigger. We tried a vari-ety of medications, stress reduction techniques, referral to a headache specialist who recommended the newest injectable medications and more sophisticated tests. The headaches that wouldn't quit prompted a series of "just to be sure" tests to eliminate an incubating brain tumor or pulsating arterial aneurysm from the list of potential medical issues. Alicia went through a battery of scans, from CT, to MRI, PET, and an electroencephalogram or EEG. They were normal. The medica-tions had only a temporary effect, and I started to feel they were mak-ing her worse. Alicia became a paragon of alternative treatments and

Googled advice: trips to Chinatown for homeopathic cures, acupuncture, qigong to tai chi. These measures were testimony to the persistence of her symptoms and my utter inability to help her. The feeling that the medical "arsenal" might be part of the problem and not part of the solution nagged at me.

Months later her complaints shifted subtly, and then abruptly, to chest discomfort. Heaviness with effort, a tightness that came with a cough. New-onset asthma, I thought. We went over her living conditions, allergies, pets, dust, and travel. Medication trials were mixed, and the persistent symptoms prompted me to send her to a pulmonary specialist. The standard workup included pulmonary function tests, inhalation provocation tests, a CT scan, and invariably different combinations of the newest asthma medications. No change. After exhausting all the possible pulmonary possibilities, the lung specialist felt the symptoms might be refluxing stomach acid irritating her upper airways, so he made a referral to a gastroenterologist.

The GI specialist slipped a black flexible tube through her mouth to view the lining of her stomach and esophagus. The normal endoscopy was followed up with a "swallow" of liquid chalk-like contrast to look for acid reflux, also normal. Alicia left the office of an über-specialist with a wire from her esophagus poking from her nose and duly recorded her symptoms in a diary for seventy-two hours. The acid readings were normal.

"I can't seem to get better," she would sigh. "It would be nice to know what's going on with me."

Ditto, I thought. What next?

The senior physician entered possible cardiac disease into the diagnostic equation, having been burned by a recent missed case. He took the liberty of arranging for a cardiologist "to be on the safe side."

After a brief history and physical in the doctor's office, an echocardiogram showed detailed anatomic pictures of the beating heart with normal valve and muscle function. The stress test that followed added no abnormalities on the repetitive squiggly lines of the EKG that poured off the machine. The cardiologist gave her a thumbs-up.

The tuna sandwich remained in its wrapper and the room-temperature

Dr. Brown's cream soda sat on my clinic desk late one afternoon a few months later as Alicia related her lower abdominal cramping, diarrhea alternating with constipation, and some blood in her bowel movements. Directed by a vegan-disposed dietitian, she had switched her diet to slurries of fruit and vegetable shakes fortified with assorted powders.

I wondered what was going on with Alicia. How had she become caught up in the web of technological probes and rays? What were her symptoms trying to tell me?

Some years earlier, sitting at lunch with Diana and my mother on our porch, we started talking about these odd symptoms. The view of the valley from our old farmhouse in New Hampshire was stunning. My parents had brought us a large cooler of food from Zabar's, the ultimate food emporium in Manhattan, convinced there was no food in the Upper Valley. We never told them otherwise. Why spoil the spoiling? We were enjoying the smoked salmon, sable, scallion cream cheese, and fresh bagels with crisp chilled white wine while some Andalucian *coplas* sung by Martirio filtered from the living room. I began talking about the frustrations of caring for many of my patients who seemed to have ever-shifting symptoms.

"I didn't know what the problem was at all. The diagnosis, that is."

"What do you mean?" my mother, May, asked me point-blank, her dark eyes focused on me. She was very direct and always came to the point. My family assumed it was from a life-threatening illness as a young teenager. Did that make her so no-nonsense? Who knew?

"After all my years looking after patients, I realized that half of the people who come in to see me have nothing physically the matter with them."

"What do the patients complain of when they come in?" May was curious now.

"A stew of different things. There is no single pattern. That is part of the puzzle. The symptoms morph, they change. I mean a patient may have stomach or intestinal symptoms and then later back pain.

Headaches and then tiredness or profound weakness. Chest pain. Things that sound like allergies, insomnia, food sensitivities. It goes on and on."

"Somatization." Diana put the name on the transformation of psychic distress to physical symptoms.

"Exactly. You have to work your way backward. The patient has the symptom, say, chronic back pain. After testing you see there is no physiological *there* there. Everything is normal, from the point of view of the medical establishment. Some patients are reassured momentarily. The evaluation relieves them. Others bail and seek all the alternative therapies and healers. For others, it's frustrating because we have not found the underlying problem. The pain remains unexplained."

"So now what?" May asked.

"Well, several possibilities. There are many layers, like an archaeological dig. On the top layer we have the physical complaint—say, back pain or headaches. The patient goes to the doctor and, hopefully, gets the diagnosis. Many doctors stop there after running some tests or prescribing some medication. Or they kick the ball to another specialist. For the patient, though, this label has a real function. *I can't go to work because I have a back spasm. I need to be alone because I have a migraine.* The label offers legitimization; it carries rights and privileges. Others might even look after them or help them out.

"A deeper evaluation, however, reveals depression and anxiety, the most common expressions of psychic distress. This is an almost universal manifestation of dis-ease—thus the huge market in antidepressants. The fastest-growing market.

"But another level down we see the effects of self-medication—alcohol abuse, drugs, and often violence in the home. This is harder to talk about, and to treat. Most doctors don't go near this.

"The next layer down reveals a lack of love and intimacy. These go hand in hand with a lack of self-esteem, shame, and a deep sense of humiliation. Humiliation is the well that everything comes from. The anger comes from that humiliation and underlies everything else. It's the propellant."

"But men will express that anger and humiliation in a different way than women do, right?" Diana asks.

"Yes, women tend to internalize their anger. They're not allowed to express it, so they turn it on themselves with depression, cutting, eating disorders, suicide attempts, and trips to the doctor. Men usually turn their anger outward, as aggression," I said.

"They externalize?" Diana said.

"With alcohol and drugs, and often physical stuff like hitting, abuse, domestic violence, inflicting pain on one hand, and on the other withholding feelings. Like a bank account. No withdrawals today, this month, or ever. Partner punishment. Men are more likely to kill themselves, though women attempt suicide more frequently. And homicide is the perfect expression of the humiliated disrespected male. They find it better to kill and be incarcerated than suffer the pain of shame, a form of non-being, social death, or soul death. I am thinking that humiliation is the common denominator, the deepest linkage of them all.

"But you know, there is another level. Think of the reigning myths in the United States about individual responsibility, making it on your own. We all live in a complex grid of social relations, class and race structures, economic and political histories. We are not tabula rasas, blank slates. The connections to a much deeper and in many cases darker reality are obscured in the daily medical world. It sort of reinforces the main national story."

We all sat there for a few minutes and didn't say anything. The afternoon light slanted through the huge sugar maple that air-conditioned the house in the summer and shed its leaves in brilliant colors every October.

"So let's go back to all the women who seek care in your office. They express neglect, you think?" Diana asked.

"Many of these women are neglected. Emotional neglect is so powerful. The fact that people are married for forty years, or have partners, doesn't begin to explain what is happening under the covers. I don't mean that only literally. The temperature of the relationship can be pretty close to zero degrees." We all turned at the same time as a posse of kids, ours and their friends, emerged from an apple orchard completely covered in dirt jabbering away.

"Unloved Woman as a diagnostic category," Diana summed up. "Is that what you are talking about?"

"Yes, precisely." I took a pause. "Strange. What you never see as a diagnostic category: the absence of love. Abuse manifesting itself as backache. Neglect resurfacing as chronic, unexplained pain. You have to go to the artists to find the emotional depth I am talking about."

"So women turn the emotional pain in on themselves and get physical symptoms?" my mother asked rhetorically. "That is what you are saying, Ricky." She always used my childhood nickname. She was sitting upright. She was small of stature but "mighty," we all conceded.

My father had joined us by this time after a visit with my brother in Norwich, Vermont. My mother filled him in on the conversation. His own doctor career began during World War II in Okinawa after an internship in Boston City Hospital; by now he had been in medical practice for decades. "Bob, do you see the kinds of things Ricky is talking about? I mean with your patients. We haven't ever talked about these issues," my mother asked my dad.

"No, I haven't," he said thoughtfully. He knew his patients very well, and they stayed with him for a long time. He was a doctor's doctor, living and breathing medicine with full enjoyment of his chosen profession. This was a generational issue in medicine if ever there was one. It was like him asking someone about their sexual orientation. He just didn't go there. Never. He could have a herd of elephants in a room and swear he was at Lincoln Center and not the Big Apple Circus.

A few days after my parents had returned home, my mother called me. "I can't believe it. I just can't believe it. I've known her most of my life." By this time I had forgotten what we'd been talking about. "Helen. She was sexually abused as a young woman. Raped by a family friend. Can you believe that? I told her my son the doctor has this new crazy theory and had she ever heard anything like it and she just told me. She'd never put it together with all her symptoms, and no doctor had ever asked her."

After thinking back on that phone call, my thinking shifted—from symptom to person. I realized how little I really knew about Alicia Rittner. I had focused on her physical complaints and been technically thorough with a full slate of specialists and testing capabilities. But I had been treating her as a specimen rather than a human being. I knew next to nothing about this young woman in front of me. The balance of when to look and how hard to pursue is a complex one. Different patients require different strategies.

I rethought the case as it evolved over time, questioning Alicia when she came back to see me over the next few visits about the possibility of depression, anxiety, drug or alcohol use, the most common culprits. Then a deeper dive into the wider circles around her—children, her partner(s), income and expenses, the neighborhood, her friends and network of social supports and family. I was trying unsuccessfully to get at her feelings. A hint, a whiff, an opening, in her safe public persona that might give me a clue about where her symptoms came from. She handled me like a tennis pro running me from baseline to baseline.

Everyone has secrets, private fears and fantasies. They may share them with a special person or keep them behind walls and off-limits. Sometimes they are the small humiliations and hurts that dully persist into adulthood and rob us of the full range of feelings and intimacy, like color blindness or a phantom limb. In one case something is missing and you don't know what it is. In the other something is gone but it feels like it is there. For some people there are unspeakable demons. Vigilance may be needed to keep them from overwhelming the walls we build to protect ourselves. Denial is a first-responder strategy, but it is not adequate for all emotional situations. Dissociation or splitting a personality into pieces develops in childhood as another level of strategic coping with intolerable anxiety. It is effective, and like many coping strategies it becomes a way of living, part of who you are. At some point it can interfere with intimacy and building and maintaining relationships. Hair triggers, seemingly inconsequential and nearly invisible, can send someone into another zone in a moment.

"Alicia, something doesn't add up. Your tests are fine. You are healthy from every point of view. Yet I feel something is going on. Do you have an idea what it might be?" The visits reassured her. I stopped doing more than taking my stethoscope out of my coat pocket, making a quick reassuring check of blood pressure, heart, and lungs, and listening. Low tech and high touch.

When she left the office one day, I had a few moments of downtime while we were hunting for a Fulani translator for my next patient. The Fulani, a widely distributed West African people, had a language with many dialects, as complicated as the regional politics. My mind drifted to other patients in other times. A woman in her seventies reappeared like a daydream. She was in a long-term marriage to a pillar of the community, a banker, who was highly respected for both his financial sagacity and his public generosity. She had been to see me for over a dozen years with multiple complaints that changed with the seasons or orbits of the moon. Slight, formal, and superficially friendly, she was always immaculately dressed.

One night she was hospitalized with chest pain. We worked her up for a heart attack. But nothing.

I sat by her bedside in the stillness of a hard New Hampshire winter and asked her what was going on. Quietly, and with great precision, she told me a long story about how her husband sexually abused her young granddaughter over years. She put a stop to it immediately when she found out. But she could not bring herself to go to the police or even her priest for fear of destroying her family's reputation and their standing in the community. She reviled her husband. A savage intensity radiated from her eyes, and the tension in her body ionized the exam room. It had taken years for these words to be spoken out loud to another human being. Her family life was a vortex of anger, guilt, rage, impotence, and bottomless shame. The secret was poisoning the next generations. She was dying of a broken heart.

My patients were like persistent afterimages, burned into my retinas. I could channel them into the consultation room. Marilyn, for example, who came in for her monthly blood checks. She was on clozapine injections and needed to have her white cells measured before her next injection. It worked better than the other anti-psychotics. Her chart was in three volumes and full of visits, hospitalizations, trips to the emergency room, crisis team outreach checks, and a zillion tests and workups. The diagnosis changed over time. I had spent a long entire afternoon reading through it and outlining the case. I was doctor number ten or twelve. The new guy in town, a handoff patient, part of the medical "economy." She weighed 250 pounds. Medication side effect, I thought.

"You know, Marilyn, this is our anniversary," I told her when she'd settled in and begun some random chatter.

"What do you mean, anniversary?" She looked at me quizzically.

"Two years now. We have been together for two years. Two years ago today to be precise you came to see me."

"You are right, Eric, it is two years. I have collected doctors like stamps or buttons. I think you win the award for the longest," she said and promptly continued.

"All my other doctors got sick of me. I could tell. They would refer me and refer me trying to get rid of me, making up some kind of excuse or other. It was a game. I would tell them a symptom I made up and the predictable referral would appear. Plus I got side effects all the time from the meds they were handing out like candy. A conjuring trick you doctors do, you know." I knew.

"You have not ordered anything on me in two years. Not one test, nothing. Just my high blood pressure that we play around with. And you never said a word about my weight or my smoking. How come? You don't play the game, how come?"

"I don't think you have anything worrisome. I think you are a pretty healthy woman. I am here to listen and offer something when I think I have something to offer you. I think you have suffered a lot at some point in your life. You are talking to me with your body, and listening is my treatment."

"I never told anyone this. Since it is our anniversary, you should be the first to know. My older brother raped me for ten years. From when I was five years old. Until he went to prison for extra-family sexual abuse of minors. Why do you think I got so fat and ugly?" She said it out loud, crystal clear, and looked at my reaction. I had first thought of her as the Toad in *The Wind in the Willows*. After a couple of visits, her wit and cutting sarcasm made me look forward to seeing her. She had come in one time for a checkup. I had started her on a new blood pressure medicine and read her the usual side effects and a throwaway "plus it can turn your hair green." When I looked up from my desk, she was sitting in the chair cool and calm with her hair dyed green. "Doc, great medication. No side effects this time!" She was a safety hatch from the "worried well" auto-monitoring their bodies for the slightest whisper of an infirmity after every news article and morning TV or radio report.

These experiences made me sense that Alicia's parrying and avoidance pointed to a dark force somewhere. I was aware she had been born in Argentina during the Dirty War or what is called El Proceso—an era that lasted from 1976 to 1983 when the country was run by a military dictatorship. It was global Cold War politics that had gone viral in a South American test tube. I had tried to engage Alicia to talk about her time there, her family, and the experiences she had as a young girl, a teenager before having an affair with an American hippie who was backpacking in South America. She hitchhiked with him to Tierra del Fuego, got pregnant, and left the country precipitously. My wife had written a book about the dictatorship, and Diana and I had spent hours talking about the long-term effects of violence. Many survivors fled Argentina to other safe havens in Mexico or Spain or the United States just as Alicia's family had once fled fascist Europe for Peronist Argentina. Safe havens that were not safe anymore. Multiple packings and fleeings: You slept with your passports under your pillow and sniffed the political winds continuously.

Years later, I still didn't know what had happened to Alicia Rittner except that now she had been admitted in a near-fatal condition, and the head nurse was escorting me to newborn Naomi Rittner's room in the NICU. Baby Naomi had done well despite the emergency C-section. She was on the road to recovery. I stopped and chatted with the nurses and other mothers nursing their newborns. It was a complete medical universe in miniature. A small baby was being evaluated by a pediatric surgeon wearing blue-green scrubs. His large index finger exerted an ounce of pressure on the tiny abdomen. Black formfitting eyeshades protected the yellow-tinged baby from the light therapy he was receiving for the high bilirubin levels in his blood. Blue light converted the dangerous variety of bilirubin into a benign molecule that could not cause damage to the delicate brain tissue in development.

The preemie's X-ray showed small black air pockets around the intestinal lining. This was a sign of inflammation of the intestinal wall or NEC, necrotizing enterocolitis, a treacherous complication of prematurity. With luck and patience it resolved on its own with a decrease in feedings and less stimulation of the intestine. Life-threatening infections requiring surgery, decompression with a tube, or removal of part of the intestine was the other trajectory. This was watch-and-wait-and-hope therapy.

Nurses in colorful scrubs padded around softly adjusting their tiny charges, calming them with strokes and caresses while many mothers sat by incubators with their babies strapped to their chests rocking them back and forth. A few volunteer Kangaroo moms had tiny kitten-size preemies squeezed tight between their breasts and chatted quietly to one another. The neonatal intensive care unit deliberately created an environment to soothe the vulnerable, rapidly developing and maturing brain's neuronal connections for its tiny patients. Overstimulation was toxic for nervous systems making their connections. Low-tech or reverse migration of simple solutions was making its way back to a medical universe high on technology and innovation. A couple of neonatologists in Bogotá in the 1970s, unable to afford the latest incubators, made the mothers surrogate incubators, skin-to-skin. Kangaroo care had arrived, was successful, saved lives, and cost nothing.

Naomi was out of her incubator swaddled to a Kangaroo volunteer mom who had her wrapped tightly against her chest. Naomi's eyes were wide open. She had a small pink cap on and was receiving protein feedings from an IV pump into an umbilical blood vessel. There was a tiny oxygen tube connected to her nostrils. The first two weeks had been stormy as she began to adjust to life outside a uterus before her organs had matured. The team was ready to pull the feeding catheter and switch Naomi entirely to breast milk pumped from her mother upstairs in the ICU. Lorie pointed to the oxygen levels on the computer screen above my head and said quietly, "She doesn't like us talking here." As our voices had risen, her blood and pulse went up and her oxygen levels dropped slightly. "We should leave."

A few mornings later I bought a coffee with heavy cream and a couple of croissants at the Au Bon Pain in the lobby of the hospital early in the morning. The day shift was coming on—walking in from Penn Station, the ferry slip on the East River, the express-bus stops at 23rd Street, and the six-train station at Park and 28th. Thousands of people threaded their way to the hospital a few blocks south of the United Nations building. I took the elevator up to the surgical floor, said hello to the nurses coming on, and knocked on the door of Room 28 before walking in. Two distinct Spanish dialects filtered through the open door. Laura, the Mexican from the crime victims unit, sat in a chair with her back to me talking to Alicia.

They invited me to pull up a chair, and I laid out the breakfast I had brought Alicia. I also bought her a copy of the *New York Times* and brought her my faded college copy of *Ficciones* by Borges.

"Sorry to interrupt, ladies," I said.

"No, join us for a few minutes before the surgical team arrives and I am booted out of here." Laura pulled over a chair for me. "We were talking about what happened."

"Okay, Alicia, if I sit in?"

"*Claro que sí*, Eric, of course," she said clearly.

Laura continued her conversation with Alicia as if I weren't there. "Your parents fled Europe and by chance ended up in Argentina. Survivors can sometimes feel that it is better to have perished. There is a lot of guilt attached, Alicia. Does this make any sense to you?"

"I deserve the punishment I got," she said, looking at her hands.

"Nobody deserves what you got. Nobody," Laura said. "You are not responsible for what happened. The man who did this seduced you and then stole parts of you, little by little. You couldn't see it coming."

"He didn't take anything from me, Laura. Those parts you mention were stolen long before I ever met him."

The knock on the door was perfunctory as the white lab coats descended on us to check Alicia's progress. Laura and I beat a quiet retreat. I headed back to my office.

I was preoccupied with a phone call from two days earlier. Alicia's common-law husband, Gregory Annas, had been transported from his cell at Rikers Island to Bellevue for the standard forensic psychiatric evaluation. He sat in a single cell on suicide prevention watch. It was not rare for us to have the victims in our ICUs as their attackers were being looked after in the prison unit.

The general profile of Gregory Annas was in the public record. His role in a self-perpetuating cycle of violence was familiar fare to our psychiatric teams. He had grown up in a lower-middle-class family on Long Island with six brothers and sisters. They had been home-schooled, and the family had been investigated several times. Neighborhood vigilantes, alarmed by the identical uniforms the kids wore on the rare occasions they went outside accompanied by their father, called 911. One report from a social worker who did several home visits indicated that he brought a soccer ball for the kids one time and they had no idea what to do with it. A sign that read "Order and Progress" hung from a wall.

There was no evidence of corporal punishment or physical abuse, no evidence of malnutrition. There was no television, radio, or Internet access visible. The children were managed by their stay-at-home mother. No visitors came, and no one could leave the apartment or go outside except under the direct supervision of the father when he came home from work. There was a phone that had been rigged to only receive calls. Every child had a typed list of responsibilities, tasks to complete that were recorded in neatly checked-off boxes. The operating family philosophy, summed up by the investigating social worker, was, "Society is toxic and dangerous. It is our responsibility as parents to protect our children from the social influences that will damage them. We accept total responsibility for their growth and development and ask no help from any government or private organization." There was no evidence of a cult affiliation. This was merely one man's control over his family, within the boundaries of the law and the rules of the child welfare agencies.

After several days of questioning, it became clear that Gregory had incorporated his father's pathological control issues. His father died suddenly. He did not come home one day. The police showed up at the door. His wife showed no emotion and thanked the officer. His maternal grandparents pieced together the family's ability to function over time with great care and sensitivity and the injection of resources. The grandparents had been shut out of their daughter's life by edict but not by lack of love. They had considerable means and ensured that all of the children went to private schools close to the grandparents' Long Island estate, where they built a house for their long-lost daughter and grandchildren. Gregory went off to college and became involved in a drug scene and a variety of religious groups from ultra-Orthodox Judaism to Scientology to evangelical Christianity to Hinduism and back. He experimented relentlessly and kept a live feed of the Western Wall (or "Kotel") on his computer desktop as a screensaver. The rest of his story was the repetition of control and abuse.

Patty silently entered my office, startling me. A lingering side effect of my platinum chemotherapy was hearing loss and a high-pitched tinnitus or buzzing. My wife strongly suggested hearing aids. I said I would have a Seeing Eye dog first. Great help that will be, she said.

"There is a young man here to see you. Isaac Rittner. His mom is in the hospital." Patty handed me some important paperwork I'd neglected. She had telepathically completed half and tagged with colored stickies options and question marks without being asked. After more than a dozen years working together, we were in sync. I heard Patty's teenage daughter laughing outside with Jan, our newest office recruit. I didn't know how Patty managed with three kids in public schools all on the verge of collapse, the neighborhood a veritable gang training ground, trains that worked half the time making the commute from central Bronx a daily crapshoot, and on it went. When she wasn't haranguing the board of education, nearly a full-time job, she had started a volunteer program out of our office for kids and young adults to work in the hospital, from helping in the operating room, to conducting patient interviews, to navigating patients through their appointments. Our office overflowed. As the economy slid into a deeper recession, we had a small army of volunteers whose ranks ran from high school students to a post-retirement FBI agent.

Isaac was Alicia's teenage son. Pregnant at fifteen in Buenos Aires, she grabbed the first ticket out of Argentina with the North American hippie who'd offered her companionship, caresses, and a twelve-hour overnight flight from a country that was suffocating her. Her descent from upper-middle-class Buenos Aires affluence was relatively swift. She ended up on her own in the Bronx just off the Grand Concourse— an almost genteel Jewish neighborhood where up until the 1960s kids studied hard and went to City College for free.

"Isaac, it has been a long time. It's nice to see you. We have a lot to catch up on." I gave him a hug and motioned to a black swivel chair around the large oblong table in my office. "What's up?" I asked as he settled in and swiveled around while he surveyed the office pictures, art, books, and piles of articles and projects and the reflecting wall of glass that had become my view. From staring at the UN rectangle I had been reduced to a faux Narcissus, looking at myself courtesy of the New York City Economic Development Corporation.

"You lost your view, Doc." He didn't miss anything.

He had on jeans, new white Nike sneakers, a designer T-shirt, and facial hair Dominican-style. It had been cut with an electric razor to millimeter sideburns threaded to a trimmed beard. Every hair was gelled in place. Tight. I expected merengue from the white ear pods draped over his shoulders connected to the smartphone on his belt.

"You know I don't know much except the headlines. Your mom stopped coming here some time ago. There are big pieces missing." It was almost lunchtime, and we agreed to share some lunch while we talked. I popped my head out the main office door and asked Patty to grab some tortas and Snapple from our newest street food vendors from Puebla. I gave it two more years before New York City was completely Latinized. It wasn't just the Spanish language everywhere.

The whole city was beginning to look more like any Latin American city with its failing infrastructure and undersupported educational and health programs.

I sat back in the chair and looked at Isaac. He was different from the overweight sulking youngster I had known many years ago. Like most Bellevue kids, he tagged along with his mother to her office visits. Day care was unaffordable. Back then I would hold his small hand and walk him to the pediatrics floor where the Reach Out and Read program colonized the waiting room. Kids sat like flocks of migrating birds on blue mats surrounded by the volunteer reading instructors/coaches whose canvas bags were overflowing with books for all ages. Isaac would tentatively join a group, scrunch himself onto a corner of a mat, and listen enraptured as the young medical student in skintight blue jeans and a green Old Navy T-shirt, hair in a ponytail, worked her way through a Dr. Seuss opus and a trimmed-down version of *Around the World in Eighty Days*.

He always came back gripping a new book, his very own with his name printed on the inside cover: "ISAAC R." Most kids only had a Bible and some comic book–style self-help literature in their apartments. Depending on where the mothers were from, their cultural background and literacy, reading at home was a never event. The kids took a direct hit and ended up several years delayed at school by the time they reached kindergarten; they never made up the difference. Many mothers came to the waiting room even if they did not have appointments with their kids. Their kids lit up with the books in hand as the staff called out their names while hugging them and finding some mat space.

"You know, the last time I saw you I think you were fixated on the adventures of *The Count of Monte Cristo* in Spanish or English, I don't remember. You ignored everything else around you. It was pretty cool. So what's happened, Isaac? Last I knew you were a reader with a mother who had an apartment like a public library branch." He looked behind me at the packed bookshelves, stacks of journals, and piles of papers that were a reflection of my cerebral cortex.

He began slowly. "It was a hard ride at first. I got into some street gang stuff. Nothing much. Alicia went nuts and grounded me forever. I had the world record of time-outs. So I went underground."

"Yeah, so how did you turn your ship around?" I asked.

"Pure *suerte*, luck, Doc. I mean, I had this friend twice removed so to speak. We were walking together toward what looked like a warehouse in a sketchy part of the Bronx. There were lots of people coming in and out, all ages, races, sizes, and shapes. I mean a real carnival of humanity. Completely out of place in a neighborhood where pizza joints, bodegas, pawnshops, and liquor stores were on every block."

A safe port in the storm? I was thinking.

"We heard great hip-hop from the wide-open double metal doors. So we walked over and asked the guy at the door if we could come in and listen.

"There was a musical of sorts going on. Not like Broadway or any of that commercial stuff. But dancers, musicians, poetry, singing, some amazing hip-hop dancing, better than anything I had ever seen."

"So what happened, Isaac?"

"This woman comes up to us, Rodney and me. We had been there for over an hour, just standing and watching and listening, the time just went. Her name was Mildred, a Puertorriqueña singer who was from the neighborhood. She ran the place with Steve, her Afro-American husband, also a musician. *El Puente*, it was called. They started as pickup musicians in high school. From there they had a group and decided to start something in the high desert of the Bronx fifteen years ago. A place for kids to come and do something besides drugs."

Isaac was animated, in charge, and had pulled himself quickly out of a superficial funky younger avatar. "We got introduced to Steve and were invited back. The place has stuff going all of the time. Art, music, dance, and theater for starters. They have trips all over the city to see stuff I had never imagined except on those blue mats at the hospital waiting for my appointments. I mean I found a real *Cat in the Hat*." He smiled and shrugged with an *aw shucks* look.

"So you still involved with them?"

"I got into writing. I still do that. Like short stories, working on the

Mano newsletter, learning to edit and then into playwriting and short stories." He had safely swerved the lethal street scene.

"What was going on at home?" I asked him in a monotone.

"Home was a real disaster zone. My mother hooked up with this guy who initially was okay, cool, friendly, and seemed to care about the two of us. That lasted about a year. I don't know what came first, his drinking and acting out or the acting out and then the drinking. At any rate I was old enough to spend more time on the streets and with my friends and avoid the yelling, slapping, door slamming, throwing shit, breaking things, and then the making up. It was quiet for a few days or a couple of weeks. He'd be super considerate. A real gentleman." He paused and took a bite from the torta sandwich dripping with burnt-orange-colored sauce. Chipotle.

"They would go shopping and bring home fresh lobsters and Italian food from Arthur Avenue near the Bronx Zoo. You can hear the elephants in between cab horns and the grinding gears of delivery trucks. We ate with candles on the table stuck in empty wine bottles, fresh baguettes, bottles of red wine that did not come in the shape that fits in your back pocket, and even an embroidered tablecloth my mother bought from our Mexican neighbors upstairs. Like a real family from television. Then one day he brought my mom some roses. Real roses from the Korean place across the street. I'm not sure who said what but he reached out and slapped her across the face with a dozen red roses. The alcohol reeked from the open hole in his face.

"It was out of the movies really. Like you paid a few dollars, got some popcorn and a soft drink, and settled into one of those tall chairs that slid down as you settled in and watched your life in play for two hours. Then the credits came on, the music stopped, and the lights came on. Then the movie was over. No more candles. No more embroidered tablecloths. The wine bottles were stacked forty deep next to the fridge and the stuff would start all over again. Eventually there was no making up, and no two weeks off on good behavior. It blurred together into one bad nightmare scene. It was just pissed-off bad stuff all the time. So much for *The Count of Monte Cristo*." There was a reason Rikers was hidden on an island with a slim causeway from Queens and killing tidal currents scuffing the rocky rim. Pissed-off rage and nothing to lose is a powerful thing.

"He was a smart guy, had a decent job. Speak about books, he did have book knowledge. He read the newspapers and talked a good game. What a fucking loser.

"The worst part for me was seeing my mother grovel for the guy. I mean she lost her self-respect. To not provoke the guy she would try to be perfect. But there is no perfect in this other universe. Anything could make him angry and set him off. Dinner was late. Dinner was early. Too hot or too cold. It made no difference. But the son-of-a-bitch had stalked her perfectly and set her up to fall into his trap. He had made slow cuts, little ones, almost not noticeable, but persistent, and he stole her from herself, until he owned her." *Textbook*, I thought. *Psychopath.*

"Doc, I had two lives and kept them separate as I could. I had all this stuff to do and to think about and it was always there for me. It saved me from what was happening at home. I switched channels when I was there. Like I said, I was lucky."

"How's Alicia doing today, Isaac?" I asked.

"She is better and getting better every day. I just wonder what it will take for her to not be with these guys. I mean, why does she pick such losers? She is a needy woman who cannot bear to be by herself. These guys pick her out with built-in radar. You can see their antennas fluttering, picking up signals." He put his fingers up over his ears and wiggled them. He was soft-spoken at this point, not talking particularly to me anymore. A general statement that said it all.

I leaned forward and half whispered to him, "What happened to her? What is the story?"

It made me uneasy that I was going down this trail again. Was it just voyeuristic interest? A need to know? To prove that I knew there was something there? To prove something to myself, to Alicia? All of the above. We all had emotional vulnerabilities, hidden fears and traumas that motivated us, propelled us, compulsively drove us to do certain things again and again. Anxieties that we rationalized, that made us hate ourselves, that stalked us in the night. If trauma hit when we were young and emotionally tender, it lingered for a lifetime and we handed it off to our children. I satisfied myself that an attempted murder, lacerated liver, and near death of a fetus qualified as a reason to pursue a source—not in the perpetrator, that was another issue entirely—but in the victim. The victim who was suffering the near-lethal consequences of being a heat-seeking missile for victimizers.

He looked sharply at me and was pretty alert. The slight slouch was gone as his muscles tensed.

"Look, Doc, you have known us for a long time and seen us through a lot of stuff. To go deep and understand what is going on in my family, what family there is, is to go back to the beginning. The very beginning. Way before I came into the picture. I was part of the ticket out. I know my mother loves me very much. That's not what I mean." The conversation was entering a different place. I got up and made us a couple of espressos and put on the table some bitter dark chocolate a friend had brought back from Guatemala. We stirred the inky black coffee in the tiny hand-painted Uriarte cups. The wrappers from the chicken and beef tortas covered the table between us.

We both sipped the coffee. He had a mustache from the *crema* and looked more like the kid I knew on a blue gym mat in the pediatric clinic. He snapped off a piece of the black chocolate. "She had to leave; there was no Plan B. I asked her a lot of times as a kid where were my grandparents. I mean, my father had disappeared after a couple of years. He was one messed-up dude, from what I can make out. So there was really the two of us holding down the fort in the Bronx, literally our own Fort Apache with triple locks and window bars so people couldn't crawl in from the fire escape. We couldn't get out if there was a fire but that was secondary. You had to live long enough to have a fire to burn to death from." A piece of homegrown wisdom from the South Bronx. I had grown up on the other side of the tracks in the same borough.

"Her father was military. I mean not her real father, not my grandfather, either. The people that brought her up were military. It took her a number of years and lots of questioning and detective work. First they admitted that she was adopted. That took some time by itself.

She was very persistent once she got it in her head that they might not be her real parents. I mean biological. And she kept asking why didn't they tell her and who were her real parents." He chilled and slowed down the pace.

"*Hijos*, children of the disappeared?" I asked. The dots were lining up.

"They said she had been left as an orphan in the hospital where she was born. She had been abandoned at birth. They were alerted by nuns from their diocese and went to see her and immediately decided to adopt her. She was so precious, they loved her as their own blood daughter. They considered that she was their daughter and there was no need to tell her. They apologized for bad judgment." A dark storm cloud was descending over the household. Alicia Rittner was not then Alicia Rittner. "She was Alicia. Her biological parents had named her—she learned that much. The parents who adopted her were military as I said. This was during the *Guerra Sucia*, the Dirty War."

Isaac was having trouble at this point. This was getting close to the unspoken truth that had driven his mother from her presumed home and made her a permanent refugee unable to go find her real home and the family that she might rightfully call hers.

"Her real parents had been kidnapped—her mother was seven months pregnant with her. They were young professionals in graduate school, journalism and architecture. Jewish. They were picked up one day off the street and disappeared. They were never seen again. The military secret service had taken the baby Alicia from her mother just after she was delivered and given her to the nuns to look after her. There was an understanding that she would be offered up for adoption to high-ranking military families. They killed her mother as they had killed her father." He spoke of his grandparents in the third person. Like telling a story about someone else and not his own family member.

"Doc, I keep asking what if? What if she'd never found out? She would have skied in Bariloche, and gone horseback riding in the countryside, and learned French in Paris?"

"Too many what-ifs, Isaac. Where would you be, by the way? What if the English had lost the Battle of Britain and there was a Nazi flag on Whitehall? *What if*, Isaac, *what if...what*?" He had launched me into an alternative world of what-ifs, a counterfactual universe that did not happen. Once she suspected, she had to know or be poisoned. Already the lie had seeped into her.

"My mom did the research through the different support groups, parents' groups, children's groups, Jewish groups, and the international human rights groups that have assisted people in finding their parents, their sisters, brothers, children. The relentless march of the *Madres*, the Mothers, around the Plaza de Mayo with the pictures of their missing children brought her to this central city square. She returned every week to the marches of the mothers, talking to them and piecing together what was really happening in Argentina behind a facade secured with secret police and a city littered with clandestine torture centers. She went to the *Abuelas*, the Grandmothers who tried to identify their lost grandchildren. She found out who she was and heard that her own grandmother was dead."

The small inconsistencies of daily life multiplied and led her to the disappeared, her parents, whose final moments were blindfolded on a flight over the miles-wide Rio Plate before it disgorged a continent's effluvia into the Atlantic along with drugged men and women. When Alicia had connected all the dots she left and never looked back. She had moved out of her house some months earlier. She had been living on friends' couches and in borrowed apartments. She was a fifteen-year-old who had grown up under privilege, with a beloved Bolivian nanny, Carmen, who had been her wet nurse, and a chauffeur, Arturo.

An American grad student met her in a café. They began walking the city together and she moved in with him. She became pregnant with Isaac and they decided to move to New York City, his hometown. He found work with the help of his grandparents, and she took in other children and taught Spanish to high school students. At first it was odd that he never brought her to meet his family, and they never came to visit. There were a million excuses. Given her own flight from her "family" she didn't ask too many questions, since they had found each other and created a nest and a refuge from the world. The world gradually constricted for her as he began to monitor her activities and insisted that she stay close to home. The neighborhood was dangerous, the gangs were prolific, the city was in tough times so it all made reasonable sense on one level as a concerned loving partner. Until he hit her the first time.

She had freed herself from one set of monsters, sitting across the dinner table, sharing a meal, watching television, and pretending that normal family life was proceeding calmly. That the banal domestic routines of school, church, clubs, dinners, visiting Iguazú, were supported by caring and love. She had not freed herself from a self-hatred, a self-loathing, that she had been violated so deeply, and contaminated so profoundly by her self-proclaimed parents who loved her to death. Literally it seemed.

Diana had led me through this world step by step fifteen years earlier as she was writing a book on the Dirty War. We had walked with the Mothers of the Plaza de Mayo, visited the torture centers, talked with close friends who had lost their loved ones. The deceptively simple act of mothers meeting weekly and walking in front of the Casa Rosada, the president's house, year after year never allowed the wound to seal over. They continued to make the disappearances visible as an act of denunciation.

I walked Isaac from my office to First Avenue. We were both depleted and hardly said a word. His searching heart had found a place with people who offered him another mat to scrunch onto as he gradually spread himself out into a cosmopolitan city. All Alicia's symptoms made sense. A tormented woman looking for help and for care. The inner wounds would not light up on any scan.

A few days later my phone buzzed with a text from Patty during a jammed public meeting in the large open atrium at the main entrance to the hospital. The mayor and governor were announcing support for the public health system. "Better than the private sector" were the last words I heard as I slipped out to make a phone call.

"Lorie, what's up?" She ran the SS *NICU* like a military vessel.

"Alicia has freaked out. ACS is here about her daughter. We need your assistance on this one."

She met me at the glass doors to the NICU with Helen from social work and the attending Suzanne. "Hi, guys, let's go into the break room."

"Child protection is here to evaluate her fitness to care for her daughter. She is over the top." Helen got it out fast and to the point.

"She is breast-feeding her daughter and making a good recovery. All of the bad chemicals, drugs, antibiotics have been replaced by a flood of maternal oxytocin. I don't get it." Child protection? Who pulled the alarm?

Helen read me. "We had to file. It is the law. Automatic. They filed from the hospital where they did the C-section. Also Eric, Naomi was almost killed, remember?" Lorie added, "Can you guarantee Naomi will be safe?" My thoughts turned to sliding steel doors and electronic locks. Greg Annas having dinner at Rikers Island before being sentenced to an upstate prison. How many years?

I suddenly realized Alicia could lose her daughter. It had not occurred to me. "Let me go talk to her." They nodded in agreement, that was the plan. I walked the long corridor of permanent twilight and hushed tones.

"Laura, I need to talk to you about what to do, what is the right thing to do now." I was sitting with the crime victims social worker in her office.

"Eric, she has no insight into what is happening to her, how she gets involved with these control-freak guys. She emotionally short-circuits. We see this over and over again."

"So what can be done? She loves her son and he dodged the craziness and is thriving. She obviously loves her daughter. She is not a hopeless basket case on crack selling herself in front of her children." ACS was frequently in a tough position of when to pull the plug to put kids' safety first. There was no biopsy for this one.

"There is a lot she can do, and things are not hopeless. Believe me, I understand what is at stake here." Laura was thinking things through and coming up with a plan.

"Time out from men would be a good thing also." Laura smiled. "She is a passion junkie and her anxiety goes way down when she is feeling cared for, looked after, the seduction piece."

"First she needs to commit to treatment, I mean therapy. I can get her a really good person. We don't need to use the Yellow Pages. Then she needs to join a group of people like her and hear stories and build up some trust with other victims. It works. Like AA and other support groups, it really does work. And she will need additional therapies, like cognitive behavioral therapy or dialectical behavioral therapy, that work in the here and now on practical skills to handle her emotional ups and downs.

"I have seen it firsthand on the child psychiatric unit with Dr. Liu in kids from six to twelve. It does work. 'Think of pizza with pepperoni when you have those angry feelings.'" We were developing a plan to sell to Alicia and to ACS. They both had to buy it.

"Eric, most important for you, before you go into the deep end of the pool on this one, let her tell you in her own words what happened. She has to show you a little trust." I knew Laura was right and I had no idea what Alicia would say or could say.

Alicia was sitting in a wheelchair, her eyes rimmed in red, her shoulders covered in a hand-embroidered shawl in the unit conference room. The official from protection got up and introduced herself, "Hi, Sarah Caldwell. I have to make a couple of phone calls. Will be in the nursing station when you are done." She quietly closed the door.

Alicia switched to Spanish. "They want to take my baby away from me. They say she may not be safe in my home."

"What do you think?" I asked her.

She looked at me and said nothing for a long time. The pause said more than her words. "Eric, I want you to help me keep her. They will listen to you if you support me. You know me well, you know Isaac. I need your help now." The magic words.

Could I help her? Should I help her? I could imagine her parents. I had walked around the Plaza de Mayo with the Mothers. I had seen the pictures of their missing children. I had known the stories of *hijos*, children, and the rippling effects through families and generations. But I also saw a woman who for reasons she might not be able to control had been cycling in destructive relationships. Could she look after herself? Could she look after her children?

Was there some middle ground? A compromise position where protection's needs could be met, where the law's requirements could be satisfied? Could I guarantee that Naomi would be looked after and safe from harm? Naomi Rittner-Annas, I remembered. How many years would the sentence be?

"Alicia, I need to know what happened to you in Argentina, before you left pregnant with Isaac," I said, then realized it was a bribe, perhaps, or a necessary price she would have to pay. Did she know that I knew? Did Isaac tell her? For years I had talked about Argentina, and not just about Borges. They were finally arresting generals from the time of the dictatorship, now octogenarians, and putting them in prison. The amnesty had been repealed. Maybe her time had come?

She took a long time before she said anything. She wasn't crying. She sat in her chair and looked at me directly. She knew we weren't playing a game and there was a lot at stake now.

"My parents were killed, Eric. They were young, just married. Getting started in life. I was the family they were creating. I started to hear stories when I was a young teenager. Murders, kidnappings, children put up for adoption. Little pieces started to come together as I reached out to members of the community created by the Mothers and Grandmothers. The family that raised me and their most intimate friends dismissed the activism and publicity as showmanship and a way to blackmail the Argentine state. One cretinous man, our neighbor, said the military never finished the work it needed to do, that was the problem."

She looked down at her daughter's face on her breast. "How many generations, Eric? How many generations have to be lost to this violence?"

"You have to put an end to the cycle, Alicia. You can do it. It will be hard and take time. But you can do it."

"You think so? I have to think so, too. My daughter's life depends on it. And Isaac's. And mine."

"We'll talk," I said as I patted her shoulder good-bye. "Let's talk tomorrow."

My office mates left me alone and fielded the phone calls and endless stream of visitors who made it to Room 30 on the mezzanine floor. I walked down the back stairs and headed for First Avenue through the emergency room, avoiding the long F-Link corridor and a million contacts. I went out the emergency room automatic sliding doors and walked the length of the new asphalted driveway for ambulances to First Avenue, crossed the wide street, made a left, and took a circuitous, aimless walk in the general direction of my home.

CHAPTER 12

Collateral Damage

The drizzle had us trapped under the parking lot overhang while attendants scrambled to move the cars suspended like larvae from elevated hangers.

"Hey, Eric, what do you think will happen tonight at the legislature?" Julian, the chief of vascular surgery, asked me from under his Red Sox baseball hat and rain gear. He was referring to the proposal for health care cuts.

"Julian, it's anybody's guess," I responded.

"What do you mean?" he asked, looking down at me from his skinny six-foot-plus frame.

"We have been doing it for so long. Patching together a hospital budget year after year."

"If they vote the cuts on the table, we will be out in the deep blue sea without any oars in the water." He was right.

That's how we ran the hospital, making do through unexpected windfalls, overdue Medicaid checks, the Obama economic stimulus funds, onetime fixes, endless cycles of million-dollar cuts, lean reengineering, a wave of Fortune 500 consultants' recycled "new" ideas in shiny binders, an omnipresent whine of the slow grind of attrition in the background, the privatization of laundry, maintenance, food, and a good dose of witchcraft.

"The deck chairs can be moved around only so many times," I said. "Let's just hope the cuts aren't too deep."

I knew I hadn't answered his question and wasn't sure there was an answer. The structural money issues in health care appeared immutable. The U.S. economy and the medical industry, a full fifth of the economy, acted like an alternative universe not subject to the laws of gravity. The effects of unaffordable health care were rippling their way through the middle class.

The constant budgetary pressures over many political cycles had left a lot of people inured to the prospects of "real" damage—what I thought of as arterial blood supply blockages causing dead tissue at the core enterprise of health care delivery for our patients.

"Yeah, for sure. It certainly could happen. Other states have taken apart their education systems and health care systems, not to mention infrastructure, pensions, and union busting. How ironic we are finally seeing some shrinkage in the prison industrial complex from state budget deficits! It took the state supreme court, but even California is releasing low-risk offenders." I wasn't sure of Julian's politics on the three-strike and the Rockefeller mandatory sentencing laws, but I put my take out there anyway. Medicine and politics didn't always mix smoothly. Physicians' shared concern for patients didn't always extend beyond a diagnosis or a treatment recommendation.

"I left private practice ten years ago because of the hassles of paperwork and the gimmicks everyone was using to churn patients and squeeze income out of the system. My ophthalmologist and my wife's gynecologist advertised for Botox injections, and my partner worked in the Emirates for a year to pay for his kids' college educations. It was a relief to come and work for a salary and take care of patients without gaming the system. I took a salary hit, but my wife says I am more like the guy she married." An increasingly common story from medicine, law, and the business world as the inflexible laws of market efficiency and the Red Queen rule became the metrics of success, run faster just to stay in the same place.

I could see my car coming out from the back lot driven by a guy in an iridescent yellow slicker. Juaquin, the Colombian-born *jefe* of the parking lot, leaned out the open window as he pulled up. "*Hola*, Doc, my sister's much better. Thanks for the *ayuda*, the help." He shook my hand and gave me a bear hug slicker than the London fog.

"*De nada*, nothing, Juaquin. She is a sweetheart. Glad to help out."

I turned to Julian as I threw my bag and papers into the passenger seat. I always loved the feel of rain. "No illusions, Julian, it can get pretty ugly." Many of the country's finest public hospitals had been gutted or were in the process of evisceration. I was not prepared to preside over auto-amputation or organizational seppuku and had spent practically every waking hour since I had joined the system avoiding death by a thousand cuts. There were ways out of the tunnel. They were all politically difficult and, given Albany's monumental dysfunctionality, perhaps not realistic. In a test case former mayor Rudy Giuliani had backed privatization of the public hospital system, putting Coney Island Hospital on the block. The plan failed a court test, and he beat a quick retreat. The easiest way to close a hospital now was to let it go bankrupt. The market forces at work in a non-level playing field. The private hospitals would pick up the paying customers and high-end specialists from the leftover detritus. We would do the rest. Hardly an invisible hand in action. What was different in the post-Giuliani era was the post–Lehman Brothers collapse syndrome. When 40 percent of the economy is the financial industry, it controls everything. Even the cop at the corner is protecting Wall Street, though the threat is coming from inside. Not only were the poorest sitting in their communities without transportation, decent schools, quality food to eat, and safe parks, but the middle class was slipping and sliding into the same morass.

I got behind the wheel of my eleven-year-old Volvo—the doc car, my family calls it—and entered the converging lines to the automated gate. Forget NPR or music tonight. The rhythmic swoosh of the wipers kept me company as I tried to collect my thoughts and emotions and weaved my way home through Manhattan traffic.

The fractured U.S. health care system was like the universe in expansion, flying apart. The acceleration came with a vengeance after the market crash of 2008. The crisis was not an ordinary banking bubble with John Q. Public picking up the socialized losses and the system going on as usual. The financial crisis represented a much deeper speculative bubble that had penetrated deeply into the structure of the global economy over decades. So many factors, including the cost of wars in Iraq and Afghanistan, were taking their toll. Among these, the "waste" in the health care system—what the insurance companies and pharmaceuticals call "administrative overhead"—was bankrupting the system.

Phone calls interrupted us that night. The hospital was full, and there was no place to put the patients streaming in. Transfers were coming in from other city hospitals, a man frothing white spittle in a Midtown restaurant went into acute pulmonary edema, a young woman fell unconscious in an elevator with a heart attack, and a man with a table saw amputated his wrist. A cab had killed a woman visiting New York. A young man had committed suicide. The crammed intensive care unit forced us to use the surgical recovery room for overflow. Reluctantly, I called the fire department dispatcher for four hours of ambulance diversion. Emergency cases would be taken elsewhere during a time-out we used only with hesitation. Twenty-five patients were lined up for admission on stretchers in the emergency room like planes on the tarmac waiting their turn at LaGuardia Airport. Little red lights went off on the dashboard of my prefrontal lobe that said we were at the upper speed limit for safety. The state legislature was locked in debate and the "cuts" committee was deadlocked in an Albany hotel room with pepperoni pizza and Diet Pepsi. The lobbyists were out in full force from their two-martini lunches. The medical industry might take a symbolic cut for the front pages but I doubted anything substantial would make it into the final recommendations. The big print would suggest a fair distribution of suffering. The small print would make them whole. Pepperoni pizza and Pepsi versus martinis and medallions of tenderloin smothered in truffle sauce—not much of a contest.

The office floor was completely empty when I unlocked my office early the next day. The vote had been postponed to allow "fuller discussion of the complex competing issues." Administrative-ese for Mach 4 pressure from the private insurance companies, the hospital industry, and physician lobbyists. Patty had left me some fruit on my desk and a chocolate bobka from Todaro's on Second Avenue. I must have been withdrawn and grouchy. She could read me with ease. *You look like you needed a treat!! Hope we still have a job!!!!* read a note Scotch-taped to the plastic wrapper. I laughed when I saw it, cut myself a generous piece of the mouthwatering high-calorie cake, and made myself a triple espresso. The coffee-and-cake euphoria did not last long. I needed to go see the cases that had kept me up all night. The walk to the emergency room is two minutes from my office. I dreaded the trip and had to force myself to go down the stairs past some detectives emptying their weapons outside the adult psychiatric emergency room.

The small family room only partially contained the tears and anguish of a woman hysterical with grief, restrained by uniformed police and nurses. Her lamentation washed out over the hallways. Family members sat mute in a hyper-adrenalized stupor intensified by the lack of food, endless cups of coffee, bright fluorescent lights, hard chairs, and continuous interruptions fed by the automatic metal doors that swung open and shut. A parade of nurses, aides, doctors, policemen, attendants, cleaning staff, administrators, supervisors, wheelchairs, and stretchers went back and forth. But the family didn't seem to notice. They were lost to their grief. Even the DOC prisoners in orange jumpsuits wearing leg irons and handcuffs and the psychotic men and women escorted by physicians and security to the psychiatric treatment warren did not get through to them.

Usually heads would look up expectantly with every swing of the door, hoping a messenger would bring the status of their wife, husband, child, mother, father, sister, or neighbor. Family members would have cell phones glued to their heads. Some huddled in one another's arms for respite from the antiseptic air, the institutional colors, the white coats and rumpled scrubs and fragile anticipation, whiffs of hope mixed with the fibrillations of death's foreshadowings. Lives changed here with time suspended in midstream or in a couple of seconds. Forever.

The door to the trauma slot was open. The room was filled with the detritus of an abortive resuscitation code. Papers, cellophane, plastic wrappers, IV tubing, bandages soaked in blood lay everywhere. A nurse was huddled over an inert body of indeterminate age and sex.

She was attempting to wrap a white sheet-shroud around the corpse. Her eyes caught mine. They locked for a second. The color was drained from her face. Her black stringy hair hung down over her shoulders and touched the jeans and T-shirt. Black shiny cowboy boots poked out from the bottom of the stretcher. Two cops were completing paperwork in one corner; a clump of doctors stood silently to one side. The light blue-ish walls were covered with plastic signs, notices, equipment; huge focused operating room lights like the necks of giant cranes arced at odd angles over the stretcher. Half a dozen pieces of equipment on wheels looked like zoo animals congregating at mealtime. Marion, the head nurse, caught my arm and pulled my attention from the scene.

"Gunshot wound to the head. Self-inflicted. High school kid. *Mother.*" As she spoke, she motioned with her head toward the waiting room. She telegraphed cryptically the key elements as the staff silently and automatically continued its routine to prepare for the next case.

The sounds of the mother keening through the metal doors merged with the sounds of other mothers whose sobbing and tears interrupted my sleep decades later. Deschapelles, Haiti, was where I had heard my Ur lamentation years earlier.

The work was strenuous and satisfying in central Haiti: babies with neonatal tetanus and a new disease bringing otherwise healthy young people to the hospital with combinations of rare skin cancers, rampant tuberculosis, and a new undiagnosable lung infection. We learned later to call this HIV/AIDS. Our number one diagnosis back then was kwashiorkor or marasmus, the formal lexicon of starvation. Flour, sugar, and protein supplements were dispensed from the hospital pharmacy window to patients waving their white papers with our scribbled prescriptions for food. The days were long, blistering hot, and thrilling in the way that only a physician in the early days of falling in love with his profession can appreciate. We were witness to the natural history of a disease voracious and practically unstoppable. There was no treatment. Untouched by medication or surgery and out of reach of shamans and voodoo priests, the hospital was the last stop before internment in the tear-soaked hardpack.

A young woman presented in the late afternoon with her mother and sisters with abdominal pain. Vague, indistinct, poorly charac-terized. We went through the history of periods, pregnancies, bowel function, urinary symptoms, fever, sweats, sexual activity. Her exam was remarkable for some tenderness on the right side, and we thought she might have appendicitis or an infection in her tubes. The blood count was normal, and there was a slight elevation of her white cells. I asked surgery to see her. She arrived sweaty with dark rings for eyes. She examined the patient and recommended antibiotics for salpingitis or a tubal infection. That night the young woman's ectopic pregnancy ruptured, and while the OR was being prepared, she hemorrhaged to death.

The next morning I was in the gloaming clinic. We started early in the cool morning before the sun baked the earth. From the shadows of the courtyard I heard keening. Everything froze. It gradually grew louder, becoming intense and focused like a Greek chorus. Then it diminished as the mother and her daughter carried the body on their shoulders, retracing their steps up rock-strewn dirt paths into the clear-cut mountainsides. The primal sound still echoes in my ears and my nightmares when the world is still and the night sits heavy in the darkness. There is no statute of limitations on what invades conscious-ness when the thrum of daily routine is drowned out by your own tachycardia and fears.

CJ, the overnight social worker, brought me out of my momentary flight from reality. She had pieced together fragments of the story of Benjamin, the young man who had shot himself, now lying in the slot. We walked to an empty conference room.

"I have been talking to some family members. Benny, who was nine-teen, had a tough time for over a decade, but really took a hit when his parents separated and divorced six years ago."

"Carol, what kind of care was he getting and where—I mean a shrink, professional care?" I asked directly.

"School counselors first and later referrals to private therapists. After a drawn-out nasty divorce, health insurance became unaffordable, fifteen hundred bucks a month for a family of four with double-digit increases every year. The husband works out of his apartment in marketing if I have it right, after being downsized or right-sized, I forget what they call it this year. Marriage gone, job gone, and finances down the tubes. Mental health coverage is like a Brazilian bikini, it doesn't cover much. They went to public mental health programs. First come, first served. Long lines and high staff turnover. Pretty much prescription mills." She shrugged.

"It's a travesty. We should just Abilify the water supply and get it over with." I declared the obvious. Fluoride plus Abilify equals public health care.

Carol continued, "Look, there aren't enough trained child psychiatrists or social workers in their district. This family is rapidly going down the middle-class ladder to a not-very-genteel poverty unless there is some millionaire crazy aunt they haven't discovered. A ten-minute follow-up visit and a psycho-pharm prescription is standard now. The family makes too much money to be on Medicaid. They make more than twenty thousand dollars a year. So they are part of the increasing horde of 'uninsured' and end up in our system for the basics. I forget how much we lose with each visit but they get virtually no treatment except pills." Talk about a donut hole. You could drive through this one with a Hummer. And California had just received a waiver to pay doctors eleven dollars for a Medicaid visit. The system was being taken apart. I could sense the exasperation in her voice. She was tired from the relentless overnight shift, and I knew she had a kid the same age as Benjamin. We weren't that different from the patients we took care of, and we all knew it. Death crossed the line with impunity.

"The kid acting out his own demons as his family falls apart," I said out loud to nobody in particular.

"These kids need multiple and complicated levels of care. They're just not getting it." We both knew the system was shredded with holes and gaps. There are times nothing can be done to prevent a suicide. But it was especially painful to lose people who possibly could have been helped. The hope is to get kids through their crisis moment. I touched

her shoulder; she gave a thin smile and went out to finish her paperwork and catch the long train ride home to Long Island.

My phone rang. "Eric, hi, Levanah here. Look, you know the Ramirez
family? Right." Levanah was from the Colombian Consulate. We did
a lot of work together over a dozen-plus years on health issues, family problems, and patients who had complex needs. Her birth name
was Xiomara Vargas. A long spiritual journey had brought her from
Catholicism to quasi-Orthodox Judaism with many stops and side
journeys in between. Twice a week for years she'd attended discussion groups that parsed the Torah and Kabbalistic texts with a master
teacher trained in Cordoba, Spain, and Jerusalem. She wore a gold Star
of David around her neck.

"Sure, hi, Levanah. Long time no see. Let's have lunch soon, you
have left me behind in my spiritual development. Remember, I was way
behind before you started your rescue program. *¿Por favor?* Of course
I know Ramirez. What's up?"

"He's been in your emergency room now for two days. No beds
and the family is getting antsy. And I promise to catch you up on your
'development,' as you call it. Though you are pretty hopeless, Eric."
She laughed. She had steered Señor Abraham Ramirez and his family to me years earlier and I'd followed them through a long medical
thrash from symptoms to diagnosis, diagnosis to treatment, treatment
to side effects, the inevitable hospitalizations, and terminal slides.

"Listen, I'm in the craziness right now. Let me go find the Ramirez
clan and see what's blocking traffic." She thanked me and we agreed
to have lunch together. The lessons in Halakha and the Midrash over
french fries and spanakopita reminded me of a dear old friend, another
Diana, twice exiled from Argentina, who had run a Kabbalah group
for years during the 1990s in her apartment overlooking the zoo in
Buenos Aires. We discussed the Garden of Eden and the nature of
desire as the elephants trumpeted in the eerie darkness of the troubled
city. The ghosts of the disappeared were everywhere.

*   *   *

Every conceivable space in the emergency room had been turned into a treatment or parking area for stretchers. I weaved my way to the panopticon nursing station and checked the whiteboard for the initials *AR*. There he was "AR, Abraham Ramirez, Medical Record Number and Team 2, east side." It gave me a place to start. There were half a dozen prisoners handcuffed to stretchers with DOC officers crammed into any available square feet on the east side, but I found one curtain pulled and figured that two days in captivity here had created a mini ecological niche of privacy and family care. Another week like this and we would have a shantytown on our hands. Occupy Bellevue!

"*¿Doctor, como ha estado?* How are you?" I peered around the curtain. There was a daughter and wife, identical in so many ways and exhausted. Abraham was covered by a sheet and multiple blankets, skeletonized, his face waxy and drawn, the skin stretched tight outlining the anatomy of his facial bones, like a cadaver the first day in a gross anatomy lab. A unit of blood was dripping into his left arm. He attempted a smile.

"*Hola.* I am so sorry you folks have been stuck here. Bring me up to date, and I will get a room for Abraham." I wasn't so sure I could right away, but something would be done. The hospital was way over census, full to overflowing. *Hospital-paresis.* We were frozen—couldn't take patients in, couldn't get patients out. So many of our patients had limited options. Few places take them without insurance. Our own nursing homes were at capacity. That wasn't counting the homeless, the undocumented, and the countless patients with severe disabilities, mental health issues too numerous to count. Society in mega distress.

The youngest daughter, Claudia, a social worker, spoke to me in English. "Papa has been so weak. The transfusions only last a week now. Even less. He gets a small boost for a few days, a little energy, and can make it to the bathroom and to his favorite chair where he sleeps most of the time. But now we cannot leave him for even a moment. He fell two days ago." She was the family's point person to the medical profession and always accompanied her mother, who never left her husband.

"Claudia, I can see you're tired. But there's something else?" She was tense and strung out. Not her usual efficient machine-like self.

"My parents moved in with my sister six months ago," she said.

"I thought they had the house you guys grew up in, Cortelyou Road, right?" Tree-lined streets with large Victorian homes in central Brooklyn.

"They had the house, but Papa's illness put them over the top in expenses. They had to mortgage the house and finally sell it. The bills from hospitalizations, nursing care, medications, co-pays, co-insurance were followed by relentless bill collectors. He is not Medicare-eligible yet. So they declared bankruptcy." She was anguished, and I could see the effect on the entire family. The financial stress was bitter on top of the emotional loss inevitably coming down the tracks.

His illness began three years earlier with easy bruising. A small bump and a large black-and-blue spot appeared. Even holding him by the arm produced a thumbprint. When he came to our clinic, his platelet count was near ten thousand, twenty times less than normal. Steroids worked like magic, and in a few days he was back to normal. The family was delighted and we felt like small-town heroes. There were relapses and a switch to a stronger medication a year later. After another six months of weakness and tiredness, a relentless anemia was detected. The bone marrow biopsy showed a progressive loss of progenitor or mother cells. It was drying up. Bone marrow failure. We knew this was progressive and would continue relentlessly or burst into a leukemic flame that was hiding in plain sight. The clock was ticking faster.

The family had been so together, it functioned as one single unit. A husband and wife like Siamese twins after forty-five years of marriage, affectionate and considerate with a tenderness that left everyone around them in awe. Three children with their own full lives but still revolving around their parents, perpetually full moons. The financial calamity was attenuated by a caring family that would do anything necessary to protect one another. The house had been their savings, their life insurance, their inheritance to the children and grandchildren. Medical bankruptcy for underinsurance and no insurance was a new epidemic we were seeing more and more. I had wondered for years why the middle class or corporate America was not in open revolt.

We were at the end of the road now with what we as physicians could do for Abraham Ramirez. How many pints of blood had he received? One hundred? More? When was enough enough? How do you decide? Who decides? Home care with his family around him had been the last decision, and no more transfusions. Then panic when he was in distress urinating or defecating and the inevitable 911 call. It was too much for the family. Hospice care near their apartment in Sunset Park, Brooklyn, or we would keep him here for the last days. That is, if they hadn't changed their minds, watching the unit of blood, drip, drip, drip.

I had almost made it to the sliding doors and a momentary respite in the late-summer air. "Eric," called a voice, and I stopped in my tracks. The organ donor team leader, Yolanda, gave me a hug and asked if we could go over a case that was "hung up." The emergency ward break room was just inside its metal doors across from the trauma slot, only a few feet away. I dutifully followed her and turned a sharp right into the rectangular room. Several nurses were sitting around the rectangular table, chopsticks in hand, eating Thai food from half a dozen white paper cartons filled with brown rice, noodles, shrimp, and pineapple chicken. They nodded at me and offered me my own plate with sign language as they chewed and swallowed in silence. The air was somber; the only sound was the clock ticking on the wall.

I emptied a chair piled with paper supplies, and Yolanda sat on a table next to me. "We can't get OR time for this case, Eric. We will lose all of the organs if we don't have something by seven o'clock today, that is it. The Kaiser family has been gracious and very understanding. But they are deep in grief, and the grandparents insist unconditionally that the organs are harvested tonight. They need this to be over. Can you help me?" She looked at me and shrugged. The nurses looked up at me as one. They were caring for this patient next door. Brain death had been confirmed on two separate occasions and it was becoming unbearable to witness the family's suffering.

Of course I could and I would. The organ donor team spent a lot of time at Bellevue. Since our trauma center was the largest in the city, the knife and gun clubs and slaloming taxi drivers trained future generations of the best and the brightest surgeons. As Frank Spencer, the former chairman of Bellevue's department of surgery, reminded me on more than one occasion in his thick, intoxicating East Texas drawl, "Anyone knows, Eric, if you want to train good surgeons, you go to train in an inner city. Near where the action is. The shootings and the stabbings that is. Pick a great city hospital. I came to New York to work at Bellevue." He smiled his slightly off-center smile, pushed his metal-rimmed glasses back, and adjusted his hearing aids.

After talking to Yolanda, I made phone calls to clear the operating rooms for Miriam Kaiser. There were too many lives hanging in the balance. People on the organ waiting list, sitting with their beepers and cell phones, hoping, many in vain, for a chance to live. To empty an OR I canceled half a dozen elective cases. The cancellations were both painful and annoying to our patients but necessary.

Karina, one of the crime victims social workers, joined the group mid-discussion. She was tall, thin, ex–Peace Corps in Thailand, and had a perpetual engaged attitude regardless of the bone-chilling circumstance that paid her city salary. She'd left a banking career five years ago to become a social worker. The back-office tedium of sitting in front of a computer screen in cartoon-like cubicles to collateralize fiction into make-believe, holding sovereign states and their citizens hostage, became increasingly enervating, depressing, and void of meaning. Buying stuff, the inevitable BMW and exotic travel, had staved off career ennui for a time. But she was calm and composed when it came to rapes, assaults, homicides, and vehicular manslaughter. When I asked her how she did it, she answered, "Resilience really. Most of our patients are amazingly resilient no matter what happens to them. It isn't me at all, it is our patients." One definition of maturity in this business is when the humanity of the people that walk through our doors becomes part of your own.

"Look, I just finished talked to the 13th Precinct guys. They finished their interviews with the cabby and the husband, Marc Kaiser, and half a dozen witnesses outside Dunkin' Donuts on Second Avenue," Karina started. I wasn't sure I had the stomach, but I let her tell me of the final moments in the life of Miriam Kaiser.

Miriam had been visiting Manhattan with her husband, Marc. They had been married for a few years and were planning on having children soon. The trip was to a specialist to check for any indications they had an infertility problem. It was early in the process and they weren't too concerned at this point given their ages and excellent general health. Marc crossed the street with his wife after parking the car when she remembered she had left her cell phone on the floor of the passenger side. She squeezed his arm, turned around briskly, and crossed the street. The day was warm with a gentle breeze. A perfect New York kind of day after a period of sweltering heat and humidity that had broken with sheet lightning and a biblical downpour. Miriam beeped the doors open, reached into the passenger side, and rummaged around for her phone. Her husband stood on the far curb and watched his wife, checking his watch.

Miriam held the phone in her hand, slammed the door, and beeped it shut. The lights blinked on momentarily. She looked up at her husband and began to cross the street. A yellow cab was heading south on Second Avenue doing sixty miles an hour. The taxi's top lights indicated he wasn't picking up any more passengers; he was heading downtown to gas up his cab and switch with his Punjabi brother-in-law, who had the overnight shift. He was running a few minutes late and tried to make up time weaving in and out down the wide avenue while accelerating through yellow traffic lights.

Miriam had made it about ten feet from the curb when the slaloming yellow taxi reached her left side. The sharp crack and screeching brakes ricocheted off the walls of the buildings.

I was saved from drowning as I listened to Karina with a spirited reminder from Patty that I needed to head for my off-campus lunch meeting. I walked through the emergency room doors and reflexively tuned out the surroundings, retreating to a parallel zone to eliminate the pain, the engine noise, and the insistent whine of an exhaust fan. A helicopter was coming in low for a landing at the waterside mini terminal when I switched mental channels. I hadn't processed the day and things were hanging loose and unresolved from too many angles. How much heartache could I absorb and not turn into a robot or a madman?

My lunch was with Javie, Juan Guerra's son. We had kept in touch after his father died. He and his mother had remained close after I coordinated Juan Guerra's complex medical care over the years. This patient and I had shared the same exact cancer. He wasn't here, and I was meeting his son. Javie enlisted in the military, following his father's fateful steps decades earlier in Vietnam. I remembered overhearing the father-son conversation on the prison unit, a mini flashback, a career choice between the local gangs and IEDs—improvised explosive devices.

He stood up at a corner table when I walked into Curry in a Hurry, a few blocks west of the hospital. The military uniform gave him away. I wasn't sure I would have recognized him. Sidewise baseball cap, studied slouch, low-rider pants, perpetual music plugged in and on full volume, he had fully morphed from a street-smart kid honing domestic survival skills into a young man. We traded brief updates. He was in an intensive language program in Arabic and Persian. Military entrance aptitude tests had put him at the top of his group. In his Latino *pandilla*, gang, there were Latinos who spoke Spanish and Arabic from Caribbean nations. It had become a secret code. I had heard of prison gangs in California using Nahuatl, the Aztec language. Moorish had been around since Columbus and the expulsion of the Jews from Spain, so why not Arabic?

"Tell me about yourself. Your mom said you were tough, difficult, wild, and on the verge of some bad decisions until you went into the military."

He grabbed a bit of everything, like tapas, blended it all with a mound of basmati rice, and sipped a large mango lassi from a sweating clear plastic cup. "Doc, I was a young kid whose father spent half his life in prison. What did I know? His military experience…well, you know." Heroin, addiction, incarceration period. He paused and took a large mouthful of the curry. A group of Pakistani taxi drivers came in white shalwar kameezes, henna-dyed orange beards, and white skull-caps, talking rapidly in Urdu and Arabic and ignoring us completely. Salafi ultra-fundamentalist Muslims. You never knew who was from where and who spoke what language. Javie said they were complaining about the rise in gas prices and also discussing which Internet porn sites were the best, in that order.

I smiled and said, "Just what Osama was doing when his uninvited guests landed in his compound. Complaining about low oil prices to bankrupt the decadent capitalist West while downloading porn to his hard drive." Javier smiled and nodded in agreement as he dipped into the slurry of curries, tandooris, and raitas with a mound of hot garlic parathas.

We went back in time. Javier knew he only had a short interval in New York before he would be shipped out again for at least six months off the grid. "I was making some really stupid mistakes as a teenager," he said seriously. "The easy money was drug-related. You started as a runner or a lookout and then graduated to selling stuff. Everyone did it. Remember, there was no other employment in our neighborhood. The hood, remember." I looked at him and listened. "I went to six funerals during middle school and high school before I bailed out and enlisted. Six. All shot to death, guys my age within a year or two. Very simple stuff. Drug-related killings, revenge killings, innocent-bystander killings, stray bullet killings. Does it really matter? What they call 'collateral.' In my current line of work that is what they call people killed who are not supposed to be shot. Collateral."

"You know, Javie, you made me just wonder how much of what we see here, I mean at the hospital, is what you call collateral damage. Policies gone amok, unintended consequences, good programs high-jacked, incentives distorted beyond recognition?"

He continued: "The U.S. government apologizes, sends cash to the families, pays off the sheik in charge with more boatloads of cash and an SUV. Not that much difference between the South Bronx and South

Waziristan, Doc. I have helicopter gunships and drones directed from Nevada by video game–trained pilots in case things get too hot. Would have been handy on the Grand Concourse on summer nights when I was fifteen. Drone to Pelham Parkway, drone to Willis Avenue Bridge. Come in, drone." He took a breather and looked around the restaurant filling up with taxi drivers. The delivery guys were all young Mexicans loading up their bicycles chained outside to a "No Parking" sign.

"So the only way out of the hole and not be in a body bag is to enlist in the military. You still get a body bag, but your mother gets a folded flag, you get a burial site in Washington, and a little cash flows to your 'contingent beneficiary.'"

He looked at me as he was mopping up his plate. The horde of cab-drivers had left with their takeout to say their prayers on the sidewalks on small colorful rugs they kept rolled up in their trunks.

"It is all about respect, Doc. One hundred percent respect and its polar opposite, disrespect. If the guys feel disrespected, then it is warfare. You carry your attitude with you at all times and show no feelings and no weakness, none whatsoever at any time. The price is too high and you learn it when you are in *pañales*, diapers. Excuse my language, Doc, pre-military training for illustrative purposes only, you fuck up and that is it for real. It is school on the streets. That is why the military is not that hard. If you survived and graduated from the University of the South Bronx, then what exactly is so tough to learn about advanced weaponry and survival skills? Especially when you have billions of dollars of backup, equipment, gyms, McDonald's and Cinnabon shops, bowling, plus air-conditioned tents in 117-degree desert and everything else you want and don't need. Turkey and gravy for Thanksgiving. Stuff you never had and never thought you would have unless you were a drug entrepreneur. The workforce handing out your burgers and fries, ironing your socks and underwear, are conscripted from all over Southeast Asia. They jump on board to work in a combat zone to make some ready cash to send back to Bangladesh or the Philippines. They spoke better English than the guys in my battalion."

He slowed down and finished his lunch. Rain clouds had moved in and big fat drops were hitting the metal overhang, pinging hard. Then

a torrential downpour hit. We had the window open and were splat-
tered from the backsplash but enjoyed the gusts of fresh air through
the window, the smell of the rain, folks hustling to find corners to hide
in and overhangs filling up. The cabdrivers had rolled up their rugs,
opened their trunks in unison, shut them, and were slowly pushing
off in their yellow cabs one by one, knowing a guaranteed time to get
customers was during a downpour in NYC.

The rain eased off to a steady drizzle. We did not talk for some
time—just listened to the drops, the clatter from the kitchen, and the
Urdu, Hindi, Punjabi, and Arabic that filtered from the other room.

Javie continued. "For me it is about knowing when to get out. I just
need to learn my languages and get out alive. Being a black op is not
a marketable skill if you want an ordinary life. It's about risking your
life for skills without getting killed or addicted along the way. I learned
that much from my dad. Not in lectures, but his life and the decisions
he made. And how he got trapped and played by the system."

"Javie," I interrupted. "Your dad, why didn't he finish his treatments?"

He looked at me and took a moment to answer. "Doc, when we
finally drove him home, I carried him through the apartment door and
put him into his own bed. We had made it up with his favorite *bachata*
CDs within reach and pictures of family and friends from his lifetime.
My dad made it clear he was not leaving again. There was no discussion about it, he made up his mind.

"Mom and I knew he hadn't completed the treatments. I think
between radiation, the chemo, the plastic stomach tube, and being
locked up he had finally come to a decision about his life. He was in
another zone and we only tried a couple of times to get him back to the
hospital. My mom and I knew. He wanted to die in his own home. He
ground up a handful of pain meds, put them in his feeding tube one
night, and went to sleep."

I understood. I'd had the same illness, the same radiation and
chemo. As the weeks passed I was less convinced that I could complete
the regimen. And if I did complete it and the tumor came back, there

were no other treatment options. It was morphine and palliative care. Like Juan Guerra, I had silently designed my escape route—I would end my life myself—if the treatment was not successful. Which gave me some satisfaction and a measure of relief.

When at one point I refused further treatment, only my wife's tenacity could override my choice. Still, I understood why Juan Guerra's family did not feel they could or should do that.

We said good-bye on the sidewalk and headed in different directions back to our own lives.

The swirl of people at the Bellevue shift change had the feel of Grand Central Station when I pushed through the revolving doors into the glass atrium. I nodded and waved my way through the crowds and headed toward the emergency area. I went out the ambulance bay doors with some physician colleagues to catch up. Things changed so fast, even an hour made a difference. The depth of the cuts and layoffs was on everyone's mind. We finally fell silent as the last cumulus clouds fled the city riding the rainstorm's easterlies.

The glinting early-evening light sliced in from the west, riding small particles and exhaust fumes in the narrow crosstown gap, like a clean scalpel cut that ran from the Hudson River to the East River onto the emergency room ambulance bay. We stood outside, our backs against a warm white concrete wall, looking east across the tight fresh asphalted zigzag to the metal-and-plastic overhang and automatic sliding doors that led into a small sea of stretchers. Then more sliding doors and the pantomime bustle of inaudible women and men in blue, green, and tan scrubs performing indecipherable rituals with prostrate bodies on stretchers. It was the end of summer minus the asphyxiating heat, humidity, and Con Edison brownout alerts. A few minutes to chill and huff the gasoline.

The ER bay was yet another stage for nonstop activity. Bright orange, yellow, and green hard-plastic trauma backboards were propped against a wall like surfboards outside a café on a California beach. A scrum of boxy FDNY ambulances were backed into the unloading bay, facing outward three abreast in uneven rows, as they unloaded their human cargo, scooting their steel stretchers with their charges wrapped in white sheets. A pair of emergency management technicians navigated the shoals and chutes with dexterity like double kayaks around parked ambulances. Pairs of drivers were waiting in the cabs with their engines on, the AC running, for the last to arrive to complete their paperwork and clear an exit lane. Gridlocked into a small space, they chatted, smoked, and flirted in their dark blue uniforms. A tall EMT with a graying ponytail to his shoulders came around the side of the post-9/11 decontamination showers covered in amber-colored glass zipping up his fly and adjusting himself after urinating like a dog against a wall only partially hidden by his cab. He looked around to see who had seen him, was satisfied, and walked into the emergency room.

Clumps of Orthodox Jews with knotted tzitzis poking from white shirts over their black pants chatted in groups scattered around the lot. Some smoked, some gesticulated. A group near me talked animatedly in Yiddish. I could make out the "oh fuck" and "shit" amid the guttural German-Hebrew mixture from one overweight thirty-five-year-old emergency worker from Hatzolah, the Orthodox community ambulances. He danced small circles as he pointed with his right index finger and raised his voice decibel by decibel. Black-bearded senior community members wearing finely tailored long black coats that fell below their knees arrived to the ambulance bay on foot from First Avenue. Their plastic IDs were clipped efficiently to their lapels. They nodded at me and walked through the doors past the huge black guard slouching over his beat-up wooden lectern like an old-time Southern preacher about to raise his audience of mute stretchers like Lazarus from lethargy and slumber and sin. An elderly member of the Hasidic Orthodox community had been hit by a truck near the Williamsburg Bridge in Brooklyn. The Hatzolah ambulance arrived within a couple of minutes and screamed its way across the bridge and uptown. The patient expired on the way, bleeding out from internal injuries, ripped blood vessels, a tear in his liver, and a ruptured spleen. His heart had stopped on Delancey Street. We could see it on our monitors and our BlackBerrys as it went flatline. A modern-day app for a post-modern world. Death is a flat line regardless of the medium.

The community was turned inside out for another reason. Any death was important and resulted in the arrival of rabbis with beepers

and double-barreled smart cell phones. Rabbinical interlocutors inter-
preted for the closed Orthodox communities and the outside world.
These Orthodox communities descended from rabbis who came from
the Pale of Settlement of what is now Russia and Poland. These huge
reservations had been transplanted to Borough Park, Brooklyn. A
young boy had been kidnapped and murdered by a member of the
community. The unmentionable and incomprehensible had happened.
A Jew had killed a young Jewish child. After smothering him, the
alleged murderer cut him into pieces, putting his feet into his freezer
and disposing of the rest of the corpse in neighborhood trash bins.

It would be only a matter of two days before the alleged murderer was
transported from Rikers Island to Bellevue Hospital's nineteenth-floor
inpatient prison units for a full-bore forensic psychiatric evaluation.
Was he competent? Was he hearing voices? Command hallucinations
from passersby, buildings, dogs, aliens, the CIA, hidden microphones,
women, internal electronic devices, his penis and testicles, a uterus,
invisible umbilical cords, tormenting him for years telling him to kill
and in a sexual catharsis dismember? Were there other body parts in
the backyard? Was he mentally retarded? Had he suffered childhood
sexual abuse and now begun recycling the shame and excitement? Did
his media habits predispose him to acts of violence and desecration?
Had the boy been violated before being sacrificed to a wrathful God?
Would his urine tox screen be positive for crystal meth and a cocktail of
drugs? We had been through so many varieties of human illness, suffering, and depravity it was startling to realize that there were forms and
varieties we had not seen, that could still penetrate the formalistic gaze
of the professional forensically trained physician.

Overwhelmingly these patients had been severely abused and deprived
as children, humiliated, neglected, and disrespected to the point that
they were dead souls. It was part of the script loaded against them that
enabled us to see victimizers as part of humanity even though they had
lost their own. My first night in charge of the emergency room at Kings
County in the mid-1970s, a call came in. A man had bludgeoned his wife
and three children to death with a baseball bat and then attempted to
disembowel himself with a steak knife. We were scoffing down a pizza

and Cokes between physical exams and suturing cut tendons from an orgiastic Kristallnacht in the hood during a citywide blackout. *Do you walk or run to save that life?* we asked one another.

Back inside, I put on my scrubs and wound my way to the operating rooms on the eleventh floor to talk to the organ teams. Three nurses were hunched over a computer screen, chatting, and they turned around when the door clicked shut. The schedules were being updated for tomorrow's cases. "She is in Room 14," Jo said when she saw me. We were short both nurses and anesthesiologists for what would be at least eight hours in the OR if not more to harvest Miriam Kaiser's liver, her two kidneys, a pancreas, the small intestine, both lungs, and the heart. The liver would be split, one lobe for a child waiting in New Jersey and the larger lobe for an adult in the Bronx. There were eight operating rooms going strong. Two for orthopedics—a pelvic fracture from a fall and a cleanly broken femur in a young Asian guy whose in-line skates were not meant to go off a five-foot stairway when he lost control. An expanding abdominal aortic aneurysm in a middle-aged smoker with hypertension had cut off the circulation to the artery supplying his intestine and he was back in for a "second look" operation to make sure the surgeons had removed all of the dead gut.

The neurosurgery room was wheeling out one patient after treatment for a subdural hematoma he'd suffered from a fall while taking blood thinners for an erratic heartbeat. Anti-coagulants to prevent a blood clot had made him susceptible to a random bleed. The pressure was on to turn the room around quickly for another patient with a blood clot in nearly the same location from head trauma incurred when a drug deal had gone sour. The heart room had an overtime second case. The heart of a young Senegalese woman with undiagnosed mitral valve disease and fluid in her lungs had flipped to chaotic atrial fibrillation from the increased fluid load of a third-trimester pregnancy.

Jared from the Organ Donor Network was on his cell phone outside Room 14 and gestured toward the closed door that led into the OR suite. I pushed open the door, gingerly walked to the front of the OR table, and stood on a footstool beside the anesthesiologist. The music in the OR was a Mozart horn concerto. It smoothed the rough edges of the beeps, metal-on-metal clangs, and murmurings of the half dozen teams in place. Several surgeons were bent over the table dissecting the small intestine and its blood supply. The heart pumped vigorously covered by a dampened gauze pad, and the lungs expanded and contracted with each whoosh of the ventilator. Several steel tables were parked around the OR table. Each had several large blue plastic containers filled with ice. Teams of surgeons and their assistants from different hospitals fidgeted with receptacles and vacation-size coolers for the organs, which would be prepped and delivered by car, ambulance, or airplane to a computer-matched recipient prepped and under general anesthesia in a distant hospital.

From my little perch on a stool the crescendoing rhythm of the hospital finally caught up to me. We called it "organized chaos" when all the cylinders were firing, from the clinics to the outer reaches of the inpatient units and everything in between. We weren't perfect, we made mistakes and were frustrated and angry by moments. But I marveled at my colleagues, all of them, who were mission-driven to provide great care to anyone, no matter. It had been an exhilarating dozen-plus years. The woman's heart beat two feet beneath my surgical mask. My mind went blank.

I got home before I realized we had a dinner that night with the Matta family. Diana was changing into formal wear and getting ready to go when I walked in, depleted from the day. "You're kidding," I said as I remembered. Diana smiled. She knew I'd get my second wind. I always did. The Matta family, the entire clan, was back in New York for their annual pilgrimage to Broadway, the opera, the restaurants, the Metropolitan Museum of Art, the Guggenheim, a Yankees game, and endless rounds of shopping. I would have to change into something fancy to get into the restaurant. I had received emailed photos of Diego playing tennis on his titanium leg with his brother Augusto.

We did have a good time. It was great to see Diego doing so well—there was life after a devastating accident. He had a remarkable attitude. His girlfriend Gabriela, now his fiancée, was as gloriously decked out as ever.

His mother, the matriarch, sat in aching primness as she kept an eagle eye on her progeny. But we enjoyed ourselves. Diego gave us a beautiful silver vase, in gratitude for everything I had done for him. From then on, Diana took to calling it the one-legged vase. She can be terribly macabre in her attempts to deal with the pain associated with my profession.

The celebration was also personal. My PET scan the day before was normal. I was down to an every-six-months schedule plus the obligatory monthly endoscopies to check around my throat for a recurrence or a new primary. The fibrotic band around my neck like a dog's collar was annoying, and the choking on food left me with tears running down my face in the middle of any random meal. My emotional vibrations had equilibrated at a new set point, but I was back with my family and making up for lost time and hurt feelings on a journey no one really had a handle on except Diana. I was still putting pieces together from extreme illness. But I was walking the halls of the hospital, fielding the never-ending incoming issues, and developing new projects and new relationships. I wasn't done yet.

I realized, as if for the first time the next morning when I arrived in my office, that my window view was completely obscured by the new reflecting-glass building that had been going up in front of me. It had taken out the UN and Roosevelt Island sitting in the East River, leaving only a tiny sliver of Queens. The past day was reverberating in my head and my body as I sat back in my chair for a few moments. What would the legislature decide? How many lives would be affected by their decision? Our patients were like canaries in the coal mines, the living warning signals of the visible and often invisible lethal global transactions and tribulations. All patients came in with their medical issues and a particular history that we assembled, analyzed, and treated. They were by themselves incomplete stories of much larger and deeper events, geopolitical cataclysms, social dislocations, fraying societal contracts, tribal genocide campaigns, overpopulation, and climate perturbations. Just barely scratching surfaces opened up layers without end of diasporas, family sagas, lone narratives of victories and tragedies frequently one and the same.

I was running late. It was time to get ready for the new day.

A Note on Methodology

Because of the sensitivity of the identities of both patients and their families, the circumstances of their lives, and the impossibility of getting informed consent from many who have moved on, passed away, or whose existence is fraught, I have deliberately disguised the identities in this book while leaving intact the essential circumstances of each chapter.

Acknowledgments

This book has been fermenting for many years. Many more years than I thought when I first sat down to put pen to paper. A writer friend from my days in New Hampshire, after an evening deep in political talk, said to me casually, "Why don't you write a book?" I thought about it many times over the years, too busy most of the time to get home on time, keep up with my work, spend time with my kids, and think through a complete thought uninterrupted. Fifteen years ago I started to keep handwritten journals, a new one every three or four months. Thoughts, incidents from dozens of diverse sources, travels, conversations with friends, ideas from books, magazines, newspapers, overheard comments, fragments that triggered old memories or that clarified gestating formulations made it into these notebooks, complete with references, diagrams, and color codes. I am omnivorous in my interests so there were no entry criteria. September 11 alone became the subject of a few volumes of collected feelings and the evolution of a signature narrative as the events raced on in directions predictable only in hindsight except for a few clear-eyed Cassandras aware of the burdens of history (and empire). Several hundred pages of *Going Critical* was a first cut I began in early 2008. It was interrupted for over a year by forces beyond my control. Deep into 2010 I sat down again, determined to tell the stories of some of the remarkable human beings I have been privileged to take care of over three decades.

Several people asked me, "How did you decide who to put in the book?" I was always interested in my patients' stories. Illness was only a part of the story for each—never the entire story or even the most important one. After all, patients are not coterminous with their illnesses. For me what has always been the most important part of any story, however dramatic and compelling, is the story behind the story, the backstory. For me history, sociology, and anthropology have been essential complements to medicine. Only within a multidimensional context are a patient's stories understandable. Teasing out the ripples of the past and the blowback of apparently remote events is as satisfying as a complex diagnostic dilemma. Just why is this Fulani-speaking Mauritanian sitting on the TB ward? So my answer was that I chose the patients that illustrated different aspects of what are arguably among the critical contemporary issues in our society—those with global implications. The lens, of course, is Bellevue Hospital. By selecting a few cases out of hundreds, if not thousands, my hope is to illuminate through real lives the effects of social, political, and economic forces like moving tectonic plates, the structural elements that are so often lost in the discussion of an individual case. Most disease as we understand it is the product of these forces interacting with the genome and the episome, making nature and nurture a quaint concept.

This book literally has a cast of thousands and has been informed by innumerable conversations and events over many years. To all of the many patients I have been so fortunate to meet and to get to know under extreme circumstances, and to their families and friends, I cannot thank you enough for your generosity and remarkable resilience, which I only glimpsed through a small and often transient opening in a life.

The public hospital system in New York City is blessed with a remarkable group of dedicated individuals. I can only thank everyone who has graciously worked with me under the difficult and stressful circumstances organizing and delivering medical care in always "interesting" times.

Bellevue has an enormous number and range of physicians, nurses, social workers, aides, secretaries, technical staff, and administrators, all impressive in talent and energy. I know just about everyone and have benefited immensely from the support and sheer delight of working with a professional group of dedicated providers of care at every level. I would like to mention some of the people whose conversations and commentaries assisted me in deepening my thinking about what I was really about and what was happening to our patients. Out of the multitude, Lynda Curtis, Machelle Allen, Steve Alexander, Aaron Cohen, Lin Lombardi, Moftia Aujero, Don Lee, Howard Kritz, Ivy Natera al-Lahabi, Lindora Dickenson-Walker, Irene Torres, Liliana Rodriquez, Keith Kerr, Karen Hewitt, Barbara Else, Steven Bohlen, Minerva Joubert, Jean Carlson, Hannah Scherer, Ines Suarez, Carla Brekke, Danielle Elleman, Peggy McHugh, Benard Dreyer, Alan Mendelsohn, Linda van Schaick, Shona Yin, Mary Jo Messito, Keith Krasinski, Melissa Castro, Lauren Campbell, Amita Murthy, Ming Tsai, David Keefe, Greg Ribakove, Norma Keller, Mayra Mercado, Mera Djokic, Nafija Musovic, Belinda Nieves, Esther Ammon, Pam Pamamdanan, Sally Jacko, Omar Bholat, Spiros Frangos, Chris McStay, Marion Machado, Laura Evans, David Chong, Jeff Gold, Eric Liebert, Bill Rom, Judy Aberg, Dena Rakower, Alma Lou Brandiss, Cora Larroza, Manish Parikh, Ken Rifkin, Levon Capan, Tom Blanck, Leon Pachter, Joe Zuckerman, Noel Testa, Nancy Genieser, Mike Ambrosino, Nirmal Tejwani, Budd Heyman, Frank Spencer, Aida Yap, Rob Todd, Steve Ross, Jennifer Wu, Mary Lynn Nierodzyck, Jen Havens, Jan Nelson, Fadi Hadad, Romina Ursu, Pat Fonda, Susan Cohen, Rob Smeltz, Rob Roswell, Angelina DeCastro, Glenn Saxe, Melissa Massimo, Anil Thomas, Samoon Ahmad, Marilia Neves, Danielle Kaplan, Bob Hoffman, Elizabeth Ford, Roslyn Mayers, Randi Wasserman, Susan Marchione, Harold Horowitz, Karen Hendricks-Muñoz, Max Koslow, Steve Russell, Neal Bernstein, Mike Attubato, Lisa Park, Joan Cangiarella, Maria Aguero, Rebecca Weis, Kate Zayko, Edith Davis, Kate Hogerton, Kim Tran, Elias Sakalis, Rich Cohen, Miquel Sanchez, Helen Javier, Amit Rajparia, Diana Voiculescu, Diana Han, Cherry Siriban, Umut Sarpel, Asher Aladjem, Vivian Sun, Laura Alves, Aaron Elliot, Gary Belkin, Nathan Thompson, Ana Peña, Laura Furtansky, Manuela Birto-Fortes, Neal Agovino, Marcy Pressman, Mirian Villar, Alyssa Tsukroff, Richard LaFleur, Hawthorne Smith, Allan Keller.

Life being what it is made me a patient in my own book, not by design, but by chance. I was the recipient of the most professional caring support any patient could hope for from a team that I knew and respected, making it easy to choose to be treated by the "home team." I never had to worry about trust, competence, or mutual respect. Thank you, Bobby Bearnot, David Hirsch, Nick Sanfilippo, Silvia Formenti, Beverly Smith, Stuart Hirsch, Jamie Levine, Cathy Lazarus, Bob Glickman, Deirdre Cohen, Sally Habib, Dan Roses, Rena Brand, Kepal Patel, John Golfinos, Bill Cole, Bill Carroll, Leon Pachter. You cannot find better doctors or better people.

Turning an idea that could have been three or more books into a focused manuscript took some great advice and editing. I am very fortunate to have both extremely capable and fine people as agents in Jim Levine and Lindsay Edgecombe. They had the imagination to see where this book was coming from and where it could go. My editor John Brodie helped a new writer stay focused and not feel that vital organs were being excised when a cut was suggested. There would be other opportunities.

It has never been clear to me exactly where my work begins and ends or for that matter why I should be worried about that imaginary line. This is also true for my amazing polyglot friends, who are as immersed in their life's work and work life as I am in mine. We all share enthusiasm for exquisite meals, theater, movies, a worship of great books, incessant travel to distant lands, telling stories and hearing tales about battles fought and won, lost, or drawn. We learned to celebrate often since you never know. To Faye Ginsberg, Fred Myers, Leo Spitzer, Marianne Hirsch, Barbara Kirshenblatt-Gimblett, Max Gimblett, Alexis Jetter, Annelise Orlick, Silvia Spitta, Gerd Gemunden, Renato Rosaldo, Mary Louise Pratt, Diana Raznovich, Jesusa Rodriquez, Liliana Felipe, Mario Bronfman, Sylvia Molloy, Catharine Stimpson, Liz Woods, Eduardo Zarate, Milada Bazant, Margo Krasnoff, Sue Varma, Alyshia Galvéz, Josana Tonda, Ben Chu, Donna Moylan, Sandy Petrie, Nancy Miller, Lorie Novak, Arnie Arnison, Ed Fishkin, Marcial Godoy, Teresa Anativia, Marléne Ramirez-Cancio, Mary Brabeck, Mike Brabeck, Richard Schechner, Carol Martin, Nina Bernstein,

Andreas Huyssen, Agnes Lugo-Ortíz, Diane Miliotis, David Brooks, Susan Meiselas.

My brothers, Dean and Josh, and their families have been supportive and rooting for this to happen. My wife's family has been a fan club for a long time between trips to Antarctica: Susie, Jim, and Erin, plus the Canadian side of the family, Randy, Wendy and George, and Marga Taylor. The Zantops, Veronica, Eric Ames, Max and Isaac and Mariana, Dan, Mia are extended family. We go back a long way. My parents passed away some time before this book was written but they are very much a part of every page and every story.

My family came to my rescue in many ways. When I was too doctorly they grounded me in their reality. As I became a little wiser, I realized increasingly what I did not know and learned to go with the flow of Alexei and Marina becoming warm and caring people, great friends deeply involved in so many things with love and passion. Our dinners are legendary, and they now are breaking in the next generation, Mateo and Zoe. They generously watched me disappear for a year to complete this manuscript—and not long after I had disappeared down a dark hole, they helped pull me out of it. Gladys and the Lowe family have been warm additions to an expanding family. Diana has been my life partner for many years. She read and reread the manuscript many times and with her amazing critical eye made innumerable additions and subtractions that were based on her own deep knowledge of where I had been, who my patients were, and what their stories meant in the deepest and widest sense. She has been part of everything I have done for a long time with her generous love through everything.

Index

About the Author

Eric Manheimer is a clinical professor of medicine at the New York University School of Medicine. He was the medical director at Bellevue Hospital for fourteen years and previously was on the faculty at the Dartmouth-Hitchcock Medical Center in Lebanon, New Hampshire. He trained as an internist at Kings County Hospital in Brooklyn, New York, after receiving his medical degree at Downstate Medical School. He lives in New York City and Tepoztlán, Mexico, with his wife, Diana Taylor.